MW01144355

Promoting

The Primary Health Care Approach

third edition

Promoting Health

The Primary
Health Care Approach

third edition

Lyn Talbot

Department of Health and Environment
School of Public Health
Faculty of Health Sciences
La Trobe University, Bendigo

RN, Grad Dip HlthSc, LUCNV
MHlthSc, La Trobe
Grad Cert Higher Education, La Trobe

Glenda Verrinder

Department of Health and Environment
School of Public Health
Faculty of Health Sciences
La Trobe University, Bendigo

RN, Midwife, Cert CHN, RDNS
Grad Dip HlthSc, LUCNV
MHlthSc, La Trobe
Grad Cert Higher Education, La Trobe

First and second editions
written by Andrea Wass

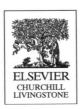

ELSEVIER
CHURCHILL
LIVINGSTONE

Sydney   Edinburgh   London   New York   Philadelphia   St Louis   Toronto

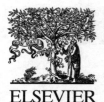

ELSEVIER

Churchill Livingstone
is an imprint of Elsevier

Elsevier Australia
30-52 Smidmore Street, Marrickville, NSW 2204
(a division of Reed International Books Australia Pty Ltd)
ACN 001 002 357

3rd edition © 2005 Elsevier Australia
2nd edition © 2000 Elsevier Australia
1st edition © 1994 Elsevier Australia

Previous editions published as *Promoting Health: The Primary Health Care Approach*
by Andrea Wass.

National Library of Australia Cataloguing-in-Publication Data

---

Talbot, Lyn.
Promoting health : the primary health care approach.

3rd ed.
Includes index.
For tertiary students.
ISBN 0 7295 3755 2.

1. Health promotion. 2. Health promotion - Australia. 3.
Primary health care. I. Verrinder, Glenda. II. Title.

613

Publisher: Vaughn Curtis
Publishing editor: Meg O'Hanlon
Publishing services manager: Helena Klijn
Project coordinator: Emma Hutchinson
Editor, project manager and indexer: Forsyth Publishing Services
Proofreader: Pam Dunne
Cover and internal design: Design Animals, Sydney
Typesetter: Egan-Reid Ltd
Printed in Australia by Southwood Press

Contents

Contents

Preface

In the years since the early 1990s, when this book was first written, two major changes have occurred that spurred us on to write a new edition. First, we now have better evidence than we did then about what determines health and illness and, secondly, there has been a significant change in the political context in which health-promotion workers operate.

Over the last 50 years, average life expectancy at birth has increased globally by almost 20 years. However, there are major disparities in the health of people around the world and these disparities are growing. Neo-liberal thinking fuels these inequities. Neo-liberal thinking has enabled vast quantities of money to be moved each year from poor countries to rich countries, in order to service debt repayments and from poor people to rich people within countries to service their status anxiety. This thinking is the dominant force influencing government policy. Support for principles such as social justice, equity and community participation can no longer be assumed to be part of the espoused values of governments or international bodies. The principles of comprehensive Primary Health Care are looking increasingly at odds with the dominant paradigm.

These changes have served to highlight how very important the principles of the Primary Health Care approach are and how vital it is that they continue to have a place in contemporary society. The role of health workers in implementing these principles is thus even more important than when this book was first written. It is hoped that this updated edition will contribute to the process of enabling and supporting health workers in their endeavour to promote the health of their communities.

This edition builds on the sound philosophical approach of the first two editions. There has been a good deal of reordering of the text and overlaying of current policy initiatives on health-promotion frameworks introduced in the first two editions. This edition introduces robust theoretical concepts and provides and strengthens answers to the following questions, regularly put to health workers:

- Why are the principles of social justice, equity and community participation of importance to the public's health?
- Why should we address the determinants of health?
- How best do we provide accessible and socially acceptable health services?
- How do current and future public health workers need to practise?

The major frameworks that have been used to present the material and guide health workers are the principles of Primary Health Care, the action areas of the Ottawa Charter for Health Promotion and a continuum of health promotion interventions.

Lyn Talbot and *Glenda Verrinder*

Introduction

This book examines the Primary Health Care approach to health promotion. It does so from the position that health promotion is an important component of Primary Health Care, and that health promotion is a more potent force if it is driven by the Primary Health Care philosophy.

Primary Health Care was formally endorsed in 1978 as an important framework for improvement of the world's health, when the Declaration of Alma-Ata provided the blueprint for Primary Health Care and 'Health for All by the year 2000'. This declaration, supported by representatives from 134 nations, emerged from international concern that health care systems had developed with a focus on costly high-technology care, usually at the expense of the provision of even basic health services for the majority of the world's people.

Primary Health Care was seen as a solution to the inadequate illness management systems which had developed. By providing a balanced system of treatment and disease prevention, through affordable, accessible and appropriate services, it was hoped that Primary Health Care would address some of the major inequalities in health observed both within countries and between countries. At the same time, though, there was recognition that new health services alone were not the answer, and that a major reorientation was needed in the way in which we think about and act on issues which impact upon health.

Primary Health Care is therefore about much more than the provision of new health services. Central to Primary Health Care is the Primary Health Care philosophy or approach, which should guide all action on health issues. It is the Primary Health Care approach which tells us *how* we should do what we do. The Primary Health Care approach emphasises social justice, equity, community participation and responsiveness to the needs of local populations. It emphasises using approaches which are affordable, and therefore sustainable. It emphasises the need to work with people, in order to enable them to make decisions about which issues are most important to them and which responses are most useful, and to work with other sectors and groups to address the root causes of ill health. This Primary Health Care approach, to be effective, needs to be applied at all levels of the health system and in every interaction between health workers and community members. Such a comprehensive approach is so much more than the delivery of primary-level services. With the use of the term 'Primary Health Care' to refer to such services, the term is used throughout this book to reflect this comprehensive Primary Health Care approach.

The Ottawa Charter for Health Promotion, developed in 1986, reflects the same principles seen in the Declaration of Alma-Ata, and builds on the declaration by providing a clear framework for action by health workers. This same approach has been reaffirmed time and again by health promoters worldwide. This approach to health promotion recognises that action to promote health must work to change the environments that structure health chances, as well as to help individuals to change those things over which they have control. As a result, these documents present a comprehensive definition of health promotion.

Health workers will need a broad range of skills not traditionally regarded as central to the health system if they are to effectively implement the Primary Health Care approach to health promotion. This book focuses on those strategies which have emerged as central to health promotion practice, but which have been largely neglected in the education of health workers until the recent past. It is designed to provide both a theoretical introduction and practical strategies for action.

Health promotion is not the responsibility of any one discipline in health or even of the health professions as a whole. Health promotion is everyone's responsibility. Health promotion is a broad-ranging activity which must be embraced by as many people as possible if it is to be effective. Much health promotion work occurs outside the health sector, and therefore requires the active involvement of people who would not regard themselves as health workers at all. Teachers, police, road safety workers, engineers, mediators, human rights investigators and many more play a central role in health promotion. Similarly, all health workers, no matter where in the health system they find themselves, have opportunities to promote health, whether it be to lobby for changes to reduce the socio-environmental dangers to health, to work to make health services more health-promoting settings, to assist individuals to learn about health-enhancing behaviour or to engage people meaningfully in the decision-making processes that affect their health.

Members of the community have a central role to play in using the democratic process to work for change at a societal level, and where possible to make choices at an individual level to promote their health. Their role, through a process of participatory democracy, as a broad constituency for change, is potentially a very powerful one.

Within this context, though, it is worth focusing to some extent on the particular roles which health workers have to play. Firstly, they have an espoused commitment to improving the health of people, a goal which is fundamental to all health professions. Secondly, they are able to advocate for a health perspective on issues outside the health sector which have an impact on health. They are also able to work with community members, encouraging and supporting them where necessary, or providing expertise and advice where that is needed.

By virtue of these issues, health workers can take up a leadership role in the promotion of health. Multidisciplinary health associations, such as the International Union for Health Promotion and Education, have an enormously important role to play, both in advocating for the health of the community and in modelling the effectiveness of a true multidisciplinary approach.

The professional associations of the various health disciplines have an important role to play too. Each association has the opportunity as part of a multidisciplinary team to contribute to health promotion.

Of course, many health workers are still working out how they see their role in Primary Health Care and health promotion, and many others are still unaware of Primary Health Care and its implications. Hopefully this book will encourage health workers to take up the challenge to work as health activists, to promote health in a way which enables communities and individuals to live their lives to the full.

If we continue to support a burgeoning illness management system, the costs to the health of the community will be immense. If, on the other hand, the Primary Health Care challenge is taken up by all whose work impacts on health, as well as by community members who find their health being jeopardised by the circumstances in which they live, then the effect could be quite profound.

Throughout this book, the term 'health worker' is used to refer to the person working to promote health. The term first came to be extensively used in the women's health movement, because it was regarded as a term which implied a more equal relationship between professionals and their patients or clients. The use of the term health worker, rather than professional titles, was hoped to be part of the process of breaking down the way in which professional groups related to individuals and communities, enabling the establishment of more equitable health worker–client relationships. It is in this spirit of greater equality and partnership that the term health worker is used in this book.

In this book the terms 'majority world' and 'minority world' are used. 'Majority world' refers to the life experience for the majority of the world's propulation — about 80 per cent of the people. Alternative titles sometimes include 'third world' or 'developing nations'. These 80 per cent of population consume about 20 per cent of the world's resources.

The term 'minority world' refers to the minority proportion of the world's population (around 20 per cent) who consume around 80 per cent of its collective resources (often referred to as the 'developed' or 'first' world). Nations of the minority world dominate international economic decision-making and trade, and determine the extent of the inequity between nations worldwide. An example of this can be seen in the way minority world events and preoccupations dominate news items.

Health promotion draws on many areas of expertise. This means that it is difficult to make the hard choices about what to examine, and in what depth, in a text of this size. In deciding which skills and issues need to be addressed in a book such as this, consideration has been given to which topics are usually examined in undergraduate education in health. For example, it is expected that readers will already have grounding in sociology, psychology and health and disease. Hence, a number of topics, including the structural basis of ill health, communication skills and health and disease processes, while referred to, are not examined in any great depth. Readers who are using this book without having previously examined these issues are encouraged to supplement their reading in these areas.

The book is divided into eight chapters. Chapter 1 examines health promotion in the context of the development of Primary Health Care and the New Public Health movement.

We discuss how the World Health Organization began a process of working towards achieving health for all of the world's population. We review the development of this international policy process, and the 'drivers' of current policy development. We talk about the determinants of health and illness and the role that Primary Health Care and the New Public Health movement has in addressing health inequalities. A continuum of health-promotion approaches for intervention is introduced.

Chapter 2 explores the concepts and values that underpin health promotion. The centrality of social justice and equity in the promotion of health, and directly addressing the determinants of health problems, are identified as fundamental issues for contemplation and action in public health. Given the importance of these issues, and some of the challenges they have presented, Chapter 2 presents other key concepts and values, raising a number of important questions that health workers will face as they grapple with the complexities of health promotion. Health, health promotion and community are defined.

In Chapter 3, the work to develop healthy public policy to create more supportive environments is examined. Developing public policy lays the foundation for healthy living and offers scope for developing effective long-term change with wide-ranging impact on the determinants of health and illness. This chapter explores the key issues in the development of healthy public policy at a broad social level, a local/community level, and within organisations. It examines approaches when developing healthy public policy to create health-promoting environments.

In Chapter 4 we move along the continuum from 'healthy public policy' to 'community action for social and environmental change'. The environment, rather than the individual, is defined as the target for change. The potential of community development approaches to address some of the structural issues that lead to poor health is discussed. We examine the potential of community development as a way of working with communities, on issues they identify with, to achieve changes to the environment and enable community empowerment.

In Chapter 5 we examine the continuous cycle of program development, from needs assessment through to evaluation. Research skills form the basis of the process and we outline the steps necessary to develop an effective program. Using these skills facilitates the development of a research base for health promotion in a way that both strengthens the relevance of health-promotion work and enables health workers to be accountable for their practice. A broad range of approaches can be used which are grounded in Primary Health Care and there are clear relationships between the philosophical approaches and the methods used. Community engagement in the process is fundamental to the success of program development and evaluation.

Education plays a central role in health promotion and in Chapter 6 we review some of the principles of education for health, and consider the particular approaches to education that sit most comfortably with the Primary Health Care approach.

In Chapter 7, we move to the far end of the continuum of health-promotion approaches and examine some of the medical approaches to health promotion. There are a range of interventions in this approach, including individual risk factor assessment, screening and surveillance and social marketing. These approaches are focused on disease, and control over health promotion is maintained by health professionals who do not necessarily take the social context of people's lives into consideration. We do not argue that these diseases should not be addressed but we do say that by only addressing those illnesses, we risk perpetually attempting to address the end result of the problem instead of addressing the root causes of the diseases themselves or the social conditions that perpetuate disease and other suffering.

The final chapter commences with some reflections and cautions about health promotion. The purpose of texts such as this is to set out the core principles to guide practitioners in the area. In doing this we have described an 'ideal' set of circumstances and ways of working, which are much more difficult to put into practice than they seem. The book concludes by returning to the action areas of the Ottawa Charter and using them as a framework to pose a series of rhetorical questions in order to keep Primary Health Care philosophy at the forefront, even when it may be more expedient to make decisions 'for' a community.

Included throughout this book are a number of examples of how some of the concepts presented in the book have been put into practice. These examples will add to the growing list of case studies being presented in publications which address health promotion and Primary Health Care. It is hoped that these examples will add to an understanding of the issues of relevance in health-promotion work. It is also hoped that they will encourage budding health promoters to become involved, by demonstrating that health promotion is already a meaningful part of a great many health workers' practice. However, these examples are not meant to be definitive; rather, they represent part of an evolving practice. Many of the more difficult areas of health promotion, including dealing with the root causes of ill health, are not as well represented as health education designed to prevent specific diseases, because we are still coming to grips with how to address these issues. You are encouraged to read widely and examine the great many other examples currently available, and to work with your colleagues to develop your own ways of practising.

The emergence of Primary Health Care and the New Public Health movement has provided us with a strong framework for health promotion, within which health workers, policy-makers and members of the wider community can work together. The opportunity exists for all those whose work impacts on health to take up the challenge of working in such a broad health-promotion framework. We hope that this book reflects the spirit of Primary Health Care, and that it will contribute to our growing understanding of how to work to promote the health of our communities, both local and worldwide.

Acknowledgments

In completing this third edition, there are a number of people whose contributions must be acknowledged. Andrea Wass wrote the first and second editions of this book and we pay tribute to her work and acknowledge the contribution of others to those editions, and subsequently to the third edition.

The path has been smoothed by red wine, chocolate and the ongoing support of the special people in our lives, Adrian, Lizzy and David.

We are grateful to our colleagues in the Department of Public Health at La Trobe University, Bendigo campus, for their unquestioned academic support.

Thanks are extended to the students and practitioners who have contributed to the discussion and refining of many ideas presented in this work, and who have participated in 'field testing' some of the material. Thanks are also extended to practitioners who have provided examples drawn from their practice.

Thank you Melissa Graham for checking our references and being another pair of eyes in the first draft of the chapters, and thanks also to Emma Patten for developing Appendix 5.

Finally, we would like to thank Elsevier for inviting us to write the third edition and in particular, Lou Thorn, Vaughn Curtis and Meg O'Hanlon, for supporting us throughout the process, and to Jon Forsyth for his care in editing and project management.

1

Health promotion in context: Primary Health Care and the New Public Health movement

More than 50 years ago the World Health Organization began a process to work towards achieving 'Health for All' of the world's population. This chapter will review the development of this international policy process, and the 'drivers' of current policy development. The determinants of health and illness will be outlined and the role that Primary Health Care and the New Public Health movement play in addressing health inequalities will be discussed.

There are major disparities in the health of people around the world, with serious differences in life expectancy between people living in various countries, as well as differences between groups of people within countries. Over the last 50 years, average life expectancy at birth has increased globally by almost 20 years; however, the large life expectancy gap between the 'developed' and 'developing' countries in the 1950s has changed to a gap between the very poorest developing countries and all other countries (WHO 2003). Changes to the determinants of health and illness have made the difference and, further, while some people experience better access to health and other resources than ever before, many others do not.

despite Δ's to determinants of hlth & ↑ life exp. still disparities

There are many terms used to describe the position of countries worldwide. In the past the terms 'eastern block' and 'western block' countries were used to politically differentiate countries that were aligned with either communist or capitalist philosophies. Currently, the descriptors are tied to economic status such as 'developed' or 'developing'. Similarly, 'first world' and 'third world' have been used for many years. 'Developed' countries are relatively rich and have a strong industrial base. The 'developing' countries are neither rich nor have a strong industrial base. In this book we will use the terms the *majority world* and the *minority world* because they provide a meaningful description of how the world is divided up now. The *majority* of the world's people are not rich but there is a *minority* of people who are. The United States of America for example is a very rich and powerful country and part of a small minority in the world. Bangladesh is very poor and part of the large majority in the world. However, within both of these countries are people who belong to the majority world and minority world.

The World Health Organization responds to international health problems

The World Health Organization (WHO) is an agency of the United Nations. It was established in 1948, as the major body to deal with international health issues. The WHO is made up of 192 countries who, as member states, work together to promote the health of the world's people (WHO online: http://www.who.int/country/en/).

The preamble to the constitution of the WHO makes several statements about the way to achieve health worldwide. First, the WHO definition of health is that 'Health is a state of complete physical, mental and social wellbeing and not merely the absence of disease or infirmity' (WHO 1948). The constitution then goes on to state:

- the enjoyment of the highest attainable standard of health is one of the fundamental rights of every human being without distinction of race, religion, political belief, economic or social condition;

- the health of all peoples is fundamental to the attainment of peace and security and is dependent upon the fullest cooperation of individuals and states;

- the achievement of any state in the promotion and protection of health is of value to all;

- unequal development in different countries in the promotion of health and control of disease, especially communicable disease, is a common danger;

- healthy development of the child is of basic importance; the ability to live harmoniously in a changing total environment is essential to such development;

- the extension to all peoples of the benefits of medical, psychological and related knowledge is essential to the fullest attainment of health;

- informed opinion and active cooperation on the part of the public are of the utmost importance in the improvement of the health of the people; and, finally,

- governments have a responsibility for the health of their peoples, which can be fulfilled only by the provision of adequate health and social measures.

(WHO 1948)

These principles underpin the constitution drawn up in 1948; however, in the 1970s there was growing concern that all was not well with the health of the world's people and health care systems. Since the end of World War II, there had been a rapid growth in the international health industry without an increase in the health status of many people. Minority countries invested in high technology; however, those in majority countries lacked access to even basic health care services. As medical technologies and medical knowledge developed, there had been the belief that these things would solve the health problems facing people around the world. However, it became increasingly apparent that this was not the case, and that high technology acute medical services had a limited effect on the health of populations. There was growing evidence that it was public health in its broadest sense, rather than medical care, that was responsible for most population health improvement (McKeown 1979). At the same time, there was a growing scepticism of the role and power of medicine itself and the value of medical treatment (Illich 1975). In Australia, the Labor Party began to invest in community-controlled, community-based, multidisciplinary health services in 1973, and as a result of documents such as the Lalonde Report (1974) in Canada, a different approach to health system development began to emerge worldwide.

The effects of the determinants of health and illness were beginning to be acknowledged globally. Yet, few countries had acted to improve health by reducing poverty, improving housing and food availability, and stopping political oppression, despite the wide-ranging evidence that social conditions have a great impact on health.

In 1978, the WHO and United Nations International Children's Emergency Fund (UNICEF) held a major international conference on Primary Health Care in the former USSR. It was attended by representatives from 134 nations. The outcome of the conference was the Declaration of Alma-Ata (Appendix 1). This conference is now regarded as a critically important milestone in the promotion of world health.

Primary Health Care

Primary Health Care is essential health care based on practical, scientifically sound and socially acceptable methods and technology. Primary Health Care is made universally accessible to individuals and families in the community through their full participation and at a cost that the community and country can afford to maintain at every stage of their development in the spirit of self-reliance and self-determination (WHO 1978).

The principles of Primary Health Care

There are ten fundamental principles for Primary Health Care contained in the Declaration of Alma-Ata. The declaration was seen as the key to achieving 'a level of health that will permit peoples of the world to lead a socially and economically productive life' by the year 2000. This became known as 'Health for All by the Year 2000' (WHO 1978).

Several concepts stand out in the Declaration of Alma-Ata:

- equity;
- community participation and maximum community self-reliance;

- use of socially acceptable technology;
- health promotion and disease prevention;
- involvement of government departments other than health;
- political action;
- cooperation between countries;
- reduction of money spent on armaments in order to increase funds for Primary Health Care; and
- world peace.

The Declaration of Alma-Ata challenged the world to embrace the principles as a way of overcoming health inequalities between and within countries. 'Health for All' became the slogan for a movement. It was not just an ideal, but an organising principle — everybody needs and is entitled to the highest possible standard of health (WHO 2003). The WHO (cited by Chamberlain & Beckingham 1987, p. 158) states that:

> Primary Health Care should be a philosophy permeating the entire health system, a strategy for organising health care, a level of care and a set of activities.

Each of these perspectives on Primary Health Care is presented in the following section.

Primary Health Care as a philosophy

The Primary Health Care philosophy is the foundation of Primary Health Care movement and its goal of achieving Health for All. Health for All was, and remains, fundamentally a call for social justice. It is a process that leads to progressive improvements in the health of people, and is not a single finite goal.

The Primary Health Care philosophy is based on the principles described above and works to improve the root causes of ill health. It emphasises working with people to enable them to make decisions about their needs and how best to address them. These principles reflect the Primary Health Care philosophy — using approaches that emphasise equity, participation and health promotion, and that are affordable, appropriate to local needs and sustainable.

To be effective, Primary Health Care principles need to be applied throughout the health system and in every interaction between health workers and community members. No matter where in the health system consumers find themselves, these principles need to be evident. Indeed, given the recognition of the need for action outside the health sector to improve health and the impact of social services on health, the Primary Health Care philosophy has implications way beyond the health system.

Implementation of the Primary Health Care approach is clearly a massive task involving considerable political will and major changes in health systems. This is politically significant. Given the power of the medico–industrial complex, and the urgent need for basic medical services in some parts of the world, it is not surprising that those already in power in the minority world set priorities based on the medical model of health care. With Primary Health Care approaches, the money that can be made in a technologically dependent health system, and the power that can be lost by health professionals, threatens many.

4

Selective and comprehensive Primary Health Care

The medical model has become known as *selective Primary Health Care*. It is a more limited form of Primary Health Care, but it ensures the status quo in terms of health care structures and service provision and, therefore, is less threatening. To some groups, the philosophy of selective Primary Health Care is diametrically opposed to the philosophy proposed at the Alma-Ata conference. To some groups, the philosophy underpinning Primary Health Care at this conference has become known as *comprehensive Primary Health Care*.

On one hand, comprehensive Primary Health Care is a developmental process that emphasises the aforementioned principles of equity, social justice, community control and working for social changes that impact on health and wellbeing. In comprehensive Primary Health Care, emphasis is on addressing the determinants of health; that is, the conditions that generate health and ill health. Therefore, provision of medical care is only one aspect of comprehensive Primary Health Care. On the other hand, selective Primary Health Care concentrates on treating illnesses. Thus, while comprehensive Primary Health Care focuses on the process of empowerment and increasing control over all those influences that impact on health, selective Primary Health Care operates in a way that assumes that medical care alone creates health and ensures that control over health is maintained by health professionals. In discussing the two perspectives, some have likened it to 'the individual versus the system' (Green and Raeburn 1988 in Baum 2002, p. 34).

Arguing for comprehensive over selective Primary Health Care is not to argue against the importance of addressing specific diseases. Selective Primary Health Care has produced important gains, such as immunisation. Clearly we must address those diseases that cause human suffering and death. However, by only addressing those illnesses, we risk perpetually attempting to address the end result of the problem instead of addressing the root causes of the diseases themselves or the social conditions that perpetuate disease and other suffering. Comprehensive Primary Health Care addresses these illnesses and other issues in their social context, using a process that recognises the expertise that ordinary people have and their right to exert control over their own lives. Box 1.1 provides four key areas in which selective Primary Health Care compares poorly with comprehensive Primary Health Care.

Primary Health Care as a strategy for organising health care

When the philosophy of Primary Health Care is implemented, a particular strategy for the organisation of health care becomes apparent. A balanced system of health promotion, disease prevention, rehabilitation and illness treatment can be developed, with the entire system built to meet the goals of Primary Health Care. To deal with the increasing burden of communicable and non-communicable diseases worldwide requires upstream health promotion and disease prevention in the community as well as downstream disease management within health care services. A health system based on Primary Health Care will:

- build on the Alma-Ata principles of equity, universal access, community participation and inter-sectoral approaches;

> **Box 1.1 Comprehensive Primary Health Care versus selective Primary Health Care**
>
> 1. By focusing on the eradication and prevention of diseases, selective Primary Health Care assumes that health is the absence of disease rather than, as in the broader WHO definition, a state of complete physical, mental and social wellbeing. This then locates action for health almost solely within the realms of specialists trained to treat disease.
> 2. Through its emphasis on those diseases and problems most likely to respond to treatment, selective Primary Health Care ignores the need to address issues of equity and social justice, which are at the root of many health problems.
> 3. In establishing medical interventions as the most important part of Primary Health Care, selective Primary Health Care ignores the importance of all those non-medical interventions, such as the provision of education, housing and food, which have a greater bearing on health than health services themselves.
> 4. Selective Primary Health Care limits the value of community development as a strategy for improving health to being a technique for increasing community compliance with medically defined solutions, rather than as a mechanism for community empowerment. It thus identifies expertise as residing with medical workers and denies the great expertise that people have with regard to their own lives and the issues that affect them.

(Source: Rifkin, S. and Walt, G. 1986 Why health improves: defining the issues concerning 'comprehensive Primary Health Care' and 'selective Primary Health Care'. *Social Science and Medicine.* 23(6): 12–13)

- take account of broader population health issues, reflecting and reinforcing public health functions;

- create the conditions for effective provision of services to vulnerable groups;

- organise integrated and seamless care, linking preventive, acute and chronic care across all components of the health system;

- continuously strive to improve performance.

(WHO 2003, p. 108)

Primary Health Care as a set of activities

The Declaration of Alma-Ata (WHO 1978) highlights a minimum set of activities that need to occur if Primary Health Care is to be implemented. These are:

- education concerning prevailing health problems and the methods of preventing and controlling them;
- promotion of food supply and proper nutrition;
- provision of an adequate supply of safe water and basic sanitation;
- provision of maternal and child health care, including family planning;
- immunisation against the major infectious diseases;
- prevention and control of locally endemic diseases;
- appropriate treatment of common diseases and injuries; and
- provision of essential drugs.

Other potential priorities are also acknowledged by the WHO — for example, priorities set by local communities themselves.

Primary Health Care as a level of care

The term 'Primary Health Care' is often used to refer to primary-level health services; that is, the first point of contact with the health system for people with health problems. In a Primary Health Care system, this level of care should be the most comprehensive. In this way, problems can be dealt with where they begin. Primary-level health services include community health centres, domiciliary nursing care and general medical practitioners. Non-government organisations and community groups can also be an important part of Primary Health Care services. However, these services can only be regarded as Primary Health Care services if the Primary Health Care philosophy underpins the way in which those first-level services are provided. That is, Primary Health Care practitioners' work is guided by the principles of consumer control over decision-making; collaboration with other health and welfare workers to deal effectively with health issues in their local area; equity and social justice (reflected, in part, in the case of general medical practitioners, by bulk-billing or salaried medical officers attached to community health centres); and, incorporation of health promotion into their work.

Health for All by the Year 2000 was not a goal in itself, but rather a process to improve the health of the world's population. In 2003 the WHO affirmed the philosophy that underpins Primary Health Care. The WHO continues to propose an approach to health development based on the core principles of Primary Health Care formulated in 1978. Twenty-five years on, the WHO recommends that 'Principled Integrated Care' must be built on: universal access on the basis of need; health equity as part of development oriented to social justice; community participation in defining and implementing health agendas and inter-sectoral approaches to health (WHO 2003).

In recent years there appears to have been a significant increase in use of the terms 'Primary Health Care' and 'Primary Care' by government, as a way of legitimising those services, without any actual reorientation of such services. However, as we have said, without an orientation to the Primary Health Care philosophy, such services cannot take their place as central to the achievement of Health for All. Because of the now common use of the term 'Primary Health Care' to refer to community or first-level services, notably, primary medical services, 'Primary Health Care' will be used throughout this book to reflect the Primary Health Care approach or comprehensive Primary Health Care.

Primary Health Care, the Ottawa Charter for Health Promotion and the New Public Health movement

Health promotion has been variously defined and can be broadly or narrowly practised. However, the Ottawa Charter for Health Promotion (see Appendix 2) was built on the progress made through the Declaration of Alma-Ata and defines health promotion as 'the process of enabling people to increase control over, and to improve, their health' (WHO 1986). The Ottawa Charter for Health Promotion is regarded as the formal beginning of the New Public Health movement, a term that has widespread recognition, despite having been used several times before (Beaglehole and Bonita 2004, pp. 214–17). The charter was the outcome of the first WHO International Conference on Health Promotion and was held in Ottawa, Canada, in 1986. The WHO worked to develop the notion of health promotion in concert with the Health for All program. The aim was to increase the relevance of the Primary Health Care approach to industrialised countries that had largely ignored the Declaration of Alma-Ata. The Ottawa Charter for Health Promotion (WHO 1986) highlighted the conditions and resources required for health and set out the action required to achieve Health for All by the Year 2000. Like the Declaration of Alma-Ata, the Ottawa Charter for Health Promotion was, and is, a landmark document, laying out a clear statement of action that continues to have resonance for health workers around the world.

The strength of the Ottawa Charter lies in the fact that it incorporates both selective and comprehensive perspectives of Primary Health Care. Further, the five action areas of the Charter, used collectively within any population and within any setting, have a far better chance of promoting health than when they are used singularly. The Ottawa Charter for Health Promotion highlights the role of organisations, systems and communities, as well as individual behaviours and capacities. The five action areas of the Charter (see Figure 1.1) are designed to promote health by:

1. **Building healthy public policy.** It is not health policy alone that influences health: all public policy should be examined for its impact on health and, where policies have a negative impact on health, we must work to change them. For example, if a local government has a policy of allowing industrial complexes near residential areas, this would need to change if it was having a negative impact on residents' health.

2. **Creating environments which support healthy living.** The protection of both the natural and built environment is important for health. For example, in the built environment we need living, work and leisure environments organised in ways that do not create or contribute to poor health. We also need to conserve the natural environment for health. These will come through the establishment of healthy public policy.

3. **Strengthening community action.** Communities themselves are the experts in their own community and should determine what their needs are, and how they can best be met. Thus, greater power and control remain with the people themselves, rather than with the 'experts'. Community development is one means by which this can be achieved.

4. **Developing personal skills.** If people are to feel more in control of their lives and have more power in decisions that affect them, they may need to develop more skills. This could include being provided with necessary information, training or other resources that would enable people to take action to promote or protect their health. Those who work in health must

work towards enabling people to acquire the necessary knowledge and skills to make informed decisions.

5. **Reorienting health care.** Health promotion is everybody's business and inter-sectoral collaboration is the key. Within the health system there needs to be a balance between health promotion and curative services. One prerequisite for this reorientation is a major change in the way in which health care workers are educated.

This New Public Health movement approach to health promotion differs from traditional public health as it has been practised in recent years in three important ways. Firstly, it recognises the broad nature of health promotion, and the need to work with other sectors of government and private institutions whose work impacts on health. This inter-sectoral collaboration has become recognised as a central feature of effective health promotion. Secondly, it recognises the need to work in partnership with communities to increase community control over issues affecting health and to de-medicalise the control of health care. Thirdly, it recognises the primacy of people's environments (both physical and social) in determining their health, and recognises the need to work for change to the environment rather than

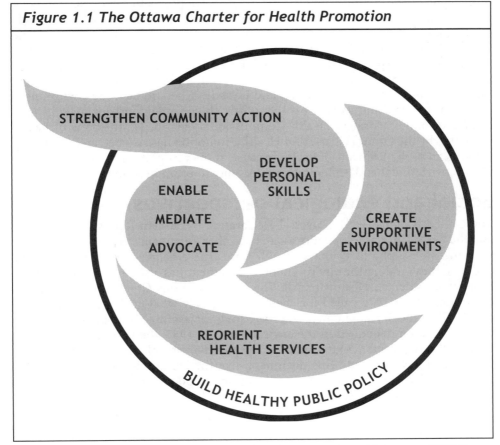

Figure 1.1 The Ottawa Charter for Health Promotion

STRENGTHEN COMMUNITY ACTION

DEVELOP PERSONAL SKILLS

ENABLE

MEDIATE

ADVOCATE

CREATE SUPPORTIVE ENVIRONMENTS

REORIENT HEALTH SERVICES

BUILD HEALTHY PUBLIC POLICY

(Source: World Health Organization 1986 *The Ottawa Charter for Health Promotion.* WHO, Geneva. Online. Available: http://www.who.org [accessed 20 January 2004])

focusing on change solely at the level of the individual (Tones, Tilford & Robinson, 1990, pp. 3–4). This means that many of the changes acknowledged as vital to the New Public Health movement may challenge existing ways of doing things. Indeed, the WHO acknowledges the need for political action in the New Public Health movement to achieve the required changes.

The New Public Health movement and the social model of health

The New Public Health movement is a conceptual framework for thinking about health. It is 'based on a clear articulation of a social model of health' (Baum 2002, p. 311) that emerges from philosophical underpinnings of the Declaration of Alma-Ata and the action areas of the Ottawa Charter for Health Promotion. Within this conceptual framework, improvements in health are achieved by addressing the many cultural, environmental, biological, political and economic determinants of health. The New Public Health movement challenges selective Primary Health Care as an approach to health promotion. In the New Public Health movement, medical and behavioural interventions have a limited role because of their failure to deliver more equitable health outcomes within and between population groups. The social model of health sets very wide parameters for health promotion practice. This is exciting because it means we can actually start dealing with health problems at the point of their origin. Indeed, a social view of health implies that we must intervene to change those aspects of the environment which are promoting ill health, rather than continue to simply deal with illness after it appears, or continue to exhort individuals to change their attitudes and lifestyles when, in fact, the environment in which they live and work gives them little choice or support for making such changes (South Australian Health Commission 1988a, p. 3). The view of health presented by the Ottawa Charter for Health Promotion has also been referred to by some as an ecological view of health because of the recognition of the importance of the environment and ecological sustainability in promoting world health.

Social and ecological perspectives

The United Nations (UN) Universal Declaration of Human Rights (Appendix 3) and the Earth Charter (Appendix 4) are two other documents that work in concert with the philosophy of Primary Health Care. The emergence of the philosophy and activities guiding the environmental movement has also been in unison with those that underpin Health for All. The United Nations Conference on Human Environments in 1972 called for changes in the way we do things. The chemical agent DDT (dichlorodiphenyltrichloroethane), for example, was banned in 1972 because it is not detoxified in the environment. In 1987, the year after the release of the Ottawa Charter, 'Our Common Future' (the Bruntland Report) called for 'sustainable development'. This document, like the Declaration of Alma-Ata and the Ottawa Charter, is considered to be a seminal document. The principles that underpin sustainable development are:

- inter- and intra-generational equity (social, economic and ecological);
- protection of biodiversity;
- practising the precautionary principle; and
- community participation in decision-making.

Globally, there was a good deal of community and political action afoot at the time of the emergence of Primary Health Care philosophy, the New Public Health movement and sustainable development. It is important to discuss both ecological and social justice perspectives and the relationship between the two. Ife (2002) asserts that the perspectives of both need to be integrated to bring about a truly sustainable society, and that the ecological perspective does not itself imply social justice principles. A major focus for those working for social justice is to challenge structural disadvantage. On one hand, without social justice principles an ecological perspective may reinforce structural disadvantage; on the other, one of the reasons a social justice perspective is inadequate without an ecological perspective is because of the conventional economic prescription for many social problems brought about through economic growth. People working for sustainability can challenge both the feasibility and desirability of continued growth, which Ife (2002) sees as contributing to the current ecological crisis. Both perspectives need to be understood in working toward enhancing health.

Affirming the philosophy: international health-promotion conferences

Each international health-promotion conference, since the first in Ottawa, has reaffirmed the philosophy that underpins Primary Health Care outlined in the Declaration of Alma-Ata. The prerequisites for health — peace, shelter, education, social security, social relations, food, income, empowerment of women, a stable ecosystem, sustainable resource use, social justice, respect for human rights and equity — have all been acknowledged. Further, the action areas of the Ottawa Charter for Health Promotion have been celebrated and built upon each time.

The theme of the second international health-promotion conference held in Adelaide in 1988 was healthy public policy. It was acknowledged at the conference that public policies in all sectors influence the determinants of health and are a major vehicle for actions to reduce social and economic inequities. In addition to making clear the importance of healthy public policy and the responsibility of all who produce public policy to observe and be responsive to the health impact of their policies, the conference urged industrialised countries to develop policies that reduce the growing disparity between rich and poor countries.

Supportive environments for health was the theme of the third international health-promotion conference. The 1991 *Sundsvall Statement on Supportive Environments for Health* stressed the importance of sustainable development. There was recognition that degradation of the physical environment was having an impact on people's health worldwide and the way forward lay in making the environment — the physical, the social, the economic and political environment — supportive to health rather than damaging it. The report from the conference was presented at the Rio Earth Summit in 1992 and contributed to the development of Agenda 21.

The theme for the fourth conference, held in Jakarta, was 'New Players for a New Era: Health Promotion into the 21st Century'. It was the first time that the private sector had been included and there was some concern expressed at the conference about the difficulties of involving the private sector in health-promotion policy development, with questions raised about the extent to which the private sector can be meaningfully involved without fundamental conflicts of interest (Hancock 1998). The conference declaration called for decision-makers in both the public and private sectors to demonstrate social responsibility by preventing harm to individuals and the environment, by restricting trade in harmful products and by integrating concern for equity into all policy development. In addition, conference delegates called for an increase in investment in health and areas that impact on health, including housing and education, demanding particular attention be paid to groups that have poor health or are most vulnerable, including women, children, older people, and indigenous, poor and marginalised populations. The conference delegates stated that effective health and social development requires collaboration between all levels of government and society to make the changes necessary to improve health chances for all and that these partnerships must be ethical and based on mutual respect. Further, as health promotion is a participatory process, communities and individuals need to be provided with the necessary skills for and access to decision-making power, to enable them to influence the determinants of health. Developing local-level expertise through education and dissemination of health-promotion experience is necessary, as is ensuring that all countries have the necessary 'political, legal, educational, social and economic environments to support health promotion' (WHO 2004b). The conference delegates called for funding to establish and maintain infrastructures for health promotion locally, nationally and globally. They believed that efforts to motivate government and non-government organisations to mobilise resources for health promotion needed to be made (WHO 1997, p. 263).

Commitment to the fundamental principles of Primary Health Care continued in Mexico at the fifth international conference, in the year 2000. The Mexico Ministerial Statement for the Promotion of Health: From ideas to Action and Framework for Countrywide Plans for Action (WHO 2000) outlines the processes to address the determinants of health, to ensure greater equity in health. The technical themes for the conference demonstrate the path that the conference delegates took, namely:

- evidence base for health promotion;
- investment for health;
- social responsibility for health;
- building community capacity and empowerment of the individual;
- securing an infrastructure for health promotion; and
- reorienting health services.

The key issues and statements arising from the meeting were:

- a focus on the determinants of health;
- a need to bridge the equity gap;
- acknowledgment of the role of women in health development;
- a restatement of the relevance of health promotion; and that
  — health promotion is scientifically sound;
  — health promotion is socially relevant;
  — health promotion is politically sensitive.

A summary of health-promotion conferences is provided in Box 1.2.

18th World Conference on Health Promotion and Health Education

In 2004 the theme for the 18th World Conference on Health Promotion and Health Education in Melbourne was 'Valuing diversity, reshaping power: exploring pathways for health and wellbeing'. Health for all (and not just for some) (Wise & Hearn 2004) was once again the focus of an international conference.

There was acknowledgment that inequalities in social, economic and environmental circumstances continue to increase and erode the conditions for health and,

Box 1.2 International health-promotion conferences		
Conference	**Theme**	**Priorities or issues**
The Second International Conference on Health Promotion — Adelaide, Australia, 1988	Healthy Public Policy	1. Support for the health of women, in recognition of their often unequal access to health and their role as health promoters within their own families. 2. The elimination of hunger and malnutrition through action that takes account of agricultural, economic and environmental issues. 3. The reduction of tobacco growing and alcohol production. 4. The creation of more supportive environments, in particular through the alliance of the Public Health, Peace and Ecological movements. (WHO/Commonwealth Department of Community Services and Health — Australia 1988)
The Third International Conference on Health Promotion — Sundsvall, Sweden, 1991	Supportive Environments for Health	1. Strengthen advocacy through community action, particularly through groups organised by women. 2. Enable communities and individuals to take control of their health and environment through education and empowerment. 3. Build alliances to strengthen cooperation between health and environment campaigns. 4. Mediate between conflicting interests in society in order to ensure equitable access to a supportive environment for health. (WHO 1991, cited by Tassie 1992, p. 28)
The Fourth International Conference on Health Promotion — Jakarta, Indonesia, 1997	New Players for a New Era: Health Promotion into the 21st Century	1. Promote social responsibility for health. 2. Increase investments for health development. 3. Consolidate and expand partnerships for health. 4. Increase community capacity and empowering the individual 5. Secure an infrastructure for health promotion (WHO 1997, p. 263).

(Continued)

Box 1.2 International health-promotion conferences (Continued)		
Conference	**Theme**	**Priorities or issues**
The Fifth International Conference on Health Promotion — Mexico City, Mexico, 2000	Health Promotion: Bridging the Equity Gap	Health Ministers who sign this statement will: 1. Position the promotion of health as a fundamental priority in local, regional, national and international policies and programs. 2. Take the leading role in ensuring the active participation of all sectors and civil society, in the implementation of health-promoting actions which strengthen and expand partnerships for health. 3. Support the preparation of country-wide plans of action for promoting health, if necessary drawing on the expertise in this area of the WHO and its partners. These plans will vary according to the national context, but will follow a basic framework agreed upon during the Fifth International Conference on Health Promotion, and may include among others: • The identification of health priorities and the establishment of healthy public policies and programs to address these. • The support of research which advances knowledge on selected priorities. • The mobilisation of financial and operational resources to build human and institutional capacity for the development, implementation, monitoring and evaluation of country-wide plans of action. 4. Establish or strengthen national and international networks which promote health. 5. Advocate that UN agencies be accountable for the health impact of their development agenda. 6. Inform the Director-General of the WHO, for the purpose of her report to the 107th session of the Executive Board, of the progress made in the performance of the above actions.

(Source: World Health Organization. Conferences. Online. Available: http://www.who.int/hpr/ncp/hp.conferences.shtml [accessed 21 January 2004])

through the conference themes, the participants explored ways of becoming more effective in health promotion. Concern for equity was at the core of this exploration as it has been for all conferences with Primary Health Care, public health and health promotion as a focus.

Our understanding of the determinants of inequities in health is improving.

> There is now a significant body of scientifically derived evidence of the causes and distribution of major public health problems across populations, and the world, and of the components of effective solutions to some (even if not all) of these.
>
> (Wise & Hearn 2004)

Determinants of health and illness

There are many factors which influence health and illness. There is generally no single cause or single contributing factor to determine the likelihood of health or illness, rather there tends to be a variety of causes. Along with health care interventions, the interaction between human biology, lifestyle and the physical and social environments impact on health.

> Environmental factors can be physical, as in landscape and climate; biological, as in vegetation, the food supply, infectious agents and other animal life; and socioeconomic, as in politics, culture, standard of living and other economic factors, and interaction within and among communities.
>
> (*AIHW* 2002, p. 4)

Within these broad parameters, factors that determine physical and mental health status include income, employment, poverty, education and access to community resources. These social factors create the life experiences and opportunities which in turn make it easier or more difficult for people to make positive decisions about their health. While there are many actions that a person can take to protect their own or their family's health, very often the social context of their lives makes it impossible to take those actions. Perhaps they may feel disempowered because they are alienated from society in some way, or perhaps they are living in poverty. These social factors therefore 'determine', to a large extent, the health or illness outcomes for people. Recent international research has highlighted the relationship between lower socioeconomic status and ill health, both within particular nations and when comparisons are made between nations (Marmot & Wilkinson 1999).

The WHO (2000) has developed ten social determinants of health, namely:

1. The social gradient
2. Stress
3. Early development
4. Work
5. Unemployment
6. Social support
7. Social exclusion
8. Addiction
9. Food
10. Transport

A range of epidemiological evidence and research outlines clearly the social determinants of health and illness. Four other areas are highlighted: poverty, ethnicity, gender and social integration (see WHO Report 1998; AIHW 2002; Couzos & Murray 2003). Health-promotion planners need to take account of all of these influences of health status, and incorporate strategies which will make a sustained difference to the context of people's lives.

A snapshot of Australia's health

The pattern of health and ill health in Australia generally reflects that which exists throughout the industrialised world. Australia has benefited from the general improvements in health that occurred in the 20th century. Over this time there has been an increase in expected years of life of almost 30 years for males and 23 years for women. In 2000, life expectancy at birth was 76.6 years for males and 82.1 years for women (AIHW 2002). The leading causes of death in Australia are coronary heart disease, cerebrovascular disease and cancer. Coronary heart disease and cerebrovascular disease account for 30 per cent of all deaths. All cancers combined account for another 30 per cent.

The health and quality of life of most Australians compares well with most of the world's population. This is not only important to celebrate, but also to bear in mind so that we might consider how we can contribute to improving the health of populations in those countries less fortunate than Australia. However, Australians are not immune to the effects of inequality in health, and some of these have become worse as income inequality in Australia has increased. While the health of Australians is on average good, there are some significant differences in the health chances of a number of population sub-groups in Australian society.

Lower socioeconomic status has been clearly shown to be associated with self-reports of poorer health overall (Wilkinson & Marmot 1998 in AIHW 2002). Even though the proportion of the population reporting good health increased overall in the 1990s, '[p]eople who are less educated, unemployed or living with low income all report poorer health status' (AIHW 2002, p. 14).

Gender is a significant determinant of health chances in Australia. Mortality rates for males are higher than those for females for all major causes of death (AIHW 1998, pp. 7–9). Men are also less inclined to seek medical assistance when they experience symptoms of poor health. At the same time, however, reported morbidity rates for women are worse than those of men (AIHW 1998, p. 16), and women's experience of the health system is often negative.

There are marked differences in health status according to ethnicity. People from different cultural or ethnic backgrounds living in the same country experience quite marked differences in health status measures such as quality of life and life expectancy. While many migrants have better health on arrival than the average Australian because of the requirements of the immigration process, this advantage disappears the longer they have been in Australia, as a result of the impact of limited job opportunities, the adoption of the health habits of the country to which they have migrated, and the lack of social support when they are far from extended family and friends (AIHW website; Bates & Linder-Pelz 1990, pp. 36–8; Minas 1990). Yet, this pattern of good health on arrival may be less likely to be the case for those migrants who come to Australia as refugees on the basis of humanitarian grounds. This group of migrants is likely to be suffering both physical and psychological trauma as a result of the often brutal experiences they have endured.

It is Australia's Aboriginal and Torres Strait Islander people, however, who have the most serious health inequalities (AIHW 2002). The infant mortality rates are three times higher than the national average and life expectancy for Aboriginal children born in 1998–2000 is 19 to 21 years less than for other Australians (Couzos & Murray 2003, p. 45; Thomson 2003; AIHW 2002). As a result, Aboriginal and Torres Strait Islander hospitalisation rates are more than 50 per cent higher than for other Australians (AIHW 1998, p. 32). As poor as these statistics are, they may actually underestimate the severity of Aboriginal and Torres Strait Islander people's poor health, as information in this area is incomplete and Aboriginal and Torres Strait Islander people are not always identified in health statistics.

This unequal access to health may sometimes be ignored if only generic national figures are used, and pockets of disadvantage may be hidden behind 'average' figures. Most of the issues that cause these health differences result from structural issues outside the traditional health care system and require health-promotion action from both within the health system and outside it, in collaboration between various levels and sectors of government and non-government bodies.

When we consider the multiple effects of these determinants it is clear that they must assume the major priority in health-promotion planning and activities. As indicated, there is generally more than one factor associated with each physical or mental illness. For instance, consider the impacts on the likely mental health status of an Aboriginal woman living in poverty who is isolated from mainstream Australian society and possibly from her Aboriginal community. Similarly, what would be the likely mental health status of a middle-aged man who has recently arrived in Australia, who doesn't speak English and has been granted refugee status?

One of the most significant social factors which influences health status in Australia and elsewhere is the effectiveness of a person's social integration or social connectedness. When people are asked about what it means to be healthy, social factors are most commonly mentioned. '[P]eople's experiences of health are more about their experiences of capacity and connectedness than about their experiences of death and disability' (Labonté1997, p. 13). Social connectedness is a prerequisite of social capital.

Social capital has been shown to be very important to a community's level of health and social and emotional wellbeing. Social capital refers to 'the processes between people which establish networks, norms, social trust and facilitate coordination and cooperation for mutual benefit' (Cox 1996 cited in Baum 1998, p. 94). Social capital helps protect people against negative effects of economic and other deprivations.

Positive health and wellbeing

To be healthy means significantly more than the absence of disease. In fact many people with disease, disability, even terminal illnesses, regard themselves as being very healthy despite the complexities in their lives that their conditions impose, or despite their impending death. To be healthy entails physical, mental and social dimensions. People need the vitality and energy to do the things they need and enjoy, bringing meaning and purpose to their lives. People gain a feeling of control over their lives through this sense of meaning and purpose and the sense of connectedness with the communities in their lives. The vital energy allows us to enjoy social relations which further enhance our sense of connectedness. These dimensions together provide our sense of wellbeing. It is clear from this discussion of wellbeing that the range of social determinants has potential to enhance or impinge on our achievement of positive health (Labonté 1997).

The relationship between social determinants of health and illness and health outcomes has been explained by Labonté (1997, Chapter 2) and is diagrammatically represented in Figure 1.2.

Risk and protective factors

Risk and protective factors at a population or community level influence the physical and mental health of individuals. Risk factors increase the likelihood that a disorder will develop or be exacerbated. Protective factors reduce the likelihood that a disorder will develop. Importantly, protective factors give people resilience. Risk factors associated with physical and mental health and illness include: biological, behavioural, psychological, socio-cultural, economic, environmental and demographic conditions and characteristics.

Physiological risk factors include factors such as genetic inheritances and hypertension. The impact of these risk factors is clearly evident in measurable or observable states of health, such as in epidemiological measures of the incidence and prevalence of certain conditions in society and in outcome mortality and morbidity measures.

Behavioural risk factors describe the individual lifestyle behaviours that people engage in. These include decisions people make about smoking and use of other addictive substances, their food choices and to what degree they are physically active. These factors have been the primary foci of many government-initiated health education and behaviour-change strategies, because of their clear link with observable health status.

Psychosocial risk factors have a significant influence on the decisions people are able to make about their health. Psychosocial risk factors describe the individual cognitive or emotional states which are often reactions to the way people try to deal with the daily living situations and stressors in their lives.

Risk conditions is the term that Labonte (1997, p. 16) uses to describe the psycho–socio–cultural determinants of illness, which are:

> the living situations that are largely structured by economic and political practices and by ideologies (dominant belief systems, e.g. that competition brings out the 'best' in people).

Living situations that include poverty, low social status, poor educational achievement and dangerous stressful work affect individuals directly in their daily lives. The health of whole populations is influenced by policy approaches which increase inequalities of access, cultural characteristics such as gender and other discriminations, resource deprivations and geographic isolation.

These risk conditions and contributing factors have been arranged diagrammatically by Labonté (see Figure 1.2). The diagram illustrates the 'causal chain' linking the social context of people's lives with health status indicators of mortality and morbidity.

Similarly, Figure 1.3 illustrates a causal chain that links the context of people's lives with their chances for health rather than illness.

Why is it important to focus on psycho–socio–cultural determinants of health and risk and protective factors? If we focus on these factors we are able to improve the health of populations rather than focusing on individual gain. If we are to provide comprehensive and successful mental and physical health care we need to apply a model of health care that includes a range of influences on health, including factors at the individual, family, community sector and society level.

[handwritten margin note: focus on psycho–socio–cult determin. + need a model.]

Understanding the relationship between social/emotional/environmental factors and common illnesses in society forms important knowledge for health workers. This knowledge should inform the activities they undertake, the communities they choose to work with, and the way in which they work. Primary Health Care philosophy provides the guiding principles for public health work in any context of practice.

The iceberg model provides a useful way to examine the determinants of health and plan activities using a variety of health-promotion approaches (see Figure 1.4). The iceberg divides into three sections. The top section refers to

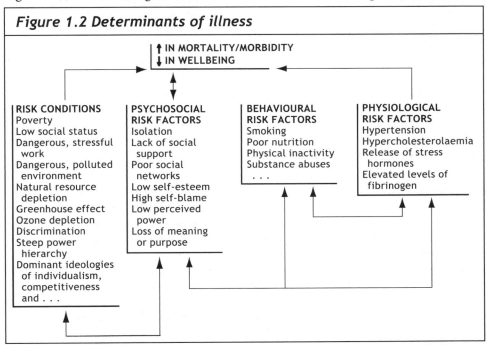

Figure 1.2 Determinants of illness

↑ IN MORTALITY/MORBIDITY
↓ IN WELLBEING

RISK CONDITIONS	PSYCHOSOCIAL RISK FACTORS	BEHAVIOURAL RISK FACTORS	PHYSIOLOGICAL RISK FACTORS
Poverty	Isolation	Smoking	Hypertension
Low social status	Lack of social	Poor nutrition	Hypercholesterolaemia
Dangerous, stressful work	support	Physical inactivity	Release of stress
Dangerous, polluted environment	Poor social networks	Substance abuses	hormones
Natural resource depletion	Low self-esteem	. . .	Elevated levels of fibrinogen
Greenhouse effect	High self-blame		
Ozone depletion	Low perceived		
Discrimination	power		
Steep power hierarchy	Loss of meaning or purpose		
Dominant ideologies of individualism, competitiveness and . . .			

(Source: Labonté, R. 1997 *Power, Participation and Partnerships for Health Promotion*. VicHealth, Melbourne, Chapter 1, pp. 13, 21)

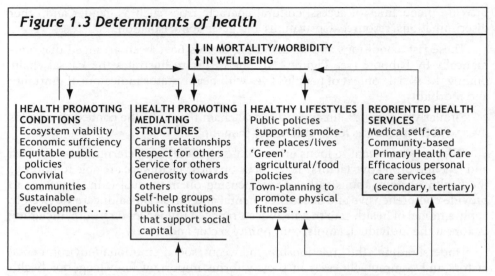

Figure 1.3 Determinants of health

↓ IN MORTALITY/MORBIDITY
↑ IN WELLBEING

HEALTH PROMOTING CONDITIONS	HEALTH PROMOTING MEDIATING STRUCTURES	HEALTHY LIFESTYLES	REORIENTED HEALTH SERVICES
Ecosystem viability	Caring relationships	Public policies supporting smoke-free places/lives	Medical self-care
Economic sufficiency	Respect for others	'Green' agricultural/food policies	Community-based Primary Health Care
Equitable public policies	Service for others	Town-planning to promote physical fitness . . .	Efficacious personal care services (secondary, tertiary)
Convivial communities	Generosity towards others		
Sustainable development . . .	Self-help groups		
	Public institutions that support social capital		

(Source: Labonté, R. 1997 *Power, Participation and Partnerships for Health Promotion*. VicHealth, Melbourne, Chapter 1, pp. 13, 21)

what is apparent; the measurable states of health or health outcomes. Using the iceberg analogy, they refer to the small section that is visible above the waterline. These could be either positive or negative states of health. These could include mortality and morbidity measures and prevalence of known risk factors related to the physiological risk factors outlined in the previous section, such as high blood pressure. The section immediately below the waterline is connected to the visible state of health and can be identified and measured without too much difficulty. This section relates to individuals' lifestyle choices and behavioural risk factors; for example, the link between smoking and lung cancer, poor nutrition and heart disease. The lowest and largest section of the iceberg, well below the surface and hard to explore, relates to the psycho–socio–cultural determinants outlined previously. Here the major factors that influence individual and population health are to be found. This diagrammatic representation is useful because it continues with the iceberg metaphor. Only a very small proportion is visible; there is far greater danger (to health status) hidden below.

It is interesting to do a simple exercise using the health iceberg model to examine heart disease. Mortality and morbidity figures indicate this is a major health issue in Australia and many other nations (AIHW 2002). What are the factors that contribute to heart disease? For example: high blood pressure, excess weight, smoking, high cholesterol, family history. What are the structural issues? For example: the overarching economic imperative to make money and consume goods leading to overtime which causes stress which leads to these physiological symptoms. What are the lifestyle behaviours that contribute to heart disease? For example: a busy life with little physical activity, poor diet — take-away food, frequenting pubs and clubs with a lot of smoking and drinking. What are the psycho–socio–cultural factors that contribute to heart disease via the factors above them in the iceberg? For example: grew up in a family where physical activity was not valued, lack of physical education at school, poor body image, no convenient

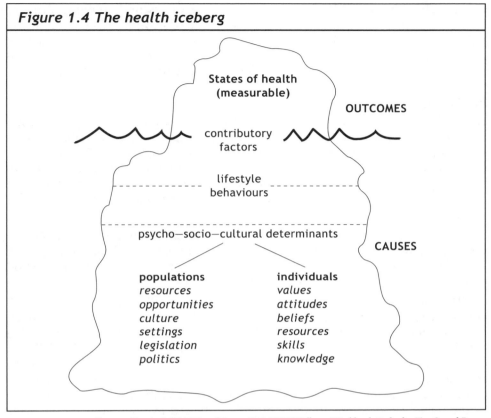

Figure 1.4 The health iceberg

(Source: Travis, J. W. MD and Ryan, R. S. 2004 *Wellness Workbook*, 3rd edn. Ten Speed Press, Berkeley, CA. © 1981, 1988, 2004 by Travis, J.W)

safe or affordable facility for activity, smoking is the normal behaviour valued among friends and family, low income so cannot afford a range of healthier foods, lack of knowledge of healthy diet, poor food preparation skills, poor use of health services to identify risk factors early.

Understanding these factors should inform the activities health workers take, the communities they choose to work with and the way in which they work. Understanding the global context is also vital.

Global and international 'drivers' in health policy

The rise of economic rationalism and the impact on health

A major threat to comprehensive Primary Health Care has been the international rise of neo-liberalism, or economic rationalism as it is more commonly known in Australia. The threat lies in the fact that the values underpinning Primary Health Care philosophy are in conflict with those of neo-liberalism. Neo-liberal philosophy is built around the belief that as much of national and international life as possible should be left to the effects of the market and that governments should minimise their involvement in public life (Baum & Sanders 1995, p. 154).

Historical overview

Australian fiscal policy was clearly underpinned in the post-World War II period through to the 1970s by the philosophy of equal rights among all citizens, with a considerable expansion of social welfare provisions (Beresford 2000, p. 45). At the same time a range of regulations were used to ensure the private sector of the economy operated to achieve broader social goals. In particular a system of import tariffs on manufactured goods was considered essential to maintain full employment.

Commencing in the early 1970s, Australian economic policy has been gradually remodelled away from a social equity agenda towards an emphasis on economic efficiency. Australia has gradually reduced its primary industry tariff protection and opened markets to international trade competition.

The election of the Australian Labor Party (ALP) Government in 1972 commenced a significant period of social and political change in Australia, which brought about changes in the fiscal policies that still underpin Australia's trading activities. The ALP Government introduced a large number of social policies in this era and social expenditure as a proportion of Gross Domestic Product (GDP) rose significantly (Castles 1989, p. 22). In 1974 the Medibank Health Scheme was commenced. The social justice purpose generated a significant increase in the size of the public service, and this was broadly criticised by conservative politicians and the business community as consuming too many scarce resources and was therefore unsustainable.

Internationally, liberalisation of trade proceeded, particularly within the development of regional arrangements, such as the European Community (EC) and the agreement between the United States and Canada. Britain commenced an innovative movement to privatise a range of public enterprises. From the early 1980s to the early 1990s the ALP Government progressively opened up the economy to the world market and liberalised market processes. Opening national markets to free and competitive trade, without government impositions increased competition on global markets, which in turn imposed pressure on primary producers to reduce overhead costs and prices.

The two policy agendas of liberalisation of trade and privatisation of government assets have been adopted since the early 1980s and are the common approaches to fiscal management adopted by many industrialised nations. The major premise is described as economic rationalism, a model of public policy where decisions are evaluated on the grounds of economic efficiency (Beresford 2000, pp. 58–9). The major policy goals of this approach are:

- reducing the size and function of the public sector;
- microeconomic reform;
- privatisation of public assets;

- corporatisation;
- deregulation; and
- introduction of competitive tendering into government service delivery.

Each of these goals is explored in more detail by Beresford (2000, pp. 61–79).

There is evidence that the liberalisation policies adopted by the successive governments in Australia have resulted in some efficiency gains, increased labour productivity and reduced costs across a number of industries (Industry Commission, cited by Henderson 1995, p. 78). However, trade liberalisation changes, including the progressive removal of primary industry tariff protection, have translated into pressure for individual producers to reduce overheads; their profit margins have been cut and work hours have increased (Tonts 2000).

The market reforms are unlikely to be reversed, particularly while economic measures continue to be almost the only criterion by which success is measured and while neo-liberal assumptions underpin governance decisions (Hancock 1999). However, it is unclear whether liberalisation has resulted in overall improvements in economic performance. The social impacts of these policy changes have not been clearly articulated either and there is acknowledgment that greater economic and social inequalities now exist than they did previously. It is also clear that market competition associated with worldwide economic liberalisation polices does have local social impacts, which are felt more in rural areas and countries whose producers are not protected by subsidies. Lower profit margins and longer work hours will have an obvious impact on the lifestyle of any family. Some social commentators have argued that global economic competitiveness is having widespread and sustained policy effects; that it has meant the end of the traditional social democracy approach underpinned by taxation and wealth distribution policies which support the philosophy of equality of opportunity (Beresford 2000, p. 91). Globalised markets ensure that nations reduce social expenditure; nations are penalised by transnational corporations who will move their industry offshore if they seek to raise taxes to support an increase in welfare payments. The rise of economic rationalism has led to a number of developments that have had a grave impact on the health of the world's population and undermined the very foundations of the Health for All movement internationally. Inequality has increased with a marked increase in the concentration of wealth in the hands of a few. As a consequence, health inequalities between rich and poor have worsened (WHO 1998b, p. 3; Labonté 2004). This is true for both industrialised and developing countries. Many multinational corporations now have larger budgets than many countries, with the world's largest 100 companies now being larger than most United Nations member countries, and the top 500 companies now controlling more than 70 per cent of world trade (Morehouse 1997, p. 4). As a result, the richest 358 billionaires together now own more than the poorest 45 per cent of the world's population (UN 1996, cited by Kawachi & Kennedy 1997, p. 1037). At least some of these consequences have resulted from the implementation of 'structural adjustment programs' in many developing countries around the world, which are contributing to the further transfer of wealth from poor to rich (Bello et al 1994).

The impact of structural adjustment programs

Throughout the 1970s, majority world countries had been encouraged to borrow large amounts of money from the major banks. With changes to the international financial situation, interest rates skyrocketed in the 1980s, resulting in those countries owing huge debts which they could not pay (Werner et al 1997, p. 81; Bello et al 1994). This situation continues today. Vast quantities of money are being moved each year from poor countries to rich countries, in order to service debt repayments. The impact of this drain on resources is felt most heavily by the poor, especially children (UNICEF 1992, cited by Werner et al 1997, p. 82).

Because of concern by the banks that these countries would not be able to repay their loans, the International Monetary Fund and The World Bank stepped in. They offered to refinance the loans, on the proviso that countries accepted 'structural adjustment programs', designed to ensure that countries serviced the debt owed, but with major consequences for their internal policies. There are four main tenets of the structural adjustment programs which debt-ridden majority countries had to agree to in order to qualify for a loan. These are, firstly, devaluation of the currency which immediately decreases the purchasing power of individuals; it makes exports cheaper, and therefore more competitive, and imports more expensive, therefore less desirable. Secondly, governments are required to make drastic cuts to its public spending, such as health, education and other social services. Thirdly, promotion of exports, through, for instance, a move away from food production to production of export goods and putting a freeze on local wages to ensure low-cost tradable items. Fourthly, countries are required to open up the economy for overseas goods and investors, such as through easing rules for foreign investment or bypassing environment legislation (Bello et al 1994; Werner et al 1997, p. 83). It is not difficult to imagine the impact that these changes have had on the health of the country's poor or how they have increased socioeconomic inequalities in and between nations. The WHO notes that 'the least developed countries faced difficulty even in maintaining basic minimum services in the social sector, including health' (WHO 1998b, p. 3). In addition, the reduction in land for food production and subsistence farming means that many of the poor can no longer get enough food to eat.

In the face of criticism that the impacts of structural adjustment packages benefited the loan agencies of the International Monetary Fund and The World Bank, but consigned the recipient nations to overwhelming debt, some reform of the programs and debt-forgiveness have been promised. To this stage there is little evidence of change (Bello 2002).

Economic rationalism in the minority world

Industrialised countries, in the meantime, have been undergoing their own self-imposed structural adjustment programs as a result of the acceptance of economic rationalism. In Australia, there have been significant reductions in real terms in expenditure on health, education and other social services (see, for example, Gardner 1995). There has also been significant support for privatisation of services, with little consideration of the consequences for those aspects of health, education and social welfare that do not fit comfortably within a market model. The gap between rich and poor in Australia has increased significantly.

In addition, publicly provided services themselves have been required to implement management techniques from the private sector. This corporatisation of the public sector has had a significant impact on the focus of public services and the philosophy that drives them (McCoppin 1995).

It can be argued that privatisation of government assets and the introduction of user-pays systems of access to services such as health care have an impact that is inequitably shared across the population (Baum 2000). Hancock (1999, p. 60) highlights the difficulty in applying the principles of economic rationalism to 'social' goods. Using commercial principles for services that are not based on discretionary decisions contradicts the philosophical assumption that public goods are distributed as a part of a national ethos of rights and fairness, and should not be purely profit-driven (Leeder 2003). Competitive capitalism may be boosting prosperity for some, but the assumption that there will be 'trickle down' benefits for all members of society cannot be sustained and there is evidence of growing inequality, which undermines community connectedness and wellbeing (Beresford 2000; Cox 1998; Labonté 1999). In addition, the public sector should serve a number of long-term human capital purposes, such as providing for training and community development. The outcomes of these may not be measurable in economic terms or they would not be measurable in usual outcome indicators or during one political cycle (Stretton & Orton, 1994). This consequence of economic rationalism, known as managerialism, or new public management, is based on a set of values fundamentally at odds with the Primary Health Care approach.

The growing impact of The World Bank on international health policy

In 1993 The World Bank in collaboration with the WHO released its annual development report, focusing on 'investing in health' (The World Bank 1993). With the power of The World Bank, particularly in poor or majority countries, this document is likely to be a significant indicator of future developments in health policy.

'Investing in Health' analysed the health systems around the world and proposed a range of health policy reforms. However, it has been acknowledged that it is a document full of contradictions, and this seems to have stemmed from the fact that it attempted to address both the WHO's Health for All agenda and the agenda of The World Bank (Baum & Sanders 1995, p. 155). 'Investing in Health' identified a range of important issues though. It identified the importance of poverty in creating ill health, and the need for effective health systems to have a strong focus on public health rather than excessive emphasis on expensive high-technology care. It also recognised the importance of education for health, and the need to change economic systems in order to change the health chances of people around the world (Baum & Sanders 1995, p. 154).

At the same time, however, it took a largely uncritical stance towards the role of markets in health, and a largely negative stance towards the value of government in service provision. It suggested greater involvement of the private sector in health services in majority and former socialist countries, without acknowledging the shortcomings of market involvement in the health systems of industrialised countries (Curtis & Taket 1996, p. 273). It recommended that governments take on the role of dealing with market failure in health care, rather than one of providing a comprehensive high-quality service themselves.

Concern has been expressed that, through investing in health, The World Bank continues to work to maintain underdevelopment in some nations, with considerable negative consequences for the poor, in order to address its own agenda, which is not primarily about health (Curtis & Taket 1996, p. 276). With its focus on providing clinical services, investing in health reflects a focus on selective Primary Health Care, an approach likely to become even narrower because of the report's focus on private provision of health and health-related services.

'Investing in Health' largely ignored the negative effects of structural adjustment programs, even though they undermine some of the very recommendations that the report made (Baum & Sanders 1995, p. 155). 'Investing in Health' may well result in health issues becoming a more visible part of the international agenda. However, its support for greater 'marketisation', its assumption that benefits trickle down to the poor, and its inadequate concern with dealing directly with inequity, seem to reflect an emphasis on health as an area for business investment rather than emphasising the inherent value in investing in people. Investing in people (and so their health) is a core value that underpins Primary Health Care. Investing in the health system is a small part of building that asset.

Health systems and Primary Health Care

In the light of these global structures, it is clear that there are enormous challenges for health professionals working within a Primary Health Care philosophy. At the Fifth International Conference on Health Promotion in Mexico, referred to earlier in this chapter, reorienting health services was one of the technical themes for the conference. The major findings of the technical report expressed the need to integrate health promotion and disease prevention into the health care delivery process and to incorporate health-promotion principles into health service management as an integral part of every stage of the system. It was acknowledged that although reorientation of health systems had been a fundamental element of the Ottawa Charter, development had been patchy and there had been no systematic analysis of what has happened and what was possible (WHO 2000). These findings are supported elsewhere. For example, the overall message of *The World Health Report* (WHO 2003) is to strengthen health systems to address health inequalities. The report calls for a reinforcement of Primary Health Care principles as outlined in the Declaration of Alma-Ata and advocates 'principled integrated care' (p. 105). The WHO also recognises the importance of collaborating with others and offers an integrated approach to improving health.

The World Health Report examines four major challenges facing health systems, namely: the global health workforce crisis; the lack of appropriate, timely evidence; the stewardship challenge of implementing pro-equity health policies in a pluralistic environment; and the lack of financial resources (WHO 2003, p. 105).

The global workforce crisis is the most urgent issue facing health care systems. There is not only a shortage of the number of people who make them work, but there is also a shortage of the right mix of skills from acute care through to health promotion and rehabilitation. Cost containment measures, changed priorities and discrimination contribute to the problem.

Cost containment measures threaten the quantity and quality of workers. In addition, government priorities have moved away from workforce issues worldwide. Traditionally, health professionals were recruited, trained and employed in health systems funded and managed by government bureaucracies. Structural reforms of the civil service in most countries no longer guarantee the numbers of skilled health professionals required. Gender discrimination in health professions continues to contribute to the workforce crisis. While men continue to occupy managerial positions in the health bureaucracy, the needs of women employees will not be met. Evidence suggests that offering workers good working conditions, adequate remuneration, the chance to work in a supportive team, the opportunity for further education and being shown respect, develops a healthy workforce. To achieve the goals associated with health care systems driven by Primary Health Care philosophy, renewed commitment and new options for education and employment of health workers are required (WHO 2003).

The lack of appropriate timely evidence also threatens health care systems. A health information system based on Primary Health Care principles can be defined as 'an integrated effort to collect, process, report and use health information and knowledge to influence policy-making, programme action and research' (WHO 2003, p. 116). The information can be used for strategic decision-making and also for program-planning, implementation, monitoring and evaluation. Integration of data, for example, from the census, epidemiological studies and health services forms part of the system as it is measuring inequalities in risk factors and key health indicators. Robust health information systems are needed in health care systems oriented to Primary Health Care principles so that the needs of the population, particularly those most in need, can be understood and addressed efficiently and effectively. Measurement of access to, and use of, health services could assist governments to perform their stewardship role more effectively.

Commitment to health equity as part of development oriented to social justice is one of the principles of Primary Health Care and an essential part of effective stewardship. Health ministries are responsible for protecting citizens' health and ensuring quality care is provided. Pro-equity health care strategies differ from country to country. Access to health care is one measure of equity. Globally this usually takes three forms. In the poorest countries most of the population have equal but deficient access to health care. The elite class in these countries find ways to obtain care. In richer countries general access is better, but the middle and upper classes benefit most and the lower class usually have to queue for care. In some countries the majority of the population has adequate access to health care but a small minority, often the poorest, are deprived (WHO 2003, p. 123). The World Health Report (WHO 2003) states that an approach based on Primary Health Care recognises the need to attack the roots of health disparities inter-sectorally and supports the notion of the Millennium Development Goals (see Box 1.3).

Primary Health Care principles and activities include community participation in defining and implementing health agendas. If governments are to perform their stewardship roles effectively they must engage the community through

> ## Box 1.3 The Millennium Development Goals
>
> 1. Eradicate extreme poverty
>   Target for 2015: Halve the proportion of people living on less than a dollar a day and those who suffer from hunger.
> 2. Achieve universal primary education
>   Target for 2015: Ensure that all boys and girls complete primary school.
> 3. Promote gender equality and empower women
>   Targets for 2005 and 2015: Eliminate gender disparities in primary and secondary education preferably by 2005, and at all levels by 2015.
> 4. Reduce child mortality
>   Target for 2015: Reduce by two-thirds the mortality rate among children under five.
> 5. Improve maternal health
>   Target for 2015: Reduce by three-quarters the ration of women dying in childbirth.
> 6. Combat HIV/AIDS, malaria and other diseases
>   Target by 2015: Halt and begin to reverse the spread of HIV/AIDS and the incidence of malaria and other major diseases.
> 7. Ensure environmental sustainability
>   Targets:
>   • Integrate the principles of sustainable development into country policies and programs and reverse the loss of environmental resources.
>   • By 2015, reduce by half the proportion of people without access to safe drinking water.
>   • By 2020 achieve significant improvement in the lives of at least 100 million slum dwellers.
>   More than one billion people lack access to safe drinking water and more than two billion lack sanitation. During the 1990s nearly one billion people gained access to safe water and the same number to sanitation.
> 8. Develop a global partnership for development
>   Targets:
>   • Provide access to affordable essential drugs.
>   • Reduce poverty.

(Source: United Nations 2003 *United Nations Development Program 2003*. Online. Available: http://www.undp.org/mdg/ [accessed 20th January 2004])

participation, empowerment and ownership strategies. 'When the right structures are in place, effective governance and vigorous community involvement support each other' (WHO 2003, p. 126).

In terms of strengthening health care systems there is great inequity in global health care spending. Globally, health care spending has grown substantially due to growth of the medico–industrial complex; however, this has occurred primarily in minority countries such as the Organization for Economic Cooperation and Development (OECD) countries. In the year 2000, the population of the OECD countries accounted for less than 20 per cent of the world's population; however, spending on health in those same countries accounted for 90 per cent of the world's health spending (WHO 2003, p. 120).

Health care spending in Australia

Health expenditure is rising in all OECD countries. Australian expenditure, for example, rose from 7.9 per cent GDP in 1990 to 9.3 per cent in 2001 (AIHW 2004). Australia spent less than the United States of America, Canada, France and Germany, but more than Japan, New Zealand and the United Kingdom during the same period (AIHW 2004). Australia maintains a predominantly publicly funded health care system; however, the public sector proportion of total expenditure is lower in Australia than in other OECD countries. For example, in 1995, the percentage in Australia was 75 per cent whereas in the United Kingdom it was 84 per cent. This compares to 46 per cent in the United States with its large private health sector (OECD 2000 in Hilless & Healy 2001, p. 39). Publicly funded health care systems have been better able to contain costs, while generating universal cover compared to more privatised systems (Mossialos & Le Grand, 1999 in Hilless & Healy, 2001, p. 39). The share of the health budget devoted to hospitals grew from the mid-1960s to the early 1980s but has since declined, while budget shares for pharmaceuticals and community-based health services have grown. About 35 per cent of expenditure goes on acute care hospitals, 18 per cent on medical services and 14 per cent on pharmaceuticals. Public health expenditure is difficult to estimate because it appears under several budgetary headings. However, disease prevention and population health promotion receives less than 2 per cent of the total recurrent health budget. If public and community health are combined, the figure comes to 5.4 per cent (AIHW 2003). However, community-based care is no guarantee of Primary Health Care principles or health-promoting activity. Public health expenditure was 'squeezed' in the early 1990s, but has been protected in joint commonwealth and state programs since 1996 (Hilless & Healy 2001). Figure 1.5 provides recurrent expenditure on health goods and services, current prices, by broad area of expenditure and Figure 1.6 provides expenditure on public health by activity.

The focus of the Australian health care system has been largely on the provision of acute illness care services to individuals. This means that attention and resources are focused on treating the end result rather than the cause of health problems, and the scope for increasing activity to prevent health problems is great. This is reflected in how Australia spends its health budget. Clearly, there is scope for Australia to focus more of its health expenditure on the promotion and protection of health. At the same time, a comprehensive whole-of-government approach is needed if we are to fully protect and maximise the health of the community. Such a whole-of-government approach would need to consider the health consequences of public policy in all areas, including the health portfolio itself.

There are three basic goals of health care system reform: equity, efficiency and quality. The major hallmarks of health system reform in Australia include the preservation of universal tax-financed health care; the dominance of 'supply-side theory' in order to contain costs; a strong stewardship role for government; some alteration in the public/private mix with attempts to strengthen the market; and a continuing commitment to social solidarity and equity (Bloom 2000b in Hilless & Healy 2001).

At the Australian Health Care Summit in 2003, a bipartisan and independent group of more than 250 consumers, doctors, nurses, allied health and other

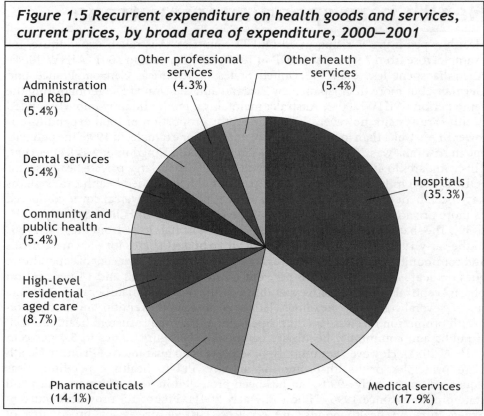

Figure 1.5 Recurrent expenditure on health goods and services, current prices, by broad area of expenditure, 2000–2001

Other professional services (4.3%)

Other health services (5.4%)

Administration and R&D (5.4%)

Dental services (5.4%)

Community and public health (5.4%)

High-level residential aged care (8.7%)

Pharmaceuticals (14.1%)

Hospitals (35.3%)

Medical services (17.9%)

(Source: Australian Institute of Health and Welfare 2003 *Health Expenditure and Funding* by Area. AIHW, Canberra)

professionals met to discuss ways of reforming Australia's health system. The *Communiqué* (http://www.healthsummit.org.au) outlined the principles that must underpin Australia's health system, and they included:

- universal access underpinned by a strong Primary Health Care system in a timely fashion based on need, not the ability to pay;
- equity of health outcomes irrespective of socioeconomic status, race, cultural background, disability, mental illness, age, gender or location;
- consumers and patients must come first in health care services;
- health promotion, preventing disease and maintaining health must be appropriately emphasised and balanced with our duty of care to those already unwell;
- personal and corporate tax contributions should fund our health care — our health insurance for each other;
- a fair balance of public and private resources and investment is needed to ensure equitable health outcomes for all Australians;
- the health outcomes of Aboriginal and Torres Strait Islander Australians must be improved so that they match those of other Australians;
- health services must be appropriate, safe and high quality;

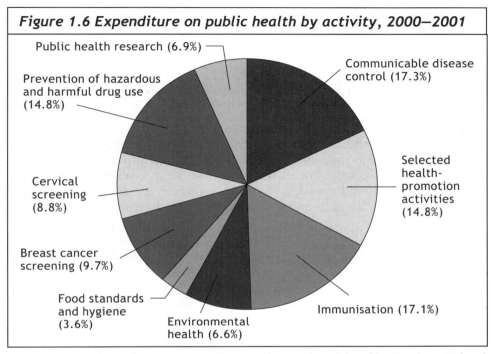

Figure 1.6 Expenditure on public health by activity, 2000–2001

Public health research (6.9%)

Prevention of hazardous and harmful drug use (14.8%)

Cervical screening (8.8%)

Breast cancer screening (9.7%)

Food standards and hygiene (3.6%)

Environmental health (6.6%)

Immunisation (17.1%)

Selected health-promotion activities (14.8%)

Communicable disease control (17.3%)

(Source: Australian Institute of Health and Welfare 2004 *Australia's Health, 2004*. AIHW, Canberra)

- the community, especially consumers and carers, must play an integral part in the development, planning and implementation of our health services; and
- the workforce must be valued.

A significant amount of money used to promote the health of the community is spent from budgets other than health. For example, money spent on safe roads, public transport systems and basic services, such as water supply, has a positive impact on health, yet is not counted as part of health-promotion expenditure. A strong health care system is essential to improve the health status of the population but it will not do it alone. There was no mention of inter-sectoral action for health at the latest summit and so while the principles are commensurate with the Primary Health Care principles, the effect on the health status of the population will not be optimised.

Reorienting health services: integrated health promotion

In *Infrastructures to promote health: the art of the possible* Moodie et al (2000) examine some of the barriers to reorienting health services and then outline the developments that are needed to integrate health promotion effectively into the health system. An effective infrastructure that promotes health relies primarily on three things, namely:

1. development of the necessary skills that ensure health promotion becomes a major issue in political and bureaucratic circles;

2. identification of existing infrastructures that could support health promotion better; and

3. the development of dedicated infrastructure for health promotion.

(Moodie et al 2000)

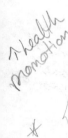

Skilled health workers in health promotion not only need knowledge and skills in the 'science' of health promotion but also the 'art' of health promotion. This means developing knowledge and skills in such things as communication, negotiation, conflict resolution, cooperation, advocacy, networking, coalition building and visioning. This will build a workforce skilled in placing health promotion on the agenda of government and its policy-making arm (Moodie et al 2000).

At the same time, the determinants of health demonstrate that inter-sectoral collaboration is essential. For health workers this means identifying the structures inside and outside the health sector that have the greatest impact on health and working with those sectors, sharing expertise, reducing duplication and ensuring development within these sectors are cognisant of health impacts (Moodie et al 2000). The public health workforce includes people who have a role in health promotion but may not have recognised this; for example, business leaders, teachers or town planners. There may be others, such as community development workers and volunteers, or there may be people working at the strategic level, such as health consultants/specialists (MacKian et al 2003).

Within the health sector, a dedicated health-promotion sector can be the 'driver' for the above activities and provide the infrastructure for dedicated health-promotion practice (Moodie et al 2000).

A continuum of health-promotion approaches

Primary Health Care and health promotion

It has already been stated in this chapter that health promotion and illness prevention are based on the principles of Primary Health Care. The Primary Health Care approach emphasises health promotion, disease prevention, equity in health status, health education, and inter-sectoral health care planning and organisation. Importantly it shifts the focus away from an individual disease-prevention approach toward the underlying influences on health.

Health-promotion practice incorporates disease prevention but extends beyond it to address broader social, environmental and cultural issues impacting on health. Health-promotion activities or service delivery can be organised from a range of different, but complementary approaches, depending on the key priorities identified in epidemiological data and in the determinants of health.

Key requirements

Key requirements for quality in health-promotion practice are that it draws on the Primary Health Care philosophical guidelines set out earlier.

1. it is done with and by the people, not for them: it encourages participation in decision-making at all levels;

2. it usually involves a range of different approaches that include structural and policy changes for people in the context of their everyday lives, not just a focus on individual behaviour change approaches; and

3. it is directed to improving people's control over the determinants of their health.

How to health promotion

A number of categories for health-promotion interventions can be envisaged. They form a continuum which illustrates how the interventions relate to each other; strategies with an individual focus at one end and those with a population socio-ecological focus at the other end. Each category on the continuum is outlined briefly below.

Community action and capacity building Community action aims to encourage and empower communities (both geographic areas and communities of interest) to build their capacity to develop and sustain improvements in their social and physical environments.

Advocacy involves a combination of individual, peer and social actions designed to gain political commitment, policy support, structural change, social acceptance and systems support for a particular goal. It includes direct political lobbying.

These are typically community development activities organised across whole communities or populations such as local community capacity-building activities, and national awareness campaigns. Examples could include Schizophrenia Awareness Week, the Shared Action Project (Beillharz 2002) or the Contaminated Sites Alliance in Western Australia (Dunnet 2004).

Settings and supportive environments Health-promotion activities are organised around particular settings, such as schools, workplaces and communities, that bring together groups of people who share common characteristics. The setting also enables structural and legislative support that cannot be implemented so readily elsewhere. Examples could include SunSmart schools. Two important strategy approaches include:

1. Organisational development strategies — aim to create a supportive environment for health-promotion activities within organisations. This strategy involves ensuring that policies, service directions, priorities and practices integrate health-promotion principles.

2. Economic and regulatory activities — involves the application of financial and legislative incentives or disincentives to support healthy choices. These approaches might include policy at various levels, guidelines, protocols or organisational plans. They typically focus on restrictions and enforcement, pricing and availability. Examples could include Occupational Health and Safety, and Environmental Protection legislation.

These two approaches (sometimes referred to as socio-ecological approaches) usually involve change being made at policy or planning level by a budget-holder, on behalf of another group of constituents, workers or population groups. They are likely to be sustained over time if community members are directly involved in identifying the need, planning and implementing an approach.

Health education and skill development Health education and skill development include the provision of education to individuals (through discrete planned sessions) or groups, with the aim of improving knowledge, attitudes, self-efficacy and individual capacity to change. Activities may be organised around population groups such as adolescents, culturally and linguistically diverse groups, same-sex attracted youth or Aboriginal people. Such groups are singled out because of higher mortality or morbidity indicators and they become the 'target' for specific health-promotion messages and strategies.

Social marketing/health information Social marketing involves programs designed to advocate for change and influence the voluntary behaviour of target audiences to benefit this audience and society as a whole. The aim is to shift attitudes, change people's view of themselves and their relationships with others, change lifelong habits, values or behaviours. Social marketing and health information typically use persuasive and cultural change processes (not just information). Health-promotion activities are organised around lifestyle factors and behaviours, such as smoking, physical inactivity and ways to improve mental health.

Health information aims to improve people's understanding about the causes of health and illness, the services and support available to help maintain or improve health, and personal responsibility for actions affecting their health.

These approaches can involve raising public awareness about a health issue through use of mass media; for example, advertising in newspapers, magazines, pamphlets, and fliers or on radio, television and so forth at local, state and national levels. It may also involve a mix of promotional strategies including public relations and face-to-face communications.

Screening, individual risk factor assessment and immunisation Screening involves the systematic use of a test or investigatory tool to detect individuals at risk of developing a specific disease that is amenable to prevention or treatment. Activities include medical and preventive approaches designed at improving physiological risk factors, such as heart disease, lack of immunisation and early recognition of psychosis (State Government of Victoria 2003, p. 45). Early detection of diseases such as various cancers are also included in these approaches.

Individual risk factor assessment involves a more comprehensive process of detecting overall risk of a single disease or multiple diseases. These can include biological, psychological and behavioural risks.

These last three approaches are most traditionally identified with health-promotion activities; however, with the exception of immunisation, these activities aim at the early detection of disease rather than disease prevention or health promotion. With early detection of a primary disease, however, complications that may further compromise the health of an individual may be prevented. Strategies usually require individuals to initiate an activity to enhance their current or future health or to change an existing lifestyle or behavioural risk. The approaches do not alter the underlying life conditions for the individual.

Figure 1.6 provides a summary of health-promotion approaches represented as a continuum which extends from a population focus on social and environmental change, through behavioural approaches to the individual focus on risk assessment and management associated with many medical approaches.

Figure 1.6 Continuum of health-promotion approaches				
Population focus ———————————————————— Individual focus				
Community action for social and environmental change	Settings and supportive environments Economic and regulatory activities	Health, education, skill development	Health information Social marketing	Screening, individual risk assessment and immunisation
Socio-environmental approach	Behavioural approach			Medical approach

(Note: These health-promotion approaches underpin the structure in succeeding chapters.)

Conclusion

The last 30 years have seen the development of numerous international, national and local policies and programs designed to reorient health systems towards Primary Health Care and health promotion. These developments occurred as a result of recognition of inequities in health and social development throughout the world. We have seen some important action based on these calls for a reorientation of our approach to health issues.

At the same time, however, commitment to the principles of social justice, equity and a responsive health system based on population need has been challenged. The impact of economic rationalism around the world can be seen in a narrower commitment to Primary Health Care and health promotion. Because of these global policies it is unclear to what extent countries around the world can renew their commitment to the Primary Health Care approach. For many of the world's poor countries, the choice seems almost taken out of their hands as a result of the global economic policies, which seems to have locked them into a system of creating markets for medical technologies through replication of the health care systems of the minority world at the expense of more affordable, sustainable and equitable Primary Health Care models. The WHO, sympathetic governments and non-government organisations with a concern for social justice have an important role to play in maintaining these principles on the international agenda.

Within the context of the policies described in this chapter, and sometimes despite them, many health workers have been working to implement the principles of Primary Health Care and health promotion in their practice. The result has been some inspiring examples of what can be achieved by working in this way. In order to do this, practitioners have been drawing on a range of skills and strategies, which have then been developed and discussed in the professional literature and have been integrated into the education of many health workers. This process has been taken up around the world by many in the health professions and has paralleled the activities of governments, who cannot alone implement the changes required in a Primary Health Care approach.

The challenge for health workers is to put into practice the principles of Primary Health Care and health promotion using a social health perspective. Many of the key strategies and skills required to do this effectively are discussed in the remainder of this book. Health workers are encouraged to take up the challenge of the Primary Health Care approach by incorporating the principles of Primary Health Care into their daily practice and developing and implementing their skills in health promotion.

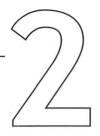

Concepts and values in health promotion

Chapter 1 identified a number of important principles in Primary Health Care and the New Public Health movement. The centrality of social justice and equity in the promotion of health and directly addressing the determinants of health problems were identified as fundamental issues for contemplation and action in public health. Definitions of health and health promotion were examined in the context of their historical development.

Given the importance of these issues, and some of the dilemmas they have presented, this chapter will explore these issues in greater depth, and present some other key concepts and values, raising a number of important challenges that health workers will face as they grapple with the complexities of health promotion. Many of these serve to reiterate the particular value base of the Primary Health Care approach to health promotion.

[handwritten margin note: social justice & equity in hltn promot'n are fundament'l issues]

Defining health

No examination of health promotion is possible without first considering what health is. The health of individuals is strongly influenced by the social and physical environments and it can never be fully considered outside that context.

[handwritten margin note: hlth strongly infl. by social & phys'l environ]

In defining health, it is not sufficient to consider only the health of the individual. If health is defined only in individual terms, then issues of power and control, and the unequal access to life chances because of socioeconomic status, ethnicity and gender, for example, are easily ignored. Two notable efforts to keep the health of individuals firmly in context have come from the Aboriginal health movement and the environmental movement, where concern for spiritual and cultural connectedness and ecological sustainability, respectively, have moved health definitions beyond the individual. And so, for example, Aboriginal health has been defined as:

[handwritten margin note: cannot def'n hlth in ind. terms.]

> Not just the physical wellbeing of the individual but the social, emotional, and cultural wellbeing of the whole community. This is a whole-of-life view and it also includes the cyclical concept of life-death-life.

[handwritten margin note: Abo hlth def'n. H do this for paper]

(National Aboriginal Health Strategy Working Party 1989, p. x)

Similarly, Honari (1993, p. 23), attempting a similar approach, provides an environ-mental definition of health by defining health as 'a sustainable state of wellbeing, within sustainable ecosystems, within a sustainable biosphere'. The WHO's definition of health, with its inclusion of social wellbeing, touches on this interrelationship by recognising the links between individuals and their social world.

Individual health is defined in different ways depending on who you are. Probably the main distinction between definitions of individual health is between those that define health as the absence of disease and those that define it more broadly as a sense of wellness. Consider the following examples. Whom would you regard as healthy:

- a person who has a chronic illness but is happy and lives an active life;
- a person who appears well but lives next to a toxic waste dump;
- a person who appears well but engages in risky behaviours;
- a person who appears well but feels a lack of purpose in their life;
- a person who appears well but is culturally isolated and psychologically depressed;
- a person who is living in poverty?

How health is defined is very important because definitions determine what are regarded as health problems and therefore what will be regarded as health promotion. If we define health as merely the absence of disease, we see health promotion as disease prevention, and ignore the determinants of health and illness that may make people's lives uncomfortable but which are not medically classified as diseases or risk factors for disease. Ignoring those problems, such as chronic back pain, discrimination, or fear for safety, for example, may leave people suffering from conditions that limit their abilities or reduce their quality of life. It is quite possible that, if we address only medically defined problems, we could be ignoring day-to-day issues that do not seem to be related to diseases, only to discover in a few years that they do, in fact, play an important role in disease causation. For example, cigarette smoking was a socially acceptable habit until recently and it is not all that long ago that sunbathing was regarded as a normal healthy activity. Furthermore, many environmental health issues are ignored on the grounds that there is no 'evidence' of a problem, when evidence may take 20 years to surface and people may have already suffered greatly during this time.

The WHO's definition of health as 'a complete state of physical, mental and social wellbeing, and not merely the absence of disease or infirmity' is probably the most often cited definition of health. It has been important for the role it has played in highlighting that health is about much more than the absence of disease, and that it is much more than a physical state. This point has been reiterated by the WHO, with the Ottawa Charter for Health Promotion stating that health is 'a resource for everyday life, not the objective of living' (WHO 1986). The extent to which people value their health depends on a wide range of factors in addition to the state of their bodies. However, the WHO definition has been criticised on a number of grounds (see, for example, Sax 1990, p. 1). On one hand, firstly, it has been argued that it is unrealistic and unachievable, because it describes a state of such total wellbeing that it is unlikely that anyone could achieve it for more than a very brief period in their lives. With its focus on perfection, too, it excludes those with disabilities or long-term medical conditions.

Secondly, it has been criticised for being unmeasurable, describing, as it does, a general state of wellbeing. Indeed, it has been pointed out that, despite health having been defined this way since 1946, health statistics still only enable us to measure death and disease and we remain without effective measures of health broadly defined (Mathers & Douglas 1998, p. 125).

On the other hand, some have criticised the WHO definition for not being broad enough. For example, a number of authors have noted its lack of inclusion of spiritual wellbeing, which is increasingly being recognised as important (Teshuva et al 1997; Raeburn & Rootman 1998). And, as noted above, those in the Aboriginal health and environmental movements have criticised its definition of individual health out of a cultural and ecological context.

Despite these difficulties with the WHO definition of health, it remains an important concept, and is an important starting point because it has pointed the way to consideration of the determinants of health. People other than health workers embedded in the medico–industrial complex often define health along the same lines as the WHO definition of health (Blaxter 1990, p. 3). That is, many people identify themselves as healthy more by a sense of wellbeing within the context of their whole lives than by the presence or absence of disease. This may be because the WHO definition of health makes intrinsic sense to many people, so it has endured as a useful definition of health, despite the difficulties experienced by scientists and social scientists in trying to measure it.

[margin note: lay people def'n hlth along the WHO's def'n of hlth.]

De Vries reminds us that a sense of wellbeing equates with a sense of wholeness, which is what the term health originally meant (de Vries 1993, p. 129). As de Vries points out (1993, p. 29):

> wholeness is not the same as being happy or living without pain, frustration or handicaps; wholeness may be achieved in the presence of disease or infirmity.

[margin note: wellbeing = wholeness even c̄ presence of disease]

This sense of wholeness, or integrity, seems to be an important dimension in health. It is interesting to note that this approach takes the WHO definition of health further, as it suggests that this sense of wholeness may be present even if disease or disability are also present.

It is out of recognition of these issues that the notion of quality of life has gained increased attention in health research. There is growing recognition of the importance of quality of life in people's experience of health, and the notion of health-related quality of life is gaining recognition (e.g. Bowling 1997, p. 36; Mathers & Douglas 1998, p. 147). Johnstone (1994, pp. 391–7) describes the range of attempts to define quality of life, which she points out is an extremely complex, perhaps indefinable, concept. She concludes that quality of life judgments can properly be made only by the individual because quality of life may be defined quite differently by different people and because only the individual is in a position to judge his or her own quality of life. This is significant because it alerts us to the importance of enabling people to make the decisions about their own health and quality of life, rather than imposing judgments on them.

[margin note: Quality of life can only be judged by ind & people must make decisions re: QoL.]

In the context of quality of life, cross-cultural studies indicate that people's experience of health can be usefully organised as follows:

- feeling vital, full of energy;

- having good social relationships;

- experiencing a sense of control over one's life and one's living conditions;

- being able to do things one enjoys;

- having a sense of purpose in life; and

- experiencing a connectedness to 'community'.

(Labonté 1997, p. 15)

It is clear that this 'experience of health' is quite a different approach to that when we consider health as absence of physical disease. How do we reconcile two such different approaches to health? The issues that arise here are so different that Mathers and Douglas (1998, p. 147) suggest that we may need to focus on two sets of information — one related to illness and another related to wellbeing or quality of life. Others suggest that they can be combined to calculate 'happy life expectancy', a combination of measures of life satisfaction and life expectancy (Veenhoven 1996 in Wearing & Headey 1998, p. 176).

The link between these two approaches appears to be becoming clearer. There is a growing feeling that this sense of wellness or quality of life may in many instances have a direct bearing on physical health. Knowledge about the inextricable relationship between physical and mental health is growing all the time, but we still have a great deal to learn in this area.

In health promotion, any contemplation of health includes thinking about collective health. In public health we often talk about population health and community health and the need for health workers working in community-based organisations to think about the health of the community. However, in order to examine the notion of community health, we need first to clarify what is meant by the term 'community', and this is by no means a simple task.

Defining community

'Community' has been variously defined but is usually characterised by geographical communities or communities of interest. Definitions that fall within the geographical definition have referred to 'community as "lots and lots of people" or community as population' (Hawe 1994, p. 200). In these definitions, communities are little more than large numbers of individuals and the term community is used to refer to society as a group of people or population. Community is also understood as 'a form of social organisation' with five related characteristics, which are: human scale, identity and belonging, obligations, 'gemeinschaft', and culture (Ife 2002, p. 80). Ife describes these characteristics as follows (p. 80):

- Human scale — this is where people know each other or can get to know each other relatively easily and as needed. Structures are small enough for people to be able to control them, facilitating genuine empowerment. There is no magic number but it could mean several thousand.

- Identity and belonging — this implies acceptance by others and allegiance or loyalty to the aims of the group. Belonging to a community gives one a sense of identity.
- Obligations — the responsibility for survival lies with the members and so membership is supposedly an active experience. It carries both rights and responsibilities.
- 'Gemeinschaft' — people interact with a relatively small number of people, whom they know well, in many different roles. Members develop and contribute a wide range of talents for the benefit of themselves and the wider community. This is different to 'gesellschaft', where we don't know the people we have contact with except for the roles they have as e.g. teacher, bus driver, shop assistant, etc.
- Culture — the valuing of locally based culture rather than the mass culture of the wider society. Members are producers of the culture rather than consumers.

Definitions incorporating these ideas define a community as 'a "living" organism with interactive webs of ties among organisations, neighbourhoods, families, and friends' (Eng et al 1992, p. 1). These dynamic definitions of communities emphasise that they are social systems (Hawe 1994, p. 201), bound together by either shared values or shared interests. In these definitions, participation in the life of the community and identification as members of the community are important and result in a sense of belonging. This sense of belonging may also be described as a 'sense of community'.

There has also been much recognition that limiting the concept of community to shared geographical location may ignore many communities of interest. A community of interest or 'community-of-common-purpose' (Falk & Kilpatrick 2000, p. 103) has been described as a group of people who share beliefs, values or interests on a particular issue. Communities of interest include such people as residents of a housing estate, groups of single parents or unemployed people, members of particular ethnic groups, and global communities, such as religious groups that span nations or social movements such as the women's movement or the environmental movement.

In addition to freeing communities from geographical boundaries by defining a community of interest around a shared perspective on a particular issue, this definition recognises heterogeneity among people and the fact that those who share an interest in one issue may have few other common interests or beliefs, and may even be sharply divided on other issues.

Examples of the way the term community is currently used include:

- A global community, with interdependent networks of trade, communication and travel and where global commons such as clean air and water and the protection of biodiversity which are important issues in health when we, as a global community are facing for example, the impacts of climate change from greenhouse gas emissions and insufficient fresh water.
- A national community, where people identify with a range of potent symbols such as Australia and the kangaroo or Australia and the idea of giving people 'a fair go'.

- A loyal community where people identify with a city or region or identify themselves as other, for example some people in Australia identifying with 'the bush'. This is a mixture of geography and emotional attachment.
- A community of identity that binds people through beliefs such as culture and religion. A local community that shares a range of living and working conditions such as climate, access to services and morale. This is often a combination of geography and interest.
- A community of interest where people share attitudes, enthusiasm, need and activities around a particular issue.
- A virtual community where people communicate online for various reasons would be included here.
- An intimate community comprising family and friends.

The term community is often romanticised, described in a way that assumes that communities are made up of close-knit groups of people who care for one another and experience little conflict (Labonté 1989a). Such an impression is far from the truth. Communities are very often not characterised by harmony and shared values on all issues and are likely to reflect elements of conflict and competing interests. Communities may be strongly divided by opposing values, and may even be built on attitudes that reflect racism, sexism or ageism, for example, rather than mutual care and concern (Minkler 1994, p. 529). In addition, the term community may often be deliberately used to take advantage of its romantic connotations, such as when governments use terms like community care or community programs (Aitkin 1985, p. i; Bryson & Mowbray 1981). Such programs may be seen positively because they are described in this way yet such programs are often under-funded or reliant on volunteer labour that, in the case of community care, is usually provided by women, with negative impacts on their own health and wellbeing.

Having considered some of the key issues that arise in attempting to define both health and community, we can now turn to the question of how we might work towards health (however defined) in a community (however defined). An examination of the values, attitudes and beliefs or the assumptions that underpin the practice of health promotion is integral to that practice.

The values, attitudes and beliefs of health promotion

Attitudes and values are 'constructs' — terms that are used to explain things that cannot be observed directly.

Values

Values refer to the concept of what a person considers desirable. They are defined in sociological terms as 'the things of social life (ideals, customs, institutions etc.) towards which the people of the group have an affective (emotional) regard. Within each culture, these values are seen as positive or negative. In Australia for example, values such as cleanliness, freedom, education, sincerity and compassion are positive, and cruelty, crime, or blasphemy' (*Macquarie Dictionary* 2001) are negative. And so, a person's individual values have a large emotional component.

Attitudes

Attitudes are positive or negative feelings about certain things. An attitude is 'an internal state that influences (moderates) the choices of personal action made by the individuals' (Gagné 1985, p. 63). They consist of cognitive, affective and motor aspects. The cognitive aspect means that we have personal understandings or beliefs about that thing, such as smoking, violence or service to the community. The affective aspect means we are influenced in forming these beliefs by our emotions or feelings such as if we have had a personal experience of someone close to us suffering lung disease, or if we have been regularly verbally and socially abused, or have had a family tradition of volunteering for community organisations. The motor component relates to our tendency or likelihood to take action (such as not smoking, taking assertiveness classes, or volunteering to work for a cause for something we believe in; Quinn 1988, p. 359). Studies have shown there is a low correlation between attitudes and behaviour. It is clear that our attitudes affect what we see and how we see it. Attitudes can also be powerfully influenced by external forces, such as media images. Yet, attitudes are personal, and sometimes irrational. They may be based on unbalanced or inaccurate information. They are derived from the diverse cultural, family and social range of experiences that make up our individual lives. Attitudes can change and be changed over time, as a result of new learning or new experiences.

Beliefs

Beliefs can be defined as 'a conviction of the truth or reality of a thing, based on grounds insufficient to afford positive knowledge' (*Macquarie Dictionary* 2001). *may A when they learn more* Depending on their culture, people may hold various beliefs about the things that contribute to health and cause illness. This may include, for example, their belief of their susceptibility to a certain disease, about the benefits of certain behaviours for preventing the disease or about certain actions they need to take to promote health. Beliefs may also vary from time to time within cultures as a result of situational changes. For instance, beliefs about one's susceptibility to a disease may change after learning one has a genetic predisposition, but there is no way of knowing in advance that one will definitely be affected. In this context, these beliefs about the value of lifestyle conditions or behaviours or about the risk of certain diseases are likely to influence personal behaviours (Becker 1974). You may believe, for example, that agricultural herbicides and pesticides being used close to your neighbourhood are contributing to increased rates of certain diseases and so you join an action group to prevent the use so close to the neighbourhood. Another example is that you believe that drinking coffee will harm your health and so you prefer to drink tea, or you believe that getting up early every day makes you 'healthy, wealthy and wise'.

Public health values underpinning practice

By its nature, public health practice involves working with a range of different individuals and communities in a diverse range of possible settings, from acute hospital wards to isolated rural schools. Wherever practice occurs there is potential for the personal values and attitudes of the health workers to be in conflict with those of the community. Professional public health practice implies a set of values underpinning the service, such as equity, mutual respect and participation.

As indicated in the introduction to this section, there can be a low correlation between a person's attitudes and their behaviour, meaning what they express in their views on a topic and their actions around the same issue are antithetical. A common example occurs with people's attitudes and actions with regard to racism. A similar pattern emerges with incongruence between attitudes and actions towards a number of other '-isms'; for example, sexism, ageism and so forth. Similarly, workers sometimes find themselves in an 'ethical dilemma' in a situation where values conflict in a practice setting. They may be forced to make a moral decision about what is the correct way to deal with a situation (Ife 2002, p. 271).

Values of public health practice may be implicit, implied in the common values and standards expected in society, such as respect for others, or they may be made explicit in the guiding principles of the health agency, perhaps set out in a mission statement or other strategic planning documents. They may also be made explicit in a formal contract that a worker enters into when they are employed, or in the 'oath' that professionals take when they are formally accepted into a professional role, such as the 'Nurses Code of Practice'. Professional practice in public health implies that a health worker's actions will be guided by the values set out in the philosophical frameworks that underpin their practice; primarily, the Declaration of Alma-Ata, but also, other complementary documents such as the Declaration of Human Rights (see Appendix 3) and the Earth Charter (see Appendix 4). Equity and social justice are key values that are common across these and other philosophical frameworks.

While it is unusual for health workers to act deliberately dishonestly or unethically, they frequently find themselves in positions of considerable power, particularly when they are working with a disempowered group or community. In these situations it is relatively easy for health workers to impose their personal values on the community, because they believe it is 'right' or 'best' for the community. They may have the 'wisdom' of experience of having worked with other, similar communities, or 'wisdom' derived from formal education. Health workers need to constantly remind themselves that their work cannot be value-free; values and attitudes are socially constructed. Communities need to be provided with opportunities to express their values through community consultation and partnerships of practice, and health workers need to take the time to examine their own values.

Equity, equality and social justice

Equity, equality and social justice are the linchpin values of public health practice. Equity is not the same as equality although the terms are often used interchangeably. Equality is about 'sameness' whereas equity is about 'fairness'. Achieving equality in service provision does not necessarily translate into equity of access or equitable opportunities for health gain. Social justice is the collective expression of the principle of equity.

Equity

Equity is about the quality of being fair or impartial. Equity is an ethical value:

> that may be operationally defined as striving to reduce systematic disparities in health between more and less advantaged social groups within and between countries . . . Equity concerns a special subset of health disparities that are particularly unfair because they are associated with underlying social characteristics, such as wealth, that systematically put some people at a disadvantage with respect to opportunities to be healthy.

(Braveman & Gruskin 2003, p. 540)

> Ethical values are closely related to human rights principles and they refer to the rights of humans everywhere to attain the highest possible standard of health. Inequities in access to health services put people who are already disadvantaged, perhaps because they are poor, female, or from a minority racial group, at further disadvantage. Equity principles are needed to address these systematic disadvantages.

(Braveman & Gruskin 2003, p. 540)

Equity is about the degree of sharing of available resources in order to provide fair access. Equity relates to the processes needed to ensure fair distribution of resources. This implies that some people, because of their life situation, will require additional support just to be able to access a service that other people take for granted. It relates to the values about providing access to services based on people's social situation. For instance, some isolated community members need transport assistance or childcare in order for them to access health services, or separate, culturally sensitive programs may be established for pregnant women from minority groups. Various 'affirmative action' and 'equal opportunity programs' have been established to ensure better access or representation of groups who have not been fairly represented. Equity principles mean consideration of the needs of future inhabitants of our communities. Thus, social health policies designed to ensure equity of access become a means of achieving equality.

Health for all people means equal opportunities for all people, whether they differ by geography, race, age, gender, language or functional capacity. People may be more or less disadvantaged, relative to other members in society, virtually everywhere in the world (Braveman & Gruskin 2003). Many strategies to enhance equitable access to health services are outside the domain of the health sector. They relate to activities in transport, housing, sanitation, water supply and education. Gender issues have been a key basis on which equity of access can be argued.

Equality

Equality implies a similarity of status. Equality policies in health provide a framework that allows people to have the same means of achieving health. This does not mean that an absolute principle of equality or sameness across a population is an ideal. It is impossible and undesirable to 'even-out' the natural differences in people's colour, shape, strengths, talents, desires, and physical and mental attributes. However, building equality into political practice and institutions such as the health care system can yield tremendous social and health consequences. Policy approaches can provide a context for people to achieve equality of capabilities, a social system where people have the capability and freedom to choose one type of life rather than another (Sen 1992; Callinicos 2000). There is a clear distinction here between policies that provide for equality of service, where people are offered the same support or services irrespective of the circumstances in their lives, and policies that ensure equality of capability, where some people are selectively advantaged in order to enable them to access services.

Equality in health care is an outcome measure; it is about the sameness of a service for all. The aim of equality as an outcome measure is to create a democratic society in which people stand in relations of equality to one another. When equality is achieved all citizens are entitled to the goods they need to function as free and equal citizens and to avoid oppression by others. Democratic equality also obliges citizens to promote equality, to be advocates for change when inequities exist. It is evident that the outcomes are equality of opportunities; equality of access is achieved when equity principles underpin allocation of resources. These can include strategies to redistribute wealth through the taxation system or a universal health insurance system such as Medicare in Australia, to provide equality of welfare. Not all disparities in health status are unfair. For instance, men and women are affected by different diseases, such as prostate and breast cancer, and female newborns tend to be naturally lighter weight at birth. Inequality exists when there is unfairness in access to education or in the way food is distributed, when distinctions in opportunities are made in gender or other grounds.

One of the major objections to the ideals of equality is that the social pursuit of equality, such as through policy approaches, inevitably violates personal liberty — the ideals impinge on a person's abilities to make individual decisions. It is true that sometimes equality policies, such as the taxation system, will be contrary to personal choice, but a society needs to have equal concern for its citizens and to create an environment where all citizens have the opportunity to achieve their goals (Sen 1992).

Equity, equality and social justice are the fundamental values that underpin public health practice. Putting these values into practice means working to reduce the systematic disparities in society by providing opportunities for disadvantaged groups to take control over aspects of their lives that would improve their health. Jeanne Daly's story of the structural and social factors influencing the lives of passengers aboard the *Titanic*, presented in Insight 2.1, provides a classic example of how such factors can be largely outside the control of people who are affected most.

Insight 2.1 Challenges in public-health promotion: a way forward

Jeanne Daly
The Titanic
The White Star Royal Mail Triple-Screw Steamer *Titanic* was the biggest ship of its time, the acme of industrial progress, designed to capture the trans-Atlantic trade from the Cunard shipping company. The 'Queen of the Ocean' was advertised as the ultimate in luxury and its maiden voyage was expected to draw on board some of the richest people of the time. In the boardroom of the White Star line the decision was taken to increase the space for the first class promenade by reducing the number of lifeboats installed on the top deck.

On its maiden voyage the ship sailed from Southampton, stopped at Cherbourg, and made its last port of call in Ireland at Queenstown. As the ship sailed away, Eugene Daly (no relation) took his Irish bagpipes to the third class promenade and played *Erin's Lament*. Despite the advertised glamour, this was an emigrant ship. In steerage (third class) were 706 people, many from the Balkans, Scandinavia, The Netherlands, England and Ireland, going to seek a new life in the New World. It was the fares of these third class passengers that helped justify the building of the luxury liners. There were an estimated 325 people travelling in first class and 285 in second class.

Life on the ship was strictly segregated, reflecting the class divisions of the time. First class passengers had the upper decks. Here the Astors, the Guggenheims and other wealthy American industrialists promenaded and socialised. Corseted women sat on deck chairs while children played. The men struck business deals in the all-male smoking room, sending messages to their companies on the revolutionary new wireless system. First class meals were served in grand dining rooms. Their day started with the enormous breakfasts that characterised the excesses of the Edwardian era. The dinner menu boasted 11 rich courses. A different wine was served with each course. This was not a healthy lifestyle.

A descent into the bowels of the liner was also a descent on the social ladder. Let us skip over second class and go to third class, the passengers travelling on the lowest decks. Here the dining room was a lot less plush, but comfortable. Dinner, served at midday, was a sensible meal of meat, vegetables and pudding or fruit. There was no alcohol served at meal times, but there was a public bar. In the general room there was a piano, and on the deck outside was a small promenade. Except for the limited space for exercise, we would find little fault with this much healthier lifestyle.

The internal structure of the liner set in place the rigid segregation of the three classes. They ate and exercised on separate decks, even had their hair cut by different barbers. Passageways connected first and third class, but these were hidden, used mainly by staff to traverse the ship without being seen by passengers. There was no lifeboat drill, so third class passengers were never shown how to negotiate their way to first class and the lifeboats. If there was conflict between the classes, it was structurally contained by geographic separation. Passengers saw only their own section of the ship.

Despite the unhealthy lifestyle of the first class passengers, on the *Titanic*, as in life, third class passengers had higher mortality rates (Table 1) [not reproduced]. The mortality rate for cooks was 94%. On the *Titanic*, as in life, it was healthier to eat first class meals than to cook them.

But, of course, the problem was not the meals eaten or the smoking and drinking, but a structural lack of opportunity. When the ship hit the iceberg and sank, there were only lifeboats for half the people on board. Women and children were to be saved first. Third class passengers were trapped below decks, although some managed to negotiate the labyrinthine passages to the top deck. There are accounts of crew making way for women and children by hauling from the lifeboats 'swarthy' men from third class who were hiding under the blankets. So intent were they on this task that some lifeboats were not filled.

On the deck, as the ship went down, a priest heard confession from those remaining on board. The band played on — according to some survivors they were playing the hymn, *Nearer, My God, to Thee* — until they were swept away as the ship went down. Perhaps the third class passengers also sang *Nearer, My God, to Thee* around the piano in the general room as the freezing water rose around their feet.

The *Titanic's* mortality statistics tell a stark story of inequality. While 62% of first class passengers were saved, 62% of third class passengers drowned. While all children in first and second class were saved, 65% of those in third class drowned. While 54% of third class women went down with the ship, 33% of first class men were saved. Included in the first class men who survived was Sir Cosmo Duff Gordon. He was later accused of bribing the crew in his half-empty lifeboat to row away from the ship, ignoring the desperate cries of survivors trying to cling to anything that would save them from the freezing water. Also saved was J. Bruce Ismay, chief executive of the White Star line. When he went on board the *Carpathia*, the ship that rescued the survivors, he sent a wireless message to New York to stop the wages of all crew rescued from the time the ship sank.

The disaster threw into stark detail social inequalities that usually remain hidden. The interpretation of these statistics gives rise to a rich variety of understandings. Early reports glorified the heroic behaviour of the 'kings of finance, captains of industry' who stood aside to save 'some sabot-shod, shawl-enshrouded, illiterate and penniless peasant woman from Europe'. Why struggle for greater social equality, the rhetoric went: all that it would achieve would be to replace these glorious Anglo-Saxon heroes with the 'frenzied mob of armed brutes' (the 'foreigners' from third class) who had to be kept out of the lifeboats at gunpoint.

This version of events found its echo in the inquiry into the sinking. The inquiry found that third class passengers were partly responsible for their own deaths. They were reluctant to leave the ship, unwilling to part with their baggage, or unable to speak English. There was a lesson, too, for women supporting the growing Suffragette Movement: equality would mean an end to preferential access to lifeboats. Images of rich and poor men dying together to save their women thus provided reassuring images of an harmonious social consensus that denied class and gender inequality but that emphasised the threat to it from the undisciplined brutes in third class.

These conservative images faded under the combined criticism of other interpretations of the event. Ben Tillett, of the Dock, Wharf, Riverside and General Workers' Union, railed against 'the vicious class antagonism shown in the practical forbidding of the saving of the lives of the third class passengers'. *The New York Evening Journal* of 16 April 1912 published an editorial on 'The Titanic Crime . . . What a satire in modern civilization! What irony of mechanical progress! . . . The steamship companies, in their hurry for the last increment of dividends, lie under the illusion that the inevitable disaster will always strike elsewhere than upon their own greed and folly.' The crew on the *Olympic*, sister ship to the *Titanic* went on strike for safer working conditions pointing out that they would be in an unenviable situation in the event of a sinking, 'even if accompanied by the band playing *Nearer, My God, to Thee*'. Women's unions pointed out that, far from benefiting from the system, 'the lives and health of thousands of women and children are sacrificed continually through their exploitation in mills, workshops and factories'.

The result was that shipping regulations were changed to make it compulsory to have a seat in a lifeboat for every passenger. Although the inquiry into the sinking failed to identify any villains on the *Titanic*, history, and Hollywood, have pilloried the owners of the White Star shipping line. Even at the time, J. Bruce Ismay became popularly known as J. Brute Ismay. He retired from public life.

(Source: *Health Promotion Journal of Australia* 2000, Vol. 10, No. 1, April, footnotes deleted)

Social justice

Social justice implies a commitment to fairness or equity of access to health opportunities for all members of society. Social justice or 'equity for all' must supersede individual goals.

When we reflect on the social determinants of health and illness, it becomes clear that a socially just society is much more likely to be a healthy society. If policy approaches, planning decisions and the strategies that are undertaken constantly seek to enhance access to those factors and situations that support health, then the society is acting in a socially just manner. If resources are allocated to those who can afford to pay, to those who are the most powerful, or most articulate, if people are not asked or their wishes are overlooked in the decision-making processes, then the decisions are not made within a social justice framework.

A case for social justice Social justice is the collective expression of equity. The concept holds that governments are instituted among populations for the benefit of members of those populations. This includes upholding the principles of social justice. The concept includes the idea that those governments which fail to see to the welfare of their citizens are failing to uphold their part in the social contract and are, therefore, unjust. Unjust societies have poorer health than just societies.

Internationally, it has long been recognised that poverty is the single biggest determinant of ill health. For millions of people around the world, in minority and majority countries alike, lack of access to sufficient basic resources is a direct cause of illness, poor quality of life and death.

What is also becoming clear is that relative poverty is also a significant determinant of ill health. That is, inequity, or lack of access to a fair share of the available resources, is increasingly being recognised as a major cause of ill health. Several major studies from around the world have demonstrated that, even in countries of relative wealth, people with lower socioeconomic status have significantly higher death and illness rates than those further up the socioeconomic hierarchy (Wilkinson 1996).

Equally important is that the strength of this link between socioeconomic status and health varies according to the degree of differences in income between people of differing socioeconomic status. Several important studies have identified recently that countries with more even income distribution have higher life expectancy (Wilkinson 1996). This seems to be the case both in countries that are relatively poor and in those that are well off. Kaplan et al (1996) have identified that states within the United States of America with greater inequality in income distribution have higher mortality rates, lower birth weight rates, higher crime rates, higher levels of expenditure on medical care and higher smoking and lower exercise rates than states with more equal income distribution. They identified that this association between poor health and income inequality was also associated with poor employment, imprisonment, social services and education levels. This work highlights the significant impact that inequality and the conditions that encourage it have on health, even in conditions of relative affluence.

Similarly, there are some significant examples from relatively poor countries of how good health has been achieved in situations in which comparatively few resources are available. In all such situations, it is the equality in distribution of resources and the related commitment to the welfare of all members of society that explains the health of the people (Beaglehole & Bonita 2004).

It is important to note that the effect of inequality in income distribution on health is not explained by effects on health caused by individual lifestyle factors, such as smoking. Rather, the death rate pattern across groups with differing income levels seems far stronger than the effect of any individual risk factors for most diseases (Wilkinson 1996, pp. 26–7). Even for diseases regarded as strongly amenable to behavioural change, such as coronary heart disease, the impact of income inequality is strong.

The increasing disregard for social inequities and their impact on the lives of ordinary people seems to be a direct result of the growth of economic rationalism and the primacy of the economy. It is ironic, then, that Glyn and Miliband (1994) have identified that inequality affects more than the health of the population — it also affects the economic health of a society. Drawing together a wide range of research, they argue that social justice is actually good for a country's economy, and that inequalities in a society have detrimental effects on a country's economic growth. This flies in the face of much rhetoric arguing that countries need to accept inequality if they wish to succeed economically and have everyone benefit by a 'trickle-down' process — it seems that the converse is the case. High levels of funding to a health care service do not guarantee equitable access to its resources. A review of several countries indicates that economic growth will not by itself improve health status in the majority world either (Beaglehole & Bonita 2004, p. 208).

This growing evidence of the impact of inequality on both individual health and the health and wellbeing of societies serves to highlight the importance of social justice to both the experience of individuals living in a society and the health and success of society as a whole. At a time when issues of equity and social justice seem to be increasingly out of favour with national governments and international agencies, this confirmation of the importance of social justice is extremely important. And, among other things, it serves to highlight and reconfirm the importance of the Primary Health Care approach.

Equity of access to public health services is a significant factor that influences the health status of the whole population of a nation. Social and public health policy directions create the context for the quality of access that is to a large extent not dependent on the total funds expended.

The following section provides a very brief overview of the health care systems of three countries/states as a way of illustrating the significance of broad public policy approaches in setting a context for equitable access to health care services.

Health Care in the United States of America

The US spends substantially more than other affluent minority nations, per capita, on health care. In fact the US spends at least 3.4 per cent more per capita than any other nation. The US has a lower life expectancy rate and higher infant mortality rate, (two key indicators of the health status of a nation), in comparison to many other countries that spend less on health care. In comparison to Australia and the United Kingdom, a very small percentage of health care services are publicly funded. The largest share of funding is through an individual's employer. The employer purchases a package of health care services on behalf of their staff. The use of health care services has a direct impact on the profitability of the business enterprise. As a consequence, businesses seek to minimise the costs associated with providing health care by entering into contracts with health insurers, in an arrangement called 'managed care'. These arrangements impose an additional, very costly, level of administration (Dudley & Luft 2001). In addition, many people who are in low paid positions, or who are unemployed, find themselves without adequate health care access. About 40 million out of a population of 300 million do not have access to funded health care. The government does provide some health care funding for the indigent and elderly persons through the Medicaid system, but the level of funding is very low compared to the Australian system. Changes towards a more socially equitable health care system have been resisted by medical professionals and health insurers who have a lot to lose financially, but also by the electorate (remembering that voting is not compulsory and the indigent tend not to vote) because greater public support for health services would come at the cost of increased across-the-board taxation (Dudley & Luft 2001).

The outcomes of this health system structure indicate that many poor people delay seeking medical care, or fail to receive the medical care they need because they cannot afford to pay privately and they are inadequately insured or uninsured. The health outcomes for Americans indicate that greater expenditure on health care does not necessarily result in improved health (Beaglehole & Bonita 2004).

Health care in Sweden

Equitable access to health care services in Sweden is made possible through the egalitarian philosophy of the government, enshrined in social and health policy decisions over a sustained period (Beaglehole & Bonita 2004). The national health service provides coverage for all residents irrespective of their nationality. No substantive private health insurance scheme operates. Users make a small payment at the time of service and for pharmaceuticals, but the out-of-pocket costs are means tested and there is a ceiling on yearly expenditure (European Observatory 2004). The proportional taxation system in Sweden ensures income differentials between rich and poor are comparatively small (Wilkinson 1994). A longstanding and strong public health program is publicly funded through the taxation system, compulsory for all those employed, and largely administered at local municipal level. Municipal councils are also responsible for social welfare and environmental health. These initiatives have provided a basis for high health status, low infant mortality and long life expectancy. Sweden spends a lower proportion of GDP on health care than the USA (8.4 per cent in 1998, European Observatory 2004), but achieves better health outcomes in terms of universal access and improved health status.

Health care in Kerala state in south-west India

The health of residents of this state is worthy of study, especially when it is put in the context of the severe overall poverty of the population and in comparison with the health status of the rest of India or other nations. Across most of India wide inequalities in access to health care services still remain, largely a product of the systems established during British rule.

Kerala state was formed in 1956, and since that time, because of state government policies, a range of health measures have become consistently better than in India as a whole. Health improvements quite clearly result from adherence to a number of principles in common with Primary Health Care philosophy and through a range of public health measures consistent with the action areas of the Ottawa Charter for Health Promotion. Despite the overall poverty, per capita expenditure on health care in Kerala is comparatively high (Beaglehole & Bonita 2004). There has been a longstanding population commitment to political and public action and social policies, including adult literacy for men and women in particular (Heller 1996). The role of education has strongly influenced the health consciousness of the population, their nutritional health, and their demands for health-promotion programs such as immunisation.

These three examples provide a strong argument for policies underpinned by the values of equity, equality and social justice. As the WHO constitution states, the enjoyment of the highest standard of health is one of the fundamental rights of every human being.

Human rights

The notion of human rights in health is closely related to the concept of equity in health and therefore also relates to equality in the sense of equality of opportunity, rather than 'sameness' of service provision. Human rights in health derives from the principle of non-discrimination '. . . and the responsibility of governments to take the necessary measures to eliminate adverse discrimination — in this case, discrimination in opportunities to be healthy by virtue of belonging to certain social groups' (Braveman & Gruskin 2003, p. 256). It is clear human rights principles are congruent with the principles of Primary Health Care, referred to in Chapter 1 (see also Appendix 4). A key aspect of these principles is that they place clear responsibilities with national governments to enshrine human rights conditions in legislation. This level of selective support for disadvantaged groups provides clear guidance and mandate for health policy-makers and program-planners to use equity as their guiding principle in resource allocation. To engage in activities that are underpinned by principles of equity and social justice requires political and social consciousness on the part of health workers. They must be advocates on behalf of communities.

Empowerment

The concept of empowerment is fundamental to any social justice strategy. Empowerment of those people for and with whom an activity is occurring is fundamental to a range of health-promotion approaches. Empowerment is an essential component of structural or social change, but in addition, empowerment is essential for health education and information-provision approaches to be effective in bringing sustained improvement in the context of people's lives.

Empowerment within the social health context has been defined as:

> a social action process that promotes participation of people, organisations, and communities towards the goals of increased individual and community control, political efficacy, improved quality of community life, and social justice.

(Wallerstein 1992, p. 198)

This notion of empowerment has been described not as an outcome measure designed to achieve power over others, but instead, a process to achieve power to act *with* others and achieve change (Wallerstein & Bernstein 1988, p. 380). The concept relates to the process involved in working with communities to achieve their goals. As the definition used above indicates, empowerment relates to increasing the power of disadvantaged individuals or groups to influence their health in a positive manner. Uneven power differentials can create and maintain disadvantage in a number of ways and, through these, health status is put at risk. Uneven power differential can be apparent in a number of ways, some of which have been presented by Ife (2002, pp. 51–62) and summarised in the three themes below.

1. Structural disadvantage expressed through distinctions made on the basis of class, gender or race/ethnicity. Mainstream health services are structured in such a way as to provide services that are less appropriate for the health care needs, and more difficult to access, for people who are, for example, poor and unemployed, or female and from racial minority groups. When these forms of oppression are combined, people suffer multiple barriers to access, such as is the case for many Aboriginal Australians.

2. Groups who are oppressed because of other personal characteristics. These groups may include those who are old, homosexual, physically or intellectually disabled, those who suffer from mental illnesses or who live in isolated rural areas. They are not singled out for structural disadvantage, such as in policy approaches; however, they are powerless because of their condition or situation.

3. Individuals who are disadvantaged or disempowered because of their personal circumstances, such as relationship issues, loneliness or grief. The issues causing disempowerment may be temporary, but they often interact with other forms of structural disadvantage, making it more difficult for those affected to access relevant support.

In a practice role, empowerment of individuals or communities is not a means for them to gain 'power over' another individual or agency. Three important points about empowerment are worth noting. Firstly, empowerment is a term that is currently popular and tends to be used quite frequently, often in a band-aid fashion without consideration of the real implications of the term. Secondly, empowerment is not about people simply feeling better about themselves, but rather about people improving their control over issues impacting on them (Hawe et al 1990, p. 115). Thirdly, empowerment is not something that can be 'done to' someone. Rather, people can only empower themselves (Labonté 1989b, p. 87) — if empowerment is forced upon people, can it rightly be called empowerment?

Power

Power is a complex concept and various perspectives on power are explored by social theorists. This text does not provide a sociological analysis. However, it is important to understand the ways that power is exercised in society (as drawn from Ife 2002, pp. 55–62 below) if community members who are disempowered are to be supported.

Assgmt 2 to spread word of program

1. Various groups, operating at a number of different levels in society, at local, state, federal and international levels, compete for power within their domains, and power over population groups and consumers. Two groups, which are particularly powerful, are political parties and media enterprises. Groups exert power by their ability to influence decision-making processes. Powerful groups may include industry groups who want to change a planning decision, union leaders and lobbyists or media owners.

2. Certain individuals can have more than their 'fair' share of power or influence, and as such they are able to influence policy directions within agencies or institutions. These 'elites' perpetuate their influence through longstanding clubs and networks, such as political parties and professional associations. They are usually powerful because of their affluence, which gives them ability to control a significant proportion of physical and personnel resources.

3. Power is expressed as a matter of 'tradition' in society, expressed through longstanding structural inequalities. Gender divisions are major causes of ongoing oppression across society, as are cultural and class distinctions. Dominant power in minority/wealthy countries such as Australia is held and strongly maintained by white, wealthy, men.

might be good for assgmt 2 — to spread word of program

4. Accepted power relations are part of the discourse, the way ideas are communicated through the use of language in words, talk or conversation, including television, books and other forms of entertainment. For instance, the accepted use of sexist language, or the portrayal of coloured people as the villains, or older people as insane, on television.

Changing power relations

how to a control of lives

If people are to gain greater power over their lives, they need greater access to information, supportive relationships, decision-making processes and resources (Labonté 1997). Health workers can play an important role in creating a climate for empowerment by enabling access to these things through the community development process. This empowerment needs to occur through both the process and the outcome of community development activity. Working to enable individuals and communities to become empowered requires particular skills in health workers. They must be willing to share their skills and time, and relinquish their need to be the expert, who holds the wisdom. That is, it is not acceptable to take over from community members in order to achieve a positive outcome for them, when in the process they are left feeling no more capable, or even less capable, of acting more independently next time. While there may be times when quick action on issues by workers is warranted, this action cannot be described as community development.

One last point is worth emphasising: empowerment is about increasing people's power over things influencing their lives, but power is rarely a neutral concept. An increase in the power that one person or group has over something in their lives will often result in someone else losing that power. This fact is extremely important because it reminds us that as long as community development concerns itself with the empowerment of people, those involved in the process risk experiencing conflict. Although consensus building is an important part of community development, conflict may sometimes be an unavoidable consequence.

Cultural safety

Cultural safety is another concept that deserves discussion and consideration by health workers across the spectrum of practice. The term has been developed by health professionals working particularly with indigenous populations in Australia and New Zealand (Eckermann et al 1995, pp. 166–8; Polaschek 1998).

> Cultural safety is the need to be recognised within the health care system and to be assured that the system reflects something of you — of your culture, your language, your customs, attitudes, beliefs and preferred ways of doing things.
>
> (Eckermann et al 1995, p. 168)

Culture can be defined as 'the sum total of ways of living built up by a group of human beings, which is transmitted from one generation to another' (*Macquarie Dictionary* 2001). Culture refers to the beliefs, knowledge, attitudes and values that determine social behaviour. Even though a culture can be moulded over time by changing knowledge and values, it provides the basis for our understanding of our own identity. Culture shapes and moulds people's perceptions of health.

Many people from different and minority groups have expressed feelings of fear and alienation about their interactions with highly structured mainstream institutions providing health and illness services. The fear and alienation stem from different definitions and understanding of 'health' derived from cultural and spiritual backgrounds.

The issue of cultural safety stems from the concept of equity, discussed earlier. Providing culturally safe services and care is not merely facilitating access to mainstream services through liaison offices which may be the link between community and the institution which, in Australia for example, is still dominated by the medical model, particularly in acute illness care services. Cultural safety relates to ensuring the system or service meets the health of the whole person and their holistic understanding of health. As we have said, for Aboriginal people, health is a spiritual concept and to maintain health means sustaining links with all forms of cultural expression; through one's language, family ties and links to the land.

> Conversely, when indigenous worth is not recognised, when one cultural system restricts the level of choice of health care facilities, health values and attitudes, clients find themselves in a position of 'cultural danger'.
>
> (Eckermann et al 1995, p. 167)

working in partnership ō people is key to PHC approach

Cultural safety is achieved when individuals and the agencies that serve them become collaborative partners in planning and delivering community-based care that is available. The notion of working in partnership with people is central to the Primary Health Care approach. This partnership approach really comes to the fore when working with people from cultures different from one's own because the expertise they bring in relation to the norms and values of their own culture is vital to the communication process and the promotion of health. However, this awareness of the norms and values of the culture with which we identify does not come automatically to health workers or community members. Culture develops within a social, political and historical context and expresses a group's preferred ways of thinking about the world. These world views permeate all social structures, and are reflected in the policies and procedures that govern the system itself. Culture defines relationships and roles within society, by describing rights and obligations. In some instances, culture constrains individual behaviour, while in others it results in shared meanings and understandings, leaving room for the beliefs and interpretations of individuals. As a result, the culture of a society, community or group is integrated into the daily lives of individuals and groups, and is largely hidden from our awareness.

how homeless value them selves. how we get that understood to reflect it in policies

The interrelationship between culture and history is reflected in the fact that the shared meanings that make up a culture have often developed from the history of that cultural group. While some of that history may be in the distant past, other history may be relatively recent and very much alive for the people concerned. The history of European treatment of Aboriginal people in Australia is a stark example of this point, and this history may be very present in determining attitudes, including wariness of mainstream health systems and wariness or stereotypical behaviour in Aboriginal–non-Aboriginal communication (Eckermann et al 1995, p. 156).

★ this is why we need to ask the homeless what their needs values etc...are

Because culturally driven beliefs and practices are so unconscious, we are often unable, unless we make a conscious effort, to recognise the culturally influenced values and behaviours we portray to others. Furthermore, because our own culture is so familiar to us, we tend to believe that the way we think, act and judge our world is shared by all others, and tend to judge unfavourably others who do not portray similar values, assuming that ours is the 'right' way. Our upbringing, our education and our own 'enculturation' make it difficult for us to reflect on and challenge notions that are considered commonsense or traditional in our culture. If we are going to work effectively with others, we need to ensure that we reflect on those beliefs and values that we take for granted, so that we can respond effectively in the face of differing values.

Language plays a key role in transmitting and reproducing the dominant culture, and can be a major barrier to effective communication. This can be the case even when communicating in English with people from another culture, as meanings and nuances can be culturally specific even when the same language is apparently being spoken. In addition, non-verbal communication is just as much culturally driven as verbal communication and so greater awareness of non-verbal communication is vital. Be mindful of the fact that other people's non-verbal communication may not mean what it appears to, and that one's own non-verbal communication may be misinterpreted.

When people find they need to work with someone from another culture, their initial reaction is often to begin to find out about the other culture, and people usually attempt to do this by reading. Certainly, reading can be an important beginning, but it is by no means the only way to learn. Books and articles are a limited way of finding out about another culture. Firstly, they tend to portray a static picture of a culture, when in fact culture is dynamic and constantly changing. Secondly, because they provide little or no room to individualise cultural beliefs and interpretation, books present an image of a culture as uniformly shared by all its members. Just as members of our own culture vary widely in the acceptance of its values, so too do members of other cultures vary in their acceptance of the values of their particular culture. Thirdly, books often represent a very limited view of the cultures they discuss. For example, many anthropological accounts of cultures ignore women's roles, and present a one-sided picture of cultural life. Therefore, reading about other cultures may be useful, but understanding will be strengthened by listening to the people themselves and coming to conclusions tentatively.

While the particular issues of relevance to communities may vary across communities and according to the concerns at hand, issues that commonly vary across cultures, and of which you may need to have an understanding, are time orientation, personal space, the interrelationship between culture and religion, family practices (such as avoidance relationships), status rules according to gender and age, philosophies and beliefs about health and illness, and forms of non-verbal communication.

Perhaps the most useful skill for a health worker working with people from other cultural backgrounds is sensitivity, including, but certainly not limited to, intercultural sensitivity. Intercultural sensitivity is built on a recognition of the value base of our own and others' cultures. It is reflected by preparedness to listen and to learn from those with whom you are working. Being culturally sensitive includes not attributing all difference to 'culture' as such, but recognising that there is scope within culture for individual difference. Indeed, there is as much variety and conflict within communities from other cultures as there is within communities generally. Being culturally sensitive therefore includes recognising the need to canvass the opinions of as many people as possible, rather than assuming that the opinions of one small group of people reflects the opinions of the community overall. This sensitivity to the people with whom you are working provides a basis on which trust can develop and effective communication can occur.

Miller identifies two important points for working with people from other cultures:

1. treat all facts you have ever heard or read about cultural values as hypotheses, to be tested anew with each [person]; and

2. remember that people can be bicultural, or engaged in the process of integrating two value systems that are often in conflict.

(Miller 1992, cited in Hopkins 1996, p. 5)

Working with people from other cultures presents a challenge for a variety of reasons. The health problems they face may be quite urgent, and the challenges of intercultural communication quite strong. The challenges to their own values can also often present a personal challenge for health workers. Nonetheless, the principles of effective intercultural work provide important guidance for health workers, both for working with individuals and groups from other cultures and for working with individuals and groups from subcultures different from their own.

Economic, human and social capital

The section on globalisation in Chapter 1 indicated how economic policy drives political agendas. Competitiveness in international trade prompts a range of policy decisions aimed at improving the balance of trade. Critics of this policy priority argue that the social agenda is sacrificed to the demands of economic success. In order to focus an analysis of social change more broadly on other dimensions of life it is useful to consider the other forms of capital.

The role of economic capital

Economic capital is perhaps the form of capital that most readily comes to mind when the word capital is used. Economic capital encompasses the monetary system and assets of commercial value and the series of financial processes that make up commercial transactions between individuals, trading partners and nations. The aim of economic capital is the accumulation of wealth.

National success and strength are generally interpreted through measures of economic activity, such as the GDP. Economic growth is seen as the ultimate aim for nations, and this aim underpins trade policy and economic primary production and industrial activities. Economic capital processes in Australia, for example, are informed by the neo-liberal or economic rationalist philosophy. A key assumption inherent in this approach is that economic growth provides a foundation for 'development'. The market is the source of social as well as economic wellbeing provided by the 'trickle-down' effect, whereby economic success of the richest and most powerful will benefit all, even those at the bottom of the socioeconomic hierarchy in society. Health enhancement is achieved as a product of continued economic growth (Beresford 2000; Hancock 1999). Coburn (2000) argues that neo-liberal or economic rationalist political and economic policies produce higher income inequality and lowered social capital, and negative social consequences follow.

At the same time as trade liberalisation policies have been implemented, Australian federal social policy has gradually been moulded to shift greater responsibility to meet social service needs back to individuals, to a user-pays philosophy in areas such as health and education in particular. This has included the introduction of means testing and cost recovery for many allied health and home-care services and measures designed to encourage people to take out private health insurance (Hancock 1999). This policy agenda has drawn on community values of communitarianism and volunteerism. Contracting, tendering and reliance on volunteers to provide essential social services move the responsibility for social provision to local communities and individual organisations.

The role of human capital

As indicated earlier, many minority nations have traditionally relied on economic growth as a means of enhancing health of their populations. Likewise they have used measures of economic productivity as indicators of development. However, more recently, they have been increasingly concerned about wellbeing and quality of life indicators as distinct from health status and life expectancy indicators. As outlined in the discussion of the social determinants of health in Chapter 1, there is recognition that the natural and social environments impact on quality of life and community processes, as well as on economic outcomes (OECD 2000, p. 9). The role that a range of human skills has on individual and community wellbeing has gained prominence in debate (Coleman 1988; Healy & Coté 2001; Productivity Commission 2003). Learning, knowledge and skills which build on inherent capabilities bring economic and non-economic returns to the individual and the wider community. The increased emphasis on the capabilities and impacts of human endeavour has given rise to the concept of *human capital*.

Human capital relates to the inherent and learned capabilities of the individual. Human capital has been defined as 'the knowledge, skills, competencies and attributes embodied in individuals that facilitate the creation of personal, social and economic wellbeing' (OECD 2001, p. 18). In a similar vein Woolcock (1998, p. 154) defines human capital as 'a society's endowment of educated, trained and healthy workers' — the capabilities that are in their head and hands.

> Human capital is multi-faceted in its nature. Skills and competencies may be general (like the capacity to read, write and speak), or highly specific and more or less appropriate in different contexts . . . Much knowledge and skill is tacit rather than codified and documented . . . Human capital grows through use and experience, both inside and outside employment, as well as through informal and formal learning, but human capital also tends to depreciate through lack of use.
>
> (Healy & Coté 2001, pp. 18–19)

[handwritten margin notes: def^n human capital & leads to social benefits see pg 60]

This quote indicates that human capital is dynamic. It includes capabilities that may be immediately obvious, such as speaking, writing, numeracy and leadership, and also less obvious personal attributes, such as perseverance, capacity for learning, making judgments and ethical decisions, problem-solving capacity and team leadership attributes (Healy & Coté 2001).

Inherent and genetic capabilities or attributes, and health status, constitute aspects of human capital because they strongly influence the outcome capabilities of an individual. Education and skills development are, to some extent, a product of these innate attributes.

Attempts to measure or quantify human capital are somewhat difficult. Human capital, as illustrated above, is formed from both formal and informal training and education activities, so measures of educational achievement fail to account for many capabilities. The quality of human capital is a product of the cultural environment of the person — valued skills in one cultural setting may seem useless in another setting. In addition, a setting that promotes a 'culture of learning' enhances more overt indicators of human capital over time. This reinforces the importance of policy support for both government investment in education expenditure and family supports. The habits of learning commenced in the family and school tend to stay with the person into adulthood in their employment opportunities, and hence the impact carries on to their health and wellbeing through secure, fulfilling employment (Bourdieu 1986; Coleman 1988). 'Societies that tend to be less equal in terms of access to education and learning outcomes also tend to be less equal in terms of income distribution' (Healy & Coté 2001, p. 26). Additional educational achievement does bring returns to the person, both in terms of the likelihood of being in employment, and the income it brings. In addition, higher educational attainment enhances creativity, technological advancement, research and innovation in workplaces, with obvious benefits for the economy and for personal health maintenance (Bartley & Blane 1997). Knowledge and human capital act as catalysts to increase productivity relatively evenly across the economy (Glyn & Miliband 1994).

In addition to the economic benefits of enhanced human capital, there are also social benefits, and these benefits may be '. . . possibly larger than the direct labour market and macro-economic effects' (Healy & Coté 2001, p. 33). Benefits are evident in lower risk-taking, such as the use and abuse of drugs such as smoking and alcohol, or 'lifestyle disease' rates such as the effects of obesity or inactivity, among the better educated. There are also family-to-child educational benefits and social benefits, such as less likelihood to rely on social welfare and unemployment benefits. Enhanced human capital reduces the risk of crime (Wilkinson et al 1998) and is associated with higher levels of volunteering. In addition there is growing evidence of the link between human capital and subjective wellbeing (Healy & Coté 2001).

There is potential for a strong positive interrelationship between human and social capital. Aspects of human capital such as education, learning and skills are associated with strong community links between people. Likewise accepted values of cooperation and collaboration at community level enhance opportunities for development of human capital.

Social capital

The term *social capital* has come to prominence in recent years. Modern usage of the term provides acknowledgment of the importance of aspects of social and community relations for both personal and community processes and outcomes. Social capital is more complex to define and understand than either human or economic capital, probably because its characteristics are less tangible and more subjective. Also, the processes of building social capital are possibly more difficult to describe than those describing building of economic and human capital.

Whereas economic capital and human capital are the property of individuals, social capital is relational at community or group levels. Similar to human capital, but in contrast to economic capital, social capital accumulates with use (Putnam 1993; Healy & Coté 2001). Social capital is a measure of community *process*, as distinct from measures of economic or physical capital, which are *outcome* measures (Cox 1995). Social capital is an indicator of people's satisfaction with the way they interact with the various communities of which they are a part. Satisfaction will generate greater participation and, in turn, stronger social capital.

A number of definitions of social capital are used in literature. There are common themes and areas of convergence in the definitions. Aspects in common derived from the various definitions of social capital include:

- being composed of a series of social norms or values, which are defined or qualified in some definitions, and not in others, and may include trust and reciprocity and aspects of communication such as fellowship and information channels;
- a descriptor which outlines the ways norms are activated in the community, such as in social relations or social intercourse or through informal or formal networks;
- an outcome measure or indicator of social capital at community level, such as social organisation or collective action.

A recent definition describes social capital as a 'broad term encompassing the norms and networks facilitating collective action for mutual benefit' (Woolcock 1998, p. 155). This definition suggests two outcomes of the shared norms, one relating to the *process* of activity of the shared norms — the 'collective action', and the other a longer-term *impact* of 'mutual benefit'. Drawing on the work of Woolcock (1998), the OECD has used the following definition: 'social capital is networks, together with shared norms, values and understanding, that facilitate cooperation within or among groups' (Healy & Coté 2001, p. 41). These, and a number of other definitions of social capital, make reference to the importance of social norms; for instance Coleman (1988) and Putnam (1993). Social norms relate to 'designated [or expected] standards of average performance by people of a given age, background, etc.' (*Macquarie Dictionary* 2001). They make up the commonly held expectations of social behaviour within a given community or group. As such, they are culturally determined, and will vary within a society. However, it cannot be assumed that all members of that community will accept the same norms about issues that are common to them. The suggestion that it is the way the norms are exercised that produces the observable outcomes is an important point within many definitions.

Norms may not be immediately apparent at community level, such as trust and reciprocity and facilitating access to other forms of capital, but the evidence of their function may be expressed in the form of fellowship, goodwill and social trusting transactions. Norms such as goodwill and sympathy, and a willingness to engage in social intercourse, are evident in their outcomes. The visibility of the activity generates stronger social norms and trustworthiness. Social capital is built in as a by-product of the social processes at the interface between individuals and communities. Social capital is built during social interactions and can be transferred into new or different interactions.

Putnam (1993, pp. 35–6), who is credited with bringing social capital to prominence, defined it as referring to 'features of social organisation, such as networks, norms and trust, that facilitate coordination and cooperation for mutual benefit'. He described social capital as the 'invisible glue' that holds society together. Commonly expressed norms enable groups of individuals to cooperate in pursuing shared objectives. In common with other social capital theorists, Bourdieu (1974) described social capital as developing during relationships, generating expectations and obligations, augmented by communication and by established explicit norms of behaviour. But Bourdieu and other authors (Portes and Landolt 1996; Portes 2000) do not see social capital as the same positive force that other theorists do. For Bourdieu, social capital is merely another form of capital, like economic capital, that exists as a form of power, particularly patriarchal power, which is used to maintain control over members of society. But because it is maintained in informal community relations, the norms are not immediately evident, and it (social capital) effectively conceals the efforts of the dominant to maintain the status quo. The institutionalised norms and mechanisms of reciprocity disguise the economic power-plays and complicities, and may in fact stifle individual economic advancement by making unreasonable demands. Therefore if one fosters a wider circle of contacts there is less need for formal guarantees or contracts, but less opportunity for individual initiatives.

In the preceding definitions, the authors refer to the characteristics and outcomes of social norms, social relations and networks at community level. Fukuyama (1995), an economist, has also theorised about the benefits of social capital. He argues that in terms of economic outcomes, the importance of human capital is gaining in importance over economic capital. Critical to the success of human capital is people's ability to associate with each other. His analysis clearly focuses on the economic benefits of positive social processes. He defines social capital as 'the ability of people to work together for common purposes in groups and organisations' (1995, p. 10). Although there a number of aspects that place this definition in common with others presented here, Fukuyama uses macro-level indicators of social capital, such as increased national prosperity and trust between nations.

The various definitions of social capital presented so far are common in their perspective that social capital, through exercise of social norms, has an effect on community social relations and networks. The essences of social capital, for Putnam (1993), are the dense networks of civic engagement in which individuals participate. These might include soccer clubs or neighbourhood associations for example. However, it isn't the nature of the associations per se that is important; rather it is what they can do for communities. Networks facilitate the generation of norms and trust among members. Putnam (1993) and Fukuyama (1995) argue that this trust then spills over into the wider society to foster greater economic success and good government. Putnam describes social capital as a resource that can be accumulated, similar to other forms of capital, but in this case, it accumulates as a community resource, rather than at an individual level, and the more that it is used, the more it accumulates (Healy & Coté 2001). In a similar way Bourdieu (1974) outlines the 'dark side' of social capital, arguing that exercise of social norms, particularly patriarchal social relations, brings about unhealthy social outcomes. Popay (2000) emphasises the lack of analysis of these dimensions of power in usage of social capital. Informal relations can be used to foster exploitation, but personalising it can reduce the risks and deceits. The intermediary network builds the social trust. It strengthens the hand in negotiation and at the same time it guarantees the deal. Other authors such as Olson (1982) and Portes and Landolt (1996) agree with this perspective, arguing that:

> long-standing civic groups may stifle macroeconomic growth by securing a disproportionate share of national resources or inhibiting economic advancement

by placing heavy personal obligations on members that prevent them from participating in broader social networks.

(Portes & Landolt 1996, p. 21)

See also Woolcock 1998. Baum (1999, p. 7) summarises the different perspectives in Box 2.1 below.

An important reason that social capital has been difficult to define is because the presence or strength of social capital only becomes evident when it is used.

Portes and Landolt (1996, p. 19) identify that social capital is the *potential* that is inhered in relations between people in communities. It is not a measure of the quantity or quality of the *outcome* of that relationship. It is the inherent knowledge that social actors have about their ability to command resources for their individual or collective purposes. It is the 'invisible glue' described by Putnam (1993), the 'sticky stuff' (Labonté 1999) which creates binding ties and which becomes evident when it serves (or doesn't serve) its purpose. Baum (1999, p. 1) supports the view of social capital as potential when she concludes that 'social capital's importance lies in the way in which it assists members of society to gain access to other forms of capital', such as economic capital, cultural capital and symbolic capital (legitimation). In this case there may be significant confidence that social capital resources are available if needed, or there may be very little confidence that this is so.

It is apparent in the definitions presented here that they reflect on the quality of social relations, but they generally fail to acknowledge the importance of social infrastructure which provides the context for the interactions. 'This leaves unresolved whether social capital is the infrastructure or the content of social relations, the "medium", as it were, or the "message"' (Woolcock 1998, p. 156). Social aspects of social capital are often described as 'civil society' (Cox 1995). Civil society has been defined as 'groups and organisations, both formal and informal, which act independently of the state and market to promote diverse interests in society' (Healy & Coté 2001, p. 47). The role of the market and the state in social capital is that they create the context for interactions and networks to function; community infrastructure creates a context for social capital as potential to be available or used (Cox 1995). Provision of infrastructure that supports and lubricates community relations fosters civil society. The quality and number of networks of association are to some extent dependent on appropriate infrastructure support. In turn, strong social infrastructure creates and fosters civil society because it provides a positive context for strong supportive networks. This point was made by Kawachi et al (1999) in their study illustrating higher rates of violent crime in less cohesive communities.

Box 2.1 Healthy and unhealthy uses of social capital	
Healthy uses of social capital	**Unhealthy uses of social capital**
• Trust	• Distrust of strangers/differences
• Cooperation	• 'Them' and 'Us'
• Understanding	• Tight-knit but excluding
• Empathy	• Fear of the unknown
• Alliances across differences	• Dislike change and new ideas
• Questioning and open to new ideas	• Racism

Natural capital and environmental justice

Economic, human, social and natural capital are inextricably linked. Natural capital refers to the natural assets of the earth such as land, air, freshwater, oceans, fish and forests. Human, social and economic capital *depend* on natural capital. We have abundant evidence of the changes to the environment and the reduction of these assets wrought by human activity and the consequences for the health of humans and other species (McMichael 2001). Globally there has been a call for change in the way we think about these problems and the way we do things (AtKisson 1999; McMichael 2001; Brown 2002; Suzuki 2002; Wilson 2002; Brown et al 2005). The way we are living is not only unhealthy for many now, but unsustainable for all in the future. Boyden (1987) suggests that for cultural adaptation to take place, that is, change, firstly we need to recognise that an undesirable state exists. Secondly, we need knowledge of the cause of the threat or the ways and means of overcoming it. Thirdly, we need the means to do something about it, and finally, we need the motivation, or political will, to take action.

The interrelationship between health and economic, human, social and natural capital are complex. However, we recognise the problem. The WHO estimates that poor environmental quality contributes to 25 per cent of all preventable illnesses (Towards Earth Summit 2002). We have the knowledge of some of the causes. Giving people a fair chance to break out of poverty and providing basic education will go a long way in improving health now and ensuring a sustainable future. Discrimination is also a major risk condition when we are looking for determinants of health. Environmental discrimination poses particular types of health risk.

> Environmental discrimination is defined as a group of people being exposed inequitably to environmental hazards in their communities, workplaces and schools.

> (Public Health Association of Australia 2003)

The groups of people most at risk of environmental health discrimination are those groups who suffer a disproportionate impact from exposures to environmental hazards and decreased access to environmental health services. These hazards can be biological, chemical, mechanical, physical and psychological. The exposures can come via land, air or water (natural capital). As a result, these groups suffer higher than average levels of morbidity and mortality. There should be no second-guessing as to who these groups are. People who are poor are often at the forefront. Many poor communities are exposed to multiple sources of environmental hazards while others lack the most basic environmental health infrastructure.

The communities of course include children, who have little control over their own lives, where they live and play, what they eat, and their financial circumstances are determined by others. According to the Public Health Association of Australia (2003), children of socioeconomically disadvantaged families are exposed more frequently than other children to potentially dangerous chemicals and other environmental hazards that can affect health. Further, in-utero exposures to environmental health hazards may constitute a source of inequity between generations. Environmental health justice demands strategies and processes in the resolution of inequalities related to environmental discrimination.

Human rights and environmental rights are inextricably linked. Environmental rights include a right to live in an unpolluted environment and to experience 'nature'. Action must ensure safeguarding natural capital for now and for future generations. This is a circular argument. Human and social capital are necessary to protect natural capital and working for community connectedness forms part of the strategy.

Social connectedness, community connectedness and community engagement

Social capital is a highly theorised construct. Due to this fact, and also because of its less tangible nature, community practitioners may find it an intimidating or confusing area in which to demonstrate effective practice. Because of these difficulties, terms such as social or community connectedness and community engagement are often used because they are overt and measurable indicators of the process of social capital.

Social connectedness is a way of describing the relationships people have with others and the benefits those relationships bring to the individual as well as to society. It includes informal relationships with family, friends, colleagues and neighbours, as well as relationships people make through participating in sport or other leisure activities, paid work, or through contributing to their communities through voluntary work or community service.

The nature and quality of links people have with all forms of other communities can be significant for their quality of life and sense of wellbeing (Labonté 1997; 1999). The links of community connectedness or community engagement are important at the interpersonal level within families, close friends and close networks, at wider community network levels and in the links people have with institutions, business and government (Woolcock 1998).

People who have limited close or community ties have feelings of isolation and hopelessness, (Labonté 1997; Syme 1997) and in addition, they are more likely to engage in anti-social behaviours such as violence (Wilkinson et al 1998). People who feel socially connected are more able to take part in volunteer community activities and are more inclined to do so (Putnam 1995). All forms of social connections with others can be positive. Working to enhance community connectedness provides an alternative framework for working with individuals and institutions to bring about positive social change. Mechanisms to enhance community connectedness will be discussed in the next chapter.

Attitudes, values and beliefs in action

Responsibility for health and victim blaming

The key impetus for the recent encouragement of community participation in Primary Health Care and health promotion has been the Declaration of Alma-Ata's call for action 'in the spirit of self-reliance' (see Appendix 1). Encouraging people to take responsibility for their own health, both individually and at the levels of the community and the country, is part of the Primary Health Care approach.

Encouraging people to take responsibility for their own health on an individual level has been the focus of health-promotion strategies since the 1970s. As the relationships between individual behaviours and illness were identified, calls for change in individual behaviours became more and more popular as an increasing number of diseases were labelled as lifestyle diseases. This recognition of the impact that individual behaviours have on health, and the role individuals have in influencing their health, is important.

There has been a slow dawning that individuals live their lives in a social context and there are many factors that influence an individual's lifestyle. As the previous discussion points out, a great many of the determinants of health are the result of the social, economic and political structures in which people live their lives. There are some real dangers, therefore, in focusing only on the role of individual behaviours in disease. People may be blamed for ill health, and for some of the determinants of ill health, when they do not have control over the factors affecting their health or the freedom to make healthy choices. This has become known as 'blaming the victim'.

Blaming the victim occurs when the structural causes of ill health are ignored and attention is focused on the individual or individuals affected by the problem, with the aim of changing their behaviour (Crawford 1977). Victim blaming is a subtle process. Ryan (1976, p. 8) has described it as 'cloaked in kindness and concern'. It occurs not only when people fail to see the structural causes of deprivation and ill health, but also when they see them but still seek to solve the problem by working to change the individual (Ryan 1976, pp. 8-9).

One of the real strengths of the Ottawa Charter for Health Promotion's five-pronged approach to health-promotion action is that it minimises the chance of victim blaming occurring: if health-promotion action occurs at the level of working for healthier public policy as well as at the level of further developing the skills of the individual, the structural barriers to ill health are likely to be addressed. It is vital, therefore, that the broad approach to health-promotion action described in the Ottawa Charter for Health Promotion is not watered down to the point where structural action disappears and is replaced by more action at the level of the individual.

Victim blaming does not happen only at the level of the individual. With a focus on community development and community-based action, when many problems stem from national or international issues, there is a danger that disadvantaged communities may be blamed if they are unable to pick themselves up by their bootstraps (Labonté 1989a, p. 88).

The issues surrounding individual responsibility for health versus social responsibility for health are complex and interrelated. It is not a case of choosing one over the other, but of what balance there is between the two. Unfortunately, because they have come to represent opposing philosophical viewpoints, many discussions present them as opposite to each other, which does not help individual workers clarify how they will address health issues and assist individuals in making changes in their lives. Health workers may need to clarify for themselves how to work with the tension between these two aspects of health promotion, to be aware of their biases, and to keep clear in their minds how both aspects of a problem need to be addressed in whatever balance is appropriate for the issue in question.

The influence of labelling

The concept of labelling is very much related to the notion of victim blaming. Our response to issues and problems that arise may well be influenced by our beliefs and expectations about particular groups of people, stages of life or illness experiences. The stereotyping or labelling of people, often because of their ethnicity, gender, age or socioeconomic status, can have a powerful impact on the way in which they are treated. For example, an older person who suffers pain when walking may be told that it is just part of getting old and is to be tolerated, while a younger person may not be treated in the same way. Similarly, stories of the development of labels, such as 'Mediterranean back', demonstrate that health workers do not always respond to a migrant working in a factory who develops back pain in the same way as they respond to non-migrants with a similar problem, and stereotypical responses to women suffering with depression has resulted in over-prescription of addictive, so-called 'minor' tranquillisers. Many such stories demonstrate the assumptions people may make about the behaviour of others and their underlying motives. The consequences of this labelling is disempowering.

Similarly, there have been examples of disadvantaged communities complaining of the way in which they are regularly victimised, particularly through the mass media. Such communities want to be recognised for their strengths as well as their needs. Constantly being depicted in a negative light, results in these communities experiencing the negative consequences of labelling, while the positive qualities and resources of these communities are denied. The resultant disempowerment itself becomes a major health problem for the community.

Dealing with opposing values and conflicts of interest

People's view of health and health promotion reflects their broader views on the way the world works. As a result, many of the issues underpinning discussions of health promotion reflect the world views that people hold. It is therefore not surprising that some of the issues raised by health promotion create conflict between people with opposing views; after all, the difference is often not simply about an issue itself but also about the underlying philosophical framework. This is particularly so where health-promotion action challenges profit or power.

Conflict can also occur with industries whose work has a negative impact on health, and for which profit has a higher priority than health. Because health promotion in many instances directly challenges these industries, the conflicts created may be intense. It is therefore not surprising that conflict can be an inherent part of health-promotion work. Health workers need to develop skills to deal positively with potential conflict situations so that conflict is not created unnecessarily, and to deal constructively with conflict should it arise. This requires effective communication and negotiation skills, and skills in assertive communication.

It is not suggested that all communication in health promotion is adversarial. Effective communication with many individuals and groups is an important part of working for health promotion, and the greater part of this is, or can be, positive and collegial rather than confrontational. Health promotion requires communication and joint action with individuals, health workers from a variety of backgrounds, workers from a range of other sectors (for example, local council workers, teachers, police, environmental workers and road safety workers) and community groups. Much of this communication can involve building bridges between people. It is very important that barriers not be created unnecessarily between groups and that people collaborate as much as possible.

Value conflicts in health promotion do not occur just at the level of conflicts between individuals or institutions. They can also occur within individual health workers as they make choices and adopt priorities as part of their normal working lives. Different aspects of health promotion may compete for priority, and choices made to support one aspect of health promotion may result in a worker feeling uncomfortable about the implications of this choice for other aspects of health promotion. These value conflicts can occur regularly in health-promotion work, and these need to be recognised and reconciled by health workers.

Similarly, as we change and our ideas develop through experience, it is quite possible that actions that seemed acceptable in the past no longer seem appropriate. However, the past cannot be changed, and health workers may have to come to terms with their previous decisions.

Attitudes of health workers towards community members

Within the context of the discussion about enhancing community connectedness, the approach health workers take towards the people they are employed to work with can have quite a marked impact on the way in which health promotion is achieved. A health worker's approach will influence how controlling or supportive they are of community members. It can therefore stifle or encourage the development of skills that will allow people to work more effectively for what they need in the future; that is, it will stifle the process of empowerment, community engagement and community connectedness. Box 2.2 highlights the different approaches.

Participation

The importance of community participation in all stages of planning, implementing and evaluating policies and services that impact on health is recognised in the Declaration of Alma-Ata, the Ottawa Charter for Health Promotion, and the complementary documents previously referred to. Since the development of the Health for All movement, community participation has been increasingly reflected in the rhetoric of health policy documents and health workers are being urged to incorporate participation strategies into their practice.

> ### Box 2.2 Working in communities
>
> **The authoritarian approach**
>
> People with an authoritarian approach believe that the experts and power holders know best, and are right in imposing their decisions on their 'target', whether this is an individual, a group or a community. They believe that, because of their expertise and status in the community, they do not need to involve community members in the decision-making process.
>
> **The paternalistic approach**
>
> The paternalistic approach is very similar to the authoritarian approach except that decision-makers believe it is important to consult with the community. However, there is a strong sense of the decision-makers being wiser than the community, and if people's wishes do not match professional opinion, it is assumed that they do not understand, and so efforts are made to explain the decision-makers' views before they are imposed.
>
> **The partnership approach**
>
> In the partnership approach, it is assumed that members of the community have a great deal of expertise regarding their own lives and the issues of concern to them. Workers therefore involve community members actively in the decision-making and implementation process, so that instead of merely being consulted, community members become joint decision-makers. Generally, people who use this approach believe that the process of involving community members in the decision-making process is just as important as the actual decision made. They also believe that the decision made is likely to be more valuable because of the involvement of the people themselves in the process. Workers are regarded as having expertise in their particular field, rather than expertise in all aspects of their clients' lives.

The importance of community participation has been recognised both for the process of participation and the outcome of that participation. Through the process of meaningful participation, people can gain a sense of confidence in their ability to work for change in the world around them. At the same time, this participation enables people to develop a wide range of skills in such areas as working effectively with groups, organisation, negotiation, submission writing and working with the mass media. The confidence and improved skills developed through this process then also increase these people's ability to work effectively for change on future issues; that is, the conditions are right for people to become empowered. However, the notion of participation is not simple or value-free. Rather, community participation is often regarded in a rather romantic manner. 'The idea of citizen participation is a little like eating spinach: no one is against it in principle because it is good for you' (Arnstein 1971, p. 71). However, in many instances community participation may be used more to control people than to encourage empowerment. Decisions about what types of participation are relevant in a particular situation are not necessarily straightforward, but are important. If there are no opportunities for people to participate in decisions which affect them, they are likely to feel disenfranchised and powerless. If, however, too much participation is expected or people are required to participate in order to obtain access to health care or other services, they are equally likely to feel powerless and the participation may feel like manipulation. It may also give the impression that the 'cost' of health-related

69

services is compulsory participation in the development of those services. Such an approach can be tantamount to victim or community blaming for disadvantaged communities.

Health workers therefore have a fine line to walk in providing opportunities for participation by community members, to make those opportunities meaningful and appropriate, and to get on and do the job themselves when that is what is required. Some discussion of the different approaches to participation is therefore valuable. Arnstein (1971) has suggested that there are at least eight types of participation, ranging from forms of manipulation and co-option through to shared decision-making power. It is worthwhile examining her 'Ladder of Citizen Participation' (Figure 2.1) because it provides quite a useful framework for the forms of participation that can operate. Although other models of participation exist, Arnstein's model provides the most useful one for the purposes of this discussion.

Arnstein describes two forms of community participation as 'non-participation', because they involve either placing people on committees in order to gain their support ('manipulation') or because they are seen as opportunities to change people's behaviour rather than give them any involvement in decision-making ('therapy'). 'Informing', 'consultation' and 'placation' are described as forms of tokenism because, while people may be heard, there is no guarantee that their ideas will be acted upon, because they have no power. It is only at the levels of 'partnership' and above that people have decision-making power. There is 'delegated power' when citizens have most of the decision-making power, while with 'citizen control' citizens have total control (Arnstein 1971, p. 73). Using Arnstein's ladder as an analytical tool, it is possible to see that a great many instances of participation are actually non-participation or tokenism and few cases of participation actually result in shared power or power being handed over to community members. However, it is this power sharing that we are aiming for in a Primary Health Care approach. In many instances, power sharing will result only from the decentralisation of decision-making.

Baum (1998, pp. 322–5) urges us not to assume that shared decision-making power is the only form of participation that is worthwhile. There may be times, for example, when consultation with a community is a valuable exercise that increases the relevance of the activity being developed. Clearly, community members cannot be partners on every health-related decision, but providing opportunities to hear their views may still be valuable. What is important is not to 'dress up' lower levels of participation as shared decision-making, and to work for real shared decision-making wherever possible. Rifkin (1986, p. 246) suggests three questions that we can ask about participation to determine the extent to which it is likely to strengthen or deny people's access to power in any one instance. They are 'Why participation?', 'Who participates?' and 'How do they participate?'.

Why participation?

There are several reasons why participation by members of the community may be encouraged by health workers, although not all of these may actually benefit those being encouraged to participate. Before we start working to increase people's participation, we need to clarify just why we want them to participate. What approach do we take to participation, and are we intending that the process

70

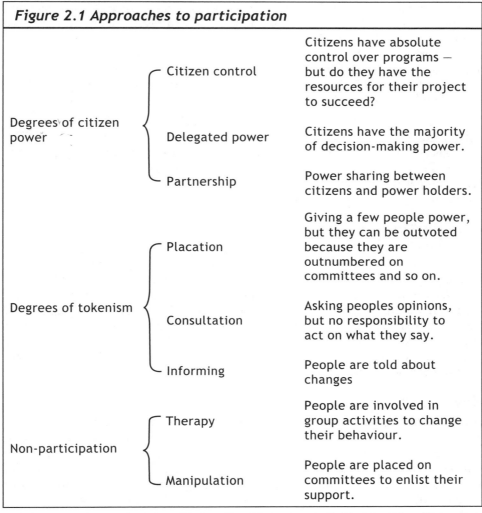

Figure 2.1 Approaches to participation

Degrees of citizen power	Citizen control	Citizens have absolute control over programs — but do they have the resources for their project to succeed?
	Delegated power	Citizens have the majority of decision-making power.
	Partnership	Power sharing between citizens and power holders.
Degrees of tokenism	Placation	Giving a few people power, but they can be outvoted because they are outnumbered on committees and so on.
	Consultation	Asking peoples opinions, but no responsibility to act on what they say.
	Informing	People are told about changes
Non-participation	Therapy	People are involved in group activities to change their behaviour.
	Manipulation	People are placed on committees to enlist their support.

(Source: Arnstein, S. 1971 'Eight Rungs on the Ladder of Citizen Participation', in Cahn, E. S. and Passett, B. A. (eds), *Citizen Participation: Effecting Community Changes*. Praeger Publishers, New York, p. 70)

will be empowering or do we want them to support our own ideas for health improvement?

Not all reasons for encouraging participation are driven by a recognition of the value of community members' contributions. People may be made to feel that they are playing an important role even when their ideas are not being given serious consideration, in the hope that the feeling of involvement will 'make them feel better'. People may be encouraged to participate because of the likely health benefits of the participation itself, rather than a belief in the value of what they may contribute. For example, members of a local support group may be permitted to have a representative on a committee looking at mental health services in the region, but this may be because it is considered to be 'good for' the members of the support group, and no real heed is taken of their opinions and ideas. This, then, is a fairly manipulative use of participation.

Participation may also be used to 'buy' people's acceptance of a pre-planned change. There is evidence that people are less likely to resist a change if they have contributed to its development. Thus, in some instances, people may be encouraged to participate, not because their ideas are highly regarded and will be implemented, but because it is hoped that their involvement will prevent them from complaining about the final result. These reasons for encouraging participation are clearly in parallel with the lower levels of Arnstein's ladder of citizen participation.

However, in the Primary Health Care approach, participation is encouraged out of recognition that community members bring their own perspective and their own expertise to issues, and these may contribute a great deal more to the quality of decisions than if decisions are made by health workers alone. There is also growing evidence that this participation may itself be directly beneficial to health when it results in empowerment of community members (Wallerstein 1992).

Who participates?

In the Primary Health Care approach to health promotion, the short answer to this question is 'as many people as possible'. However, it is of particular importance to make sure that everyone has the opportunity to participate, not just the most articulate. Equitable access to participate is as important. This may mean that it is particularly important to ensure that people for whom services are supposedly planned have real opportunities for participation in decision-making. Examination of participation processes to see exactly who is involved provides an opportunity to consider which avenues for participation currently exist and whether they are enabling people to participate fully.

How do they participate?

Dwyer (1989, pp. 60–1) outlined five forms of participation in common use in Australia. They were client feedback and evaluation, voluntarism, consultation and public discussion, representative structures, and advocacy and public debate. These will be discussed in Chapter 3. These remain the main models of participation, although many health workers have been working at the local level to adapt them to suit particular situations, providing opportunities for community members or consumers to participate more fully in issues of concern to them. In recent years, some of the more active forms of participation have become less popular with government, challenging health workers to come up with more innovative ways of ensuring that community members have meaningful opportunities to participate. Boxes 2.3 and 2.4 outline elements of the participation process which are essential for its success

Weighing up the good of the community versus the rights of the individual

In the discussion so far, the importance of people being actively involved in deciding what they want and health workers acknowledging the expertise that people have in the issues that impact on their lives has been examined. Unfortunately, there are times when this principle alone cannot guide health workers in their judgments. In many situations there are competing interests at stake, and health workers

---

Box 2.3 Prerequisites for effective participation

Skills and resources

In many respects, community members are not adequately prepared to participate effectively. Although Australia is regarded as a democratic society, we do not learn that we should actively participate or how we should do it. Therefore, if people are to be encouraged to participate, they need to be provided with an opportunity to develop the skills and resources they will need.

Power sharing

Unless people feel that they are likely to have an impact, they may decide that it is not worth the effort of trying to participate. Organisations that decide they want to encourage participation must therefore decide to prevent manipulative tactics that exclude community members from effective decision-making and to instigate affirmative action techniques in meetings and decision-making so that all participants have a fair say. Otherwise, only those people who are most comfortable with meeting procedure, and are therefore the most dominant within the group, may have their voices heard and their ideas acted upon. As Arnstein (1971, p. 72) has said, 'participation without redistribution of power is an empty and frustrating process for the powerless'.

Appropriate agendas

If people are going to participate, then obviously the agendas of the organisations concerned must be relevant to them. This has an added advantage: if organisations adjust their agendas so that they are more relevant to the community and people are therefore more willing to participate, it is likely that their activities will more effectively meet the needs of their community. Consequently, organisations are made increasingly accountable to the public, which goes hand in hand with the power sharing discussed above.

It is quite apparent that the five forms of participation described above may be put into effect more often than they currently are, as do the three prerequisites for community participation. We also need to establish more effective participation and decision-making processes if we are to enable people to participate meaningfully in the decisions that affect their lives. Health workers are currently endeavouring to develop more innovative participation strategies, and you may be able to develop some yourselves.

must choose between the wishes of different individuals, as well as between the wishes of individuals and their own professional judgment about what is 'best' for the community. At such times, health workers who are attempting to work by the principles of empowerment and community participation may experience intense personal conflict.

One related question that needs to be asked here is, who decides what is for the good of the community, and on what basis? As the discussion has demonstrated, imposition of decisions from above is problematic, but it is not always practical or possible to involve the whole community in decision-making and prepare them with all the necessary information so that they can make informed decisions. When is it acceptable for decisions to be made on behalf of the community? Do health workers have the right to manipulate the environment 'for the good of the community'? Should current manipulation of the environment (for example, by companies) be counteracted by health workers? When different parts of the community have conflicts of interest on particular issues, whose interests should

---

Box 2.4 Keys to effective participation

- Organisational policy which makes clear commitment to community participation, providing guidelines for both staff and community members on exactly what kind of participation and power sharing is supported.
- Organisational structures which include continuing community input and facilitate autonomous decision-making at the local level.
- Management, staff and community commitment to processes which respect and encourage community input.
- Recognition that the agenda of consumer and community groups may not always be the same as that of the agency.
- Commitment of resources (financial, human and material) to encourage and support community participation.
- Long time-lines during consultation processes, so that participation for community members can be meaningful.
- Use of clear, everyday language that does not exclude ordinary people.
- True support from staff and recognition of the positive outcomes of handing over power to community members.
- Training, which includes exploration of values and development of shared goals, for managers, staff and community members.
- A critical mass of enthusiastic people to enable community participation to be an ongoing process.
- Appropriate means of evaluating the effectiveness of community participation.

(Source: Auer, J., Repin, Y. and Roe, M. 1993 *Just Change: the Cost-Conscious Manager's Toolkit*. National Reference Centre for Continuing Education in Primary Health Care. University of Wollongong, Wollongong, NSW)

take precedence? These are just some of the ethical questions raised by community-wide health promotion.

Balancing responses to health problems — health promotion and illness management

As discussed in Chapter 1, Primary Health Care and the New Public Health movement represent a move to shift the emphasis from illness management to health promotion. This move does not sit comfortably with everyone, and will necessitate some shifts in power. The shift from illness management to health-promotion philosophy needs to occur on more than the individual level. Vast resources in bureaucracies, infrastructure and industry are tied up in the delivery of illness care. With the increasing privatisation of health services across the globe, this focus on an illness industry is set to increase. Moreover, many conventional health workers may have built careers around illness management and are reliant on research funds and high-technology institutions for their livelihoods.

The most important changes are those that need to occur at the level of the health system, and it is here that the notion of 'doing yourself out of a job' is most powerful. Health care systems are often one of the biggest public sector employers in the country. The impact of this system on other related industries also accounts for a great many workers. If the system is to change its emphasis and work to 'do itself out of a job', a dramatic change of focus is needed.

One of the biggest value shifts facing workers when they move from an illness management philosophy to a health promotion philosophy is in how they see themselves and their role. A common reason health workers give for enjoying their work is that they are 'needed'. Unfortunately, there is a real trap in this because, if we are really to care for those who are sick or whose health we are hoping to promote, we would hope for them that they do not need us — that they can live their lives to the full without outside interference, or in an interdependent relationship with those around them. After all, this is what we would hope for ourselves. If we really are working for health promotion, then we are working to do ourselves out of a job. Working to do yourself out of a job is not an easy thing to come to grips with, but without awareness that this is what we are trying to achieve we may be unconsciously encouraging people to be dependent on us rather than independent of us, and while this might make us feel better, it does little to really help those we are meant to be working with.

Belief in the primacy of the illness management system is not limited to health workers. Because it has been part of the dominant ideology, many people believe that science and medicine will come up with a medical solution to just about any problem. We have come to expect this and to see it as more important than the prevention of illness and the promotion of health. The mass media's use of individual emotive cases in which the state does not deliver theoretically available high-technology care, supports the expectation that it should always be available, no matter the cost.

In few of these instances is the opportunity cost of high-technology care mentioned. Opportunity costs refer to the ongoing costs of providing and maintaining a high-technology service, such as machine maintenance and parts, specialist training for staff and building of specialised spaces for equipment. In addition, lifetime health-maintenance costs for patients may be enormous, such as the cost of immunosuppressive medications after organ transplant. There may be situations where spending money on social services will do more for the health of a community than the provision of acute medical care (Labonté 1999).

Promoting your own health

As obvious as promoting your own health may sound, it is often very difficult to do. Firstly, it can be difficult to take time out when you are working on an issue that is of great importance to other people's lives. This can be particularly so for community work campaigns. Secondly, health as an issue is never neutral, and at times this can make health-promotion work stressful. Above all, health-promotion workers are more than just their profession. They are embedded in a culture with norms, values, attitudes and beliefs, that are mixed with not only professional knowledge, but also personal experience. Nevertheless, promoting our own health is a challenge we must take up. Indeed, Baum urges us to remember that conflict is an inherent part of health-promotion work (1990a) and urges us to be 'troublemakers for health' if we want to really be successful in health promotion (1990b). Therefore, it is important for health workers or community members involved in health promotion to develop healthy strategies to look after themselves and to support other members of the team with whom they are working. Unless we look after ourselves and each other, our impact on health promotion will be short-lived and more limited than we had hoped for when we first decided to take up the challenge.

Conclusion

This chapter has examined some of the key issues and concepts in health promotion, to provide a framework on which the following chapters will build. The concept of health was reviewed, with particular attention paid to the fact that health is more than a physical state and an individual phenomenon. Emerging from this was the importance of the interactivity of human beings, reflected through both the positive effects of social capital and social support, and the negative effects of inequity in personal relationships or social environments.

Some of the common potential conflicts of values in health promotion were touched on. These issues are complex and there are no easy answers to many of the dilemmas raised. Many more dilemmas arise in practice. Continuing to examine the questions raised in this chapter is important as you review the range of health-promotion issues and strategies throughout the remainder of this book.

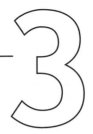

Working for change: healthy public policy to create supportive environments

In Chapter 3, developing healthy public policy to create more supportive environments is examined. In Chapter 1 we outlined a continuum of health-promotion approaches. At one end of that continuum is the population approach to health where economic and regulatory activities that create supportive environments for health become an important part of the health worker's work. Developing public policy lays the foundation for healthy living and offers scope for developing effective long-term change with wide-ranging impact on the determinants of health and illness. This chapter explores the key issues in the development of healthy public policy at a broad social level, a local/community level and within organisations. It examines strategies when developing healthy public policy to create health-promoting environments.

Work to develop healthy public policy and create more supportive environments has been identified as central to effective health-promotion practice since the development of the Ottawa Charter for Health Promotion in 1986. Developing public policy that lays the foundation for healthy living may be one of the most challenging areas of health work. At the same time, this approach offers scope for developing effective long-term change with wide-ranging impact on the determinants of health and illness. Broad social change may occur as a result of regulatory interventions. These interventions may be developed at the international, national and local levels, or all three working in concert with one another.

The challenges presented by working to build healthy public policy and create supportive environments for healthy living have resulted in development of the settings approach. In the settings approach, work for structural change occurs through partnerships. Community members and professionals from all sectors work with government to improve people's health chances.

What is healthy public policy?

The economic and regulatory activities discussed in this chapter are those activities that involve the application of legislative and financial frameworks that create opportunities for healthy living. 'Regulatory activities include executive orders, laws, ordinances, policies, position statements, regulations and formal and informal rules' (Schmid et al 1995 in McKenzie & Smeltzer 2001, p. 184). These economic and regulatory actions can be for broad activities aimed at social change, change at the local/community level or change within organisations. The Declaration of Human Rights, Local Agenda 21 and the WHO Framework Convention on Tobacco Control are all examples of policies developed at the international level and adopted at national level and local level that aim to create supportive environments for health. The WHO activities in the Healthy Cities program and Local Agenda 21 are examples of policy aimed at creating health in a particular setting. Opportunities for health are also created in organisational development where supportive environments are created in settings such as the workplace, schools and recreational clubs such as the opportunities created by VicHealth.

In these settings, health-promotion principles are integrated into the policies or service directions of the organisation. At any of these levels, healthy public policy usually requires advocacy by groups to gain political commitment, social acceptance and systems support for the change. On the continuum we outlined in Chapter 1, these activities are associated strongly with the socio-ecological approach. They are closely aligned with two of the action areas of the Ottawa Charter: building healthy public policy and creating supportive environments.

The Ottawa Charter for Health Promotion, with its emphasis on building healthy public policy as an integral component of health-promotion action, marked the formal recognition of the role that all public policy plays in influencing health and the role of the environment in shaping opportunities for health. This acknowledgment is vital because it recognises that people's social and physical environments impact strongly on their opportunities for health and that all public policies, not just those labelled as health policies, have health consequences.

Healthy public policy is central to the promotion of health because, without the support of healthy public policy, other health-promotion actions are likely to be of limited value. As Milio (1990, p. 295) has expressed it:

> by definition, even the most effective projects have limits, in time and/or the people who benefit. Projects can demonstrate, but only policies can perpetuate the effects. Projects can create oases of health, but only policies can redistribute and equalise their benefits.

Until relatively recently health workers have been concerned primarily with health policy, because it was assumed that this was the major policy that impacted on health. It is now recognised, however, that health policy may have very little impact on health by comparison with the impact of social, economic and environmental policy because it focuses largely on the structure of health care delivery. Social policy, for example, deals with such issues as income distribution, housing and transport provision, while economic policy affects such things as employment rates, inflation and taxation policies. Policies that impact on the physical environment include policies on urban planning, air quality and water quality. It is clear that all of these things do a great deal to structure the environments in which people live. The notion, then, of public policies having a substantial impact on health makes good sense, and the need for economic, social and health policies to be responsive to the requirements of the community is quite apparent. Two recent results of the growing recognition of this fact are the increasing concern for the health of the environment, and concern for the impact of economic rationalism on the quality of life of the community (Pusey 1998).

Healthy public policy 'cannot be developed in a moral vacuum' (WHO 1998, p. 210). The development of such policy requires political will and, in particular, a commitment to equity and to ensuring that all members of society receive the health benefits of social changes. However, any examination of healthy public policy and action to build healthy public policy must start with a consideration of what policy is, and how it can be influenced.

What is health policy?

Health policies are policies that have been considered as 'an authoritative statement of intent adopted by governments on behalf of the public with the aim of improving the health of the population' (Palfrey 2000, p. 3). There seem to be two characteristics common to all policies, whatever the context, and these are:

1. policy that belongs to an entity such as an organisation or a political party; and
2. policy that conveys a commitment to some form of action.

Policies imply particular values. They are driven by the values of the government of the day and organisations express their values in the mission statements, aims and objectives, which underpin the policies of the organisation. Some are very general and provide a guide to action. These might be found in the speeches of politicians before an election. Others make very specific statements or proposals implying that something definite will happen. These might take the form of a program with a specific group of people, or a process of a particular program.

'Health' policies can be *about* health or *for* health. Policies that are developed within the health system have four distinct ways of affecting people. Several authors, for example Salisbury and Heinz (1970) and Palmer and Short (2000), have found Lowi's (1964) typology useful. These policy types are not mutually exclusive.

- Distributive policies — the outcome of these policies are that services or benefits are provided to a particular segment of the population; for example, family allowances or baby bonuses provided by governments.
- Regulatory policies are specific statements that have a narrow impact. They guide or control action. They usually take the form of legislation, such as the Acts concerned with food and water quality standards.
- Self-regulatory policies are sought by organisations or groups to maintain control of their actions. Professionals often use peer review, and organisations use quality assurance processes.

- Redistributive policies are the most contested and are attempts by governments to change the distribution of income, wealth, property or rights between groups in the population. The Pharmaceutical Benefits Scheme and Medicare in Australia are good examples. Both are designed to improve access to health care to the whole population. Access to services is based on need rather than the ability to pay.

Policies are viewed differently depending on your values. Health workers working within the philosophy of Primary Health Care, for example, would support redistributive policies because of their commitment to social justice. Their work might include being an advocate for a particular group of people and lobbying government to ensure that redistributive policies are considered. It is, therefore, important not only to understand how policies affect people but how they are developed.

The process of public policy-making

Public policy-making has been described as a dynamic social and political process (Milio 1988, p. 3). Public policies result from 'a synthesis of power relationships, demographic trends, institutional agendas, community ideologies [and] economic resources' (Brown 1992, p. 104).

There are three key groups of people involved in the policy-making process — the public (including formal interest groups), political and bureaucratic policy-makers, and the mass media (Milio 1988, pp. 3–4). Some interest groups involving themselves in the policy-making process have a great deal more power than others because of their political position and their ability to influence the views represented in the mass media.

 Public comment on new and developing policies is valuable and, in health, seems to have developed as a result of two quite different phenomena. Firstly, there has been greater acknowledgement of the importance of community participation resulting from recognition of the Primary Health Care approach and the New Public Health movement, although this has been taken up to different degrees by various governments. Secondly, there has been a growing distrust of politicians to act in the community's best interest and an increasing demand by many community members to influence decisions made by governments. Nevertheless, it is usually the politicians, bureaucrats and powerful interest groups who set the agenda and decide the framework and philosophy of a policy. Members of the public commenting on a document are often in the position of trying to change the policy after the framework has been set.

Several authors have described the public policy-making process using a variety of relatively similar models. Palmer and Short (2000, pp. 32–3) describe it as a five-stage model, listed below. It is important to note, however, that this model accounts only for policies that are formally developed, not those that develop incrementally and never reach the public agenda.

1. *Problem identification and agenda setting.* A public problem is recognised as a political issue, and is placed on the political agenda. This often occurs in response to pressure from an interest group.

2. *Policy formation.* New policies are developed or existing policies are redeveloped. The social and political context in which this occurs is likely to have a significant bearing on the outcome.

3. *Adoption.* A new policy is formally accepted, through either legal enactment in parliament or approval by the appropriate minister.

4. *Policy implementation.* A policy is actually put into practice. The 'product' seen at this point may be quite different from what was imagined when the policy was first formulated. For example, its power may be eroded by the way in which it is implemented, or it may have unforeseen consequences when it is put into practice. The outcome of policies that are implemented with an inadequate budget may be quite different from that envisaged when they were originally formulated.

5. *Policy evaluation.* Policies are evaluated for their impact. Clearly, if policy evaluation is to be meaningful, it needs to be an ongoing process. Policy-making is a cyclical process, and evaluating policy in action may lead to the policy issue being put back on the policy agenda, and thus to the cycle beginning again.

Those affected by the policy concerned may be able to influence the policy-making process at any stage in its life, but this is more likely to happen during policy formation and policy evaluation. In addition, because of the cyclical nature of the stages in the public policy-making process, interested groups can be part of the process that puts issues back onto the policy agenda. With regard to issues that have never been formally discussed as policy issues but have developed incrementally, community members may be involved in the important process of getting them onto the public agenda and reviewed critically, perhaps for the first time.

Influencing public policies through social advocacy and lobbying are discussed in more detail later. It is important to note, however, that affecting public policy in this way is often a slow process, and it may take several years of concerted effort by a number of people to change the major direction of a policy process.

In health promotion, regulatory activities such as international laws that address issues such as pollution of the global commons, national laws such as immunisation requirements and local laws such as tobacco legislation, are developed for the 'common good'. These healthy public policies may be as controversial as the redistributive polices, previously described. These laws invariably infringe upon the rights of individuals. Whatever the level of policy development, the same principles apply. In health promotion, the philosophy of Primary Health Care needs to underpin the policy development process and also the policies that are developed. Ideally, the need should be identified by the community and the policy developed with community and expert knowledge combined with the experience of policy-makers. This collective wisdom will make it socially acceptable to most, and scientifically sound.

Levels of policy: from global to local

If we are to address the determinants of health and illness then we need to cast a wide net when we think about how policy affects health. As we have said, health is created outside the health system, and economic and regulatory activities are those activities that involve the application of legislative and financial frameworks that create opportunities for healthy living. These activities are developed at international, national and local levels and may be in concert with one another. Organisational development also creates supportive environments and opportunities for health in smaller settings. These include everything from international organisations to local schools.

Although healthy public policy developed at the international and national levels has a great influence on the way our daily lives are structured, a remarkably large number of policy decisions that shape our environment are taken at the local level, particularly through local government. Responsibility for such issues as land use, placement of industry, housing standards, availability of recreational areas and location of shopping areas is all exercised at the local level. Local government, therefore, is quite a powerful influence on our environments, and the health impact of public policy at the local level can be profound.

Developing healthy public policy at the local level is not without its challenges. The same tension between policy for economic development and healthy public policy exist, albeit to a lesser degree, at the local level just as it does on an international scale. As we have said, social justice and environmental justice is often compromised by a philosophy of development, which usually means expansion of industry and population. These are not necessarily conducive to health, yet they are assumed to be 'good' for the community. Recent acknowledgment of the concept of sustainable development is helping to break down this assumption. However, it is unlikely that local councils will embrace the principles that underpin Primary Health Care without considerable encouragement, both from community demand and from legislation at higher national levels, because the expansion of industry and population is highly regarded by society generally. Until it is quite clear that other approaches are more acceptable, councils may feel compelled to remain with this approach. This may mean that community members have considerable work to do in lobbying local councils to take their concerns about healthy public policy seriously.

There are many examples of healthy public policy being developed at the international level that have influenced policy development at the local level. Local Agenda 21 and the Healthy Cities project are two well-known examples.

The WHO Healthy Cities project is a long-term international development project that aims to place health high on the agenda of decision-makers in cities throughout the world and to promote healthy public policies and comprehensive local strategies to enhance health and sustainable development. The WHO project was launched in Europe in 1988 with 11 cities. It is now an international movement and a good example of how policies developed at the international and local level can work in concert to improve health. It is the most obvious example of the settings approach to health promotion.

While each Healthy Cities project will necessarily differ according to the cultural norms, needs and characteristics of the locality, all share characteristics of good governance, inter-sectoral planning, community participation and monitoring and evaluation (WHO http://www.euro.who.int/healthy-cities).

Successful implementation of this approach requires explicit political commitment, leadership and institutional change, inter-sectoral partnerships, innovative actions addressing all aspects of health and living conditions, and extensive networking between cities. These are characterised as the four elements for action:

1. Explicit political commitment at the highest level to the principles and strategies of the Healthy Cities project.

2. Establishment of new organisational structures to manage change.

3. Commitment to developing a shared vision for the city, with a health plan and work on specific themes.

4. Investment in formal and informal networking and cooperation.

(WHO 2004c)

Healthy Cities projects have been adapted by some cities in Australia. Noarlunga Healthy Cities in South Australia is one example. This project began in 1987 as a national pilot project. Among its many achievements are the clean up of a river, a community injury prevention project and a community forum taking action against drugs. Evaluations of the project conducted over a period of 16 years demonstrate the requirements that sustain a community-based health-promotion initiative. The main factors that account for the sustainability of the project are (Baum 2004, conference notes):

- ongoing resourcing and support from government;
- consistent and dedicated leadership;
- genuine community participation that has been resourced and sustained;
- participation across sectors that has accumulated credibility as initiatives gain momentum;
- consideration of both short-term achievements and working towards longer-term goals;
- gaining cross-party political support;
- a long-term relationship between a university department of public health and Noarlunga Healthy Cities; and
- a history of cooperative action in the Noarlunga region.

Internationally, Healthy Cities programs are increasingly regarded as a valuable source of experience and legitimacy for national programs (WHO 2004c). In Europe there is renewed commitment. In October 2003 WHO celebrated the 15 years of the European Healthy Cities movement with a major conference in Belfast. The conference was concluded with the adoption of the Belfast Declaration (WHO 2004c) which outlined the principles and the goals of the 2003–2007 phase (Phase IV) of WHO Healthy Cities in Europe and reinforced the political commitment towards achieving them (see Box 3.1).

The Municipal Public Health Planning Framework in Victoria, Australia overcomes the deficits in national planning for healthy cities in Australia. It is an excellent example of healthy public policy development. *Environments for Health*:

Box 3.1 The Belfast Declaration

We, the political leaders of our cities, towns and local authorities attending the World Health Organization's International Healthy Cities Conference in Belfast, Northern Ireland, United Kingdom from 19 to 22 October 2003,
Celebrating 15 years of the Healthy Cities movement in Europe and beyond;
Recognizing the power of local action;
Acknowledging city leadership in health and sustainable development;
Knowing that the key determinants of health lie outside the direct control of the health sector;
Building upon our broad experience and scientific evidence base;
Committed to the continued improvement of the health and quality of life of all our citizens;
Guided by the key principles of equity, sustainability, inter-sectoral cooperation, community empowerment and solidarity;
Understanding that health should never be the exclusive concern of any one political party or professional discipline, and that all should adhere to these guiding principles;
Drawing upon the Johannesburg Declaration on Sustainable Development 2002, which emphasises the importance of partnerships at all levels and of good urban governance.
Hereby pledge ourselves to:
• build strong partnerships, alliances and networks;
• design supportive environments to meet the needs of all citizens;
• tackle the wider determinants of health; and
• create effective policies, strategies and tools for action.

As political leaders, we commit ourselves to:

Reducing inequalities and addressing poverty, which will require local assessment and regular reporting on progress to reduce the gaps;
City health development planning, which provides our cities with a means to build and maintain strategic partnerships for health;
Promoting good governance and creating inclusive cities that ensure all citizens have a key role in shaping services and influencing city policies and plans;
Building safe and supportive cities sensitive to the needs of all citizens, actively engaging urban planning departments and promoting healthy urban planning practices;
Promoting health impact assessment as a means for all sectors to focus their work on health and the quality of life;
Taking an active role in shaping and implementing national, European and global strategies, and contributing to localization of the United Nation's Millennium Development Goals;
Demonstrating the relevance of our work and maximizing the impact and strategic standing of Healthy Cities within countries and as international players;
Systematically monitoring, documenting, evaluating and communicating our work so that we and others can learn and benefit;
Strengthening international friendship and solidarity between cities and regions, mutual support and sharing of resources, knowledge, information and experience;
Expanding national networks of Healthy Cities, as they represent a tremendous foundation of political commitment, innovation and dynamism for the whole movement;

Continued

> **Box 3.1 The Belfast Declaration (Continued)**
>
> Cities cannot act alone. We call on:
>
> Acknowledging our responsibilities for supporting Healthy Cities in other regions, enabling their pioneering work and knowledge to become globally accessible.
>
> national governments:
> - to recognise that national policies on health and sustainability have a local dimension and acknowledge the significant contribution that cities can make towards them;
> - to acknowledge that national networks of Healthy Cities have a part to play in country health development and to support their coordinating and capacity-building role; and
>
> the World Health Organization
> - to provide leadership and strategic support in work towards the goals of Phase IV (2003–2007) of the WHO Healthy Cities program/movement;
> - to strengthen inter-regional cooperation on Healthy Cities;
> - to join forces with other international organizations and agencies to meet urban health challenges.

(Source: World Health Organization 2004 *Belfast Declaration*. Online. Available: http://www.who.dk/healthy-cities [accessed 20 January 2004])

Promoting Health and Wellbeing Through Built, Social, Economic and Natural Environments is an initiative of the State Government of Victoria that is consistent with the legislative planning requirement of the *Health Act* and *Local Government Act* in that state. The framework was developed in partnership with the Public Health Division of the Department of Human Services, the Municipal Association of Victoria, Victorian Local Governance Association, local governments and community groups. It is a strategy for public health planning that aims to systematically address 'individual, organisational, community, social, political, economic and other environmental factors affecting health and well being' (State Government of Victoria website). The legislation that underpins this strategy ensures that Municipal Public Health Plans (MPHP) are reviewed annually and prepared every three years. The concepts that underpin the planning framework are in concert with the Primary Health Care approach (see Box 3.2).

At a municipal level, there is a need to develop an integrated planning approach that incorporates:

- Linkages between stakeholders' policies and plans.

- A local government governance role that provides leadership, advocacy and facilitation.

- Meaningful community participation.

(State Government of Victoria, http://www.health.vic.gov.au)

Organisational development

Health promotion has been identified as including three interrelated processes — personal development, organisational development and political development

---

Box 3.2 Environments for health: promoting health and wellbeing through built, social, economic and natural environments

Health planning concepts

The new MPHP framework uses the strengths of a number of approaches to public health planning including:

- **Strategic local area planning** A strategic and integrated approach to municipal public health planning promotes a model for integrating physical, social and economic planning, with community participation.
- **Social model of health** Participation, sense of community and empowerment are interdependent social factors contributing to individual and community wellbeing.
- **Health-promoting systems** A strong relationship exists between people and place: people's health and wellbeing reflects their socioeconomic status, and accordingly, where they live. Different locations afford varying degrees of access to healthy environments, food, services, amenities, health information, education, employment, housing and opportunities to experience a sense of community and sense of place. A holistic approach ensures that the interrelationships between all major issues impacting on individuals and families within the context of their local communities are taken into account (see Appendix 2).
- **Focusing on health outcomes** Utilising information from the Victorian Burden of Disease Study (Human Service 1999) and other sources can identify issues and areas for consideration when planning health priorities.
- **Participation and partnership approaches** People increasingly share in planning and decision-making and are empowered to affect the outcome of the process. Clients, community groups, government departments and other agencies need to participate in health planning, not only to ensure a match between local needs and priorities, but because participation itself promotes health. Clients/consumers and the wider community need to participate meaningfully to ensure appropriateness, community ownership of processes, programs and outcomes, and the promotion of accountability to the community for decisions on priorities and resource allocation.

towards health (Kickbusch 1994, p. 5). Health-promoting settings provide an opportunity to strengthen the role of organisational development as a health-promotion strategy, while also maintaining the focus on individual and political development.

As the discussion in the previous section demonstrates, the idea of implementing the Ottawa Charter for Health Promotion, with its focus on healthy public policy, at a societal level is certainly important. At the same time, though, the focus on such a broad target for change is sometimes beyond the scope of health workers unless specifically charged with the responsibilities of plans, such as the municipal health plan. However, policies operating at the institutional level can have a big impact on people's lives.

The policies of institutions, such as workplaces, schools and other community-based organisations, influence people's lives as they come in contact with these institutions and often influence the lives of community members even when they are not in direct contact with the organisation. It is vital, therefore, to work for healthy organisational policy, as part of healthy public policy.

The ways in which health workers can work for healthy organisational policy will vary depending on the institution, the ways in which the policy relates to the public, and the health workers' relationship with it. Working for change, within an organisation for which health workers work, requires following the organisation's normal lines of communication. However, working to change an organisation that sees itself as responsible to the public may require the worker to follow lines of communication similar to those for working towards change to healthy public policy; that is, in dealing with such an organisation, the worker can write to its chief executive or any people in key positions relevant to the particular issue. If requests for change come from more than one person, success is more likely. If there is no success, the request for change may need to go to others who have influence over the organisation, such as a government minister.

Fawkes (1997, p. 392) has identified several elements required of any health setting if it is to be health promoting:

- principles that inform the policies and strategies for health care service delivery, such as equity, empowerment, participation and access;
- organisational capacity to implement these principles through activities such as leadership, and through professional, technical and political skills, culture, resources, networks and partnerships;
- programs and services (core business for health care organisations) geared to promoting health; and
- facilities whose design, location and function contribute to the health and wellbeing of service users and employees, and the amenity of the local community.

Health-promoting schools

Schools play a central role in the lives of children all around the globe, and their potential as health-promoting settings is enormous. However, schools are not always positive experiences for students. Negative experiences within the social environment of the school, such as bullying, may have far-reaching effects. For these reasons, there has been considerable enthusiasm for the development of schools as health-promoting settings, with the WHO supporting and encouraging this development since the mid-1980s.

A health-promoting school is where all members of the school community work together to provide students with integrated and positive experiences and structures which promote and protect their health. This includes both the formal and informal curriculum in health, the creation of a safe and healthy school environment, the provision of appropriate health services and the involvement of the family and wider community in efforts to promote health.

(WHO 1995, p. 3)

The concept of the health-promoting school is international in its development, with many countries around the world working on programs which support schools and their communities in better health actions. For example, in Europe it is supported by the Council of Europe, the European Commission and the WHO Regional Office for Europe. Because the determinants of education and health are indivisibly linked, the program seeks to integrate the policy and practice of the health-promoting schools into the wider health and education sectors. It works at three levels: school, national and international. More than 40 countries in the European Region are members. In Scotland, for example, the national policy is to have all schools health-promoting schools by 2007. The Australian Health-Promoting Schools Association was established in 1994. This association aims to initiate and support ways of establishing in schools a broad view of health consistent with the Ottawa Charter (see Box 3.3).

A recent health-promoting policy initiative involving schools around the world is the Walking Bus. Although it is not integrated with the health-promoting schools policy it is a policy initiative that schools are taking up worldwide. There are many benefits. For example, children not only get more exercise but learn road rules, socialise and have fun going to school. There are also benefits for parents. For example, they can be assured that their children are getting to school safely, getting fitter and having the opportunity to meet new friends. If parents become a 'conductor', they can get fitter through regular exercise and feel more connected through participation in the school community. The community benefits because the bus tackles the issues of environmental pollution, transportation issues such as congestion and increases the chances of a 'sense of community' (VicHealth 2004).

Working for healthy organisational policy, while valuable, however cannot replace working for healthy public policy on a broader scale. Health workers need to ensure that they work for public policy change on issues that impact on health at the same time as they work for institutional policy change. Otherwise, we may end up ignoring the hard issues that have the biggest impact on people's health and address issues only at the level of the individual or institution.

From international to organisational: the example of tobacco

Developing healthy public policies that work in concert at all levels is obviously going to have the greatest impact on creating supporting environments for health. The policy development on the use of tobacco is a great example.

The WHO Framework Convention on Tobacco Control

The World Health Organization's Framework Convention on Tobacco Control (FCTC) will have a significant affect on the health of the population worldwide. The convention has been signed by over 100 countries and the European Community, which means that 'more than one billion people have a strong commitment from their governments to act firmly on tobacco control' (WHO www.who.int/mediacentre/releases releases/2004/pr21/en/). Once the WHO FCTC enters into force, countries that are parties to the treaty are bound by it and are expected to legislate according to its provisions.

The WHO FCTC is the first legal instrument designed to reduce tobacco-related deaths and disease worldwide. The convention has provisions that set out international minimum standards on tobacco-related issues, such as tobacco

> **Box 3.3 A charter for health-promoting schools**
>
> - Health-promoting policy — by developing coherent curricula in education for health which bring biological, ecological and social dimensions to a process of environmental health.
> - Creating supportive environments by utilising the setting of the school to encourage reciprocal support between teachers, pupils and parents.
> - Strengthening community action by drawing on existing human and material resources in the community in which the school is set and involving that community in practical aspects of the decisions, plans and actions pertaining to the project.
> - Developing personal skills by providing information, education for health and opportunities to enhance life skills in the setting of the school community.
> - Re-orienting health services by involving the school health service in project activities aimed at the promotion of health by utilising the skills of school health professionals on a broader basis than the traditional roles.

(Source: World Health Organization 1986 *The Ottawa Charter for Health Promotion*. WHO, Geneva)

advertising, promotion and sponsorship, tax and price measures, packaging and labelling, illicit trade and protection from second-hand smoke. These provisions are designed to guide governments, which are free to legislate at higher thresholds if desired (WHO www.who.int/mediacentre/releases releases/2004/pr21/en). Australia was actively involved in the development of the WHO Convention and signed it on 5 December 2003.

Australia's tobacco strategy

The Australian government has been responsible for a mixture of economic and regulatory activities in tobacco control over many years. For example, it has imposed an excise tax on tobacco products since 1901, although at that time, the tax would probably have been a revenue-raising activity rather than imposing an economic incentive to help create a supportive environment for health. More recently, the National Health Policy on Tobacco, adopted in 1991, formed the basis for the development of The National Tobacco Strategy, which has been in place since 1999. The National Tobacco Strategy comprises a range of tobacco-control initiatives developed to reduce the population's exposure to tobacco. There are six key initiatives:

1. strengthening community action;

2. promoting cessation of tobacco use;

3. reducing availability and supply of tobacco;

4. reducing tobacco promotion;

5. regulating tobacco; and

6. international action.

(National Expert Advisory Committee on Tobacco 2000)

Several strategies exist within each of these key areas. For example, within 'strengthening community action', the nationwide social marketing strategy provided Australians with television commercials about the health effects of tobacco. Under 'promoting cessation of tobacco use', preparation of best practice guidelines for smoking cessation action were prepared for medical practitioners, and within 'reducing tobacco promotion', a review of the *Tobacco Advertising Prohibition Act* was commissioned. Around the same time the *Tobacco Advertising Prohibition Act 1992* was passed to further restrict all forms of tobacco advertising, including broadcasting, the print media, and sponsorship associated with sporting and cultural events.

While the federal government has taken responsibility for a number of coordinated nationwide strategies, service delivery primarily rests with the states and territories. The State of Victoria, for example, has been an international leader in tobacco control programs.

Victoria's Tobacco Action Plan

The Victorian Tobacco Action Plan was developed to work in harmony with the national strategy. However, regulatory activities to create supportive environments for health have been part of the State of Victoria's landscape for some time. The purpose of the *Tobacco Act 1987*, for example, was to prohibit certain sales or promotion of tobacco products and to establish the Victorian Health Promotion Foundation (VicHealth). Since then, many statutory regulations have emerged to regulate sales, advertising, labelling and pricing of tobacco in Victoria. Recent developments in tobacco control in Victoria include smoke-free dining, point-of-sale tobacco advertising and display restriction and smoking restrictions in bars, clubs and gaming venues. Further, the government's work in tobacco control is supported by a number of agencies such as The Cancer Council of Victoria, The National Heart Foundation and VicHealth (State Government of Victoria 2002).

Victorian Health Promotion Foundation (VicHealth)

VicHealth works for structural change in policy development at the local and organisational level. It provides substantial funding to Quit Victoria and VicHealth Centre for Tobacco Control as well as conducting its own tobacco control activities, such as working with sports, arts and local government sectors. For example, the community is being involved through sporting associations to develop smoke-free policies within sporting associations and local clubs, and the Arts for Health Program supports agencies to develop policies and procedures to create smoke-free environments in art settings (State Government of Victoria 2002).

The development of healthy public policy for any issue at a broad social level, a local/community level and within organisations will create a supportive environment for health. The development of the policy may be 'bottom up' or 'top down' depending on the level of development. Influencing the policy may be done at any stage in its development.

Influencing policy

Community members and groups affected by the policy concerned may be able to influence the policy-making process at any stage, but this is more likely to happen during policy formation and policy evaluation. In addition, because of the cyclical nature of the stages in the public policy-making process, community members and interested groups can be part of the process that puts issues back onto the policy agenda. With regard to issues that have never been formally discussed as policy issues but have developed incrementally, community members may be involved in the important process of getting them onto the public agenda and reviewed critically, perhaps for the first time.

Because the key determinants of health are external to the individual, it is appropriate that health workers use advocacy for policy-orientated approaches to health risk factors (Atkin & Wallack 1990, p. 11). Public policies can be influenced through social advocacy and lobbying. To have maximum influence on policy formulation or policy directions health workers and interest groups work in collaboration across sectors with peak industry bodies such as the National Rural Health Alliance or the Public Health Association in Australia. Notable success in initiating or changing policy has been achieved by issue-based lobby groups ranging from conservation groups seeking to change policy allowing logging of forests, to gay men's rights groups seeking a balance in HIV and AIDS awareness and prevention programs, and the anti-smoking lobby seeking restrictions of cigarette advertising. Community members seeking to change policy at any level would be well advised to articulate their needs through the wider networks or lobby groups and peak advisory bodies, rather than acting in isolation. If health workers are to influence the direction of policy and action in a way that makes environments healthier, then clearly they need to influence policy and action in a number of sectors. They cannot do this alone, but must work with a range of other people who recognise the health impacts of actions in what are traditionally regarded as non-health areas. These people include workers in industry, transport, agriculture and education, in addition to members of the community.

It is important to note, however, that affecting public policy in this way is often a slow process, and it may take several years of concerted effort by a number of people to change the major direction of a policy process. Working with people and keeping sight of the goal is important.

It is vital, then, that health workers plan to make and maintain valuable working relationships with people in other disciplines, other agencies and other sectors in order to maximise the joint actions that are necessary to promote health. These working relationships can be very powerful, even though there may be times when conflict may arise. More often than not, though, when a working relationship exists between people, it seems much easier to deal with any conflict than when there is no previous working relationship.

Social policy advocacy and lobbying

Social advocacy and lobbying are very much recognised as part of the health worker's role, particularly since the Ottawa Charter for Health Promotion acknowledged their importance. They constitute a key strategy with which to work for healthy public policy. Health workers have two key roles to play in social or health advocacy: acting as advocates and lobbyists themselves, and encouraging and supporting other community members to take up advocacy and lobbying. Developing skills in this area, as well as assisting others to do so, is a vital part of health promotion work if health workers are to take up the advocacy role effectively.

Defining advocacy and lobbying

Advocacy occurs when a person in authority or an agency in a position of influence represents the interests on behalf of an individual, group or community in order to change or improve their situation. Advocacy activities centre on an issue that needs to be addressed, rather than about the individual or group who raises the issue. Advocacy is often necessary in community situations when there are unequal power relations, and the least powerful have been unable to get their message across or to change their situation using usual communication mechanisms.

Lobbying is the process or the activities involved in advocating on behalf of a group or an issue. The term lobbying usually describes advocacy to parliamentarians or to media sources. The term originated from the habit of policy advocates standing in the lobby of parliament in order to approach members as they entered or exited the chambers. Lobbyists may be professionals in this role, who are paid by organisations seeking policy change, who want their issue advocated directly to a minister.

People can do advocacy work as individuals, and they can do it as part of an organisation that includes advocacy and lobbying work in its activities. There are a number of key organisations that currently act to advocate for community members and consumers in the health system. Some work is specifically for community and consumer advocacy work, for example in Australia, the Consumers' Health Forum and the Health Issues Centre; others are professional organisations which include community and consumer advocacy as part of their role, for example the state-based Community Health Associations and the Public Health Association of Australia (PHAA) (see Box 3.4 for examples of PHAA advocacy on health issues). All of these organisations are among those in which health workers can involve themselves. In addition to adding their weight to the voices behind the advocacy work, a great deal can be learnt about effective advocacy work and about work being conducted by others.

Advocacy is the key to getting political commitment for an issue. We may also think of advocacy influencing the politics or the policy direction at local governance level, or within an organisation or agency, where power relations may just as effectively be obstacles to equitable access, or obstacles to change. Advocacy is an overtly political activity and to be effective advocates work across a range of sectors to bring a groundswell of engagement with a new perspective or approach. Advocacy can cause economic and political instability because it challenges the status quo. Longstanding agreements, informal arrangements and allegiances may be challenged.

Advocacy and power relations

As suggested above, people or organisations advocate on behalf of others in order to bring about change that may not be possible if the group were left to argue for change unassisted. Ife (2002, p. 248) cautions against assuming that a health worker is automatically better able to represent the views of clients, and that they

---

> **Box 3.4 Advocacy of an organisation**
>
> **Public Health Association of Australia**
>
> **ADVOCACY ISSUES**
>
> Message from PHAA President Re: Health Care Summit in Canberra
> Final Reconciling Aboriginal Health Media Release — May 2003
> Passive Smoking In Workplaces And Public Places — May 2003
> Talk given by Peter Sainsbury On: Australia-US Free Trade Agreement and the
>   Pharmaceutical Benefits Scheme (PBS) — May 2003
>
> **ADVOCACY SUMMARIES**
>
> US Attack on Reproductive Health Care — intouch December 2002
> NSW Child Health Obesity Summit — intouch December 2002
> Advocacy October/November — intouch December 2002
> Letter to: Framework Convention on Tobacco Control (FCTC)
> Reply to: PHAA's Letter to Framework Convention on Tobacco Control (FCTC)
> Letter to: The Hon Alexander Downer Minister for Foreign Affairs and Trade
> Letter to: Ms Faye L. Wong, President, American Public Health Association
> Reply to: PHAA's letter to the Minister for Foreign Affairs from the Australian
>   Agency for International Development

will naturally need to be advocated for in their efforts to bring about change or to raise an issue in public debate. Advocacy is potentially further disempowering for a client who is already in a vulnerable position. However, sometimes it is essential that 'the role of the community worker must be to enable people to represent their own interests, rather than to feel they always need someone else to do it for them' (Ife 2002). This applies with all forms of activities in working with communities. Power relations are dealt with in more detail later in this and subsequent chapters.

Why advocate?

There are four key purposes in advocating with or on behalf of a community:

1. Mobilise resources — advocacy usually argues for a different distribution of funds to what is currently in place.

2. Change opinions — advocacy may involve persuading those in decision-making positions to see an alternative perspective.

3. Catalyse change — sometimes individuals or agencies may wish to change their perspective or approach, but need guidance to commence or to implement new policies that are appropriate to another worldview.

4. Cause actions — advocates can act as mentors to guide implementation of different strategies.

Skills for effective advocacy

Advocacy involves using skills to put an issue into public and policy debate and thereby encouraging those who can influence policy to report it in such a way that the change is supported by the wider population (Egger et al 1993). Effective advocacy relates to articulating the message about an issue very clearly and repeating it as often as is necessary to change values, opinions or actions. A number of the following strategies will be useful:

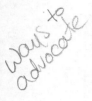
Ways to advocate

1. Be clear about what the group wants — what is the aim or goal? What is it they want to change? What do they want the agency they are approaching to do about the issue? The group or organisation seeking change needs to be very clear and precise in this statement before it is taken into a wider domain and make sure it represents the unified views of the group.

2. Establish common themes — what are the key messages about why this change needs to be made? Articulate the rationale clearly, linking it with other philosophical or political approaches. That is, use existing policy as an argument supporting the change that is being advocated for. Think about issuing messages and arguments that will appeal to a broad range of people, rather than a narrower point of view. When in the advocacy process, whether in writing or in person, keep reverting to these key themes.

3. Never stray away from the message. It is easy to be impassioned by the urgency of the change or the strong values held by the group, and this can bring advocates into argument that results in the key points being lost. Reiteration of the key message, rather than counter-argument, is a wiser strategy.

4. Use all opportunities to get the message across. 'Advocates seek to generate news coverage that will serve to reframe public debate on societal issues' (Atkin & Arkin in Atkin & Wallack 1990, p. 25). Become political in a range of forums that already operate at different levels in the community. For instance consider approaches to community-based organisations and support groups that already exist, formal community organisations such as committees of management or business networks, all levels of government (local councillors, state and federal government members), approach other advocacy or peak body groups for support, such as the Public Health Association of Australia, or environmental action groups. Use a range of media, especially targeting the ones that your audience will access.

   Publicise the message in a variety of ways in your community.

   These various approaches again reinforce the importance of having a clearly stated message and clear reasons why the change is essential. Whatever publicity option is available will entail restating the key points in more, or less, detail.

5. Develop media contacts. Keep a careful note of the approaches that are made, who is contacted and what responses are received. Be prepared to 'cultivate' those media contacts that provide rapid and positive responses.

6. Own the statistics and 'quantify' your arguments. People in positions of influence will be more readily swayed if your arguments in favour of change can be backed up with quantitative evidence. Use statistical evidence that will illustrate your argument in the starkest manner. Atkin and Wallack (1990, p. 159) describe this process as 'creative epidemiology'. 'Creative epidemiology is the use of new scientific evidence and existing data to gain media attention and clearly convey the public health importance of an issue' (p. 159). Have these statistics ready to use, and

be prepared to provide them in a printed format in all forms of publicity. Always provide valid sources for the statistical evidence. There is nothing to be gained by not being unable to back up the claims that are made — it provides an avenue for criticism.

7. Repetition is essential; be prepared to repeat the message any time an audience can be created. The message will only be 'news' the first time around, so don't expect a media outlet to keep publishing the same item — they are there to report the news, and the advocates role is to make the item newsworthy (Pertschuk in Atkin & Wallack 1990, pp. 173–6). Seek new forums for the message to be heard.

8. Find an 'attractive' internal spokesperson; that is, a person who can be the public image of the issue, a person who becomes associated with the cause. This person must be prepared to be accessible for the cause and have their name associated with the cause. This person needs also to have a positive public image, because remember, this is a very political process and some serve an agenda in opposition by discrediting the messenger, not the message.

9. Use icons with credibility. Sometimes interest groups employ persons with a public profile for another reason, to advocate for their cause (such as sports people, advocating QUIT smoking programs). Be very sure that the values and behaviours of the 'icon' are, and will remain, congruent with the issue they are advocating.

10. Be persistent. The work of advocacy requires determination and a 'thick skin'. These are the characteristics associated with all forms of political processes and social change. A refusal at one approach may mean that an alternative approach is tried, or a different person is contacted.

11. Make it OK to talk about. There are a number of issues and topics that have previously been 'taboo' or not widely spoken of in public. Sexual behaviours are key examples here. Advocates, wishing to change policy or their treatment within the health system, have been fundamental in changing social values and putting topics onto the public agenda.

12. Find corporate allies. Corporate sponsorship of an issue allows it to enter a whole new domain of influence. Sponsorship provides advocates with additional purchasing power and public profile. However, sponsorship does not come without its costs. Ensure that the values of the corporations are in line with that of the advocated agenda. Remember also that a corporation will expect some return on their investment, so be sure the demands can be met, before the contract is signed.

Lobbying

Lobbying members of parliament

Appealing to members of parliament to act on issues that impact on the health of the community can be a useful way of having certain views represented, and (hopefully) taken account of when decisions are being made at the political level.

Members of parliament have limited access to staff who can research issues for them, so they rely on constituents and lobbyists for information.

There are several possibilities. Firstly, it is worthwhile when communicating with members of parliament to emphasise the impact of the concern for the local people, as parliamentarians are elected by local people in the expectation that they will represent those people's interests. Secondly, members of parliament responsible for particular portfolios relevant to the issue at hand can be lobbied. For example, the government ministers of health may be approached regarding the concerns about a health issue. Ministers responsible for other relevant portfolios can also be approached. The transport, agriculture, sport, education and environment ministers are just some of the ministers whom it may be appropriate to approach regarding different health-promotion issues. Thirdly, the party leaders in question can be approached if you believe the issue has more serious or urgent consequences. They are best reached via their electoral offices, as their offices at Parliament House are often unattended (Beauchamp 1986, p. 122). Contacting a member of parliament by letter rather than by telephone is more likely to be successful because a written request is more difficult to ignore (Beauchamp 1986, p. 124). It really is worth taking the time to express the views, as members of parliament do use this to gauge public responses.

Lobbying members of parliament is more likely to be successful if done by a larger number of people, and much of this approach therefore involves working with other people, and informing them about the ways in which lobbying skills can be used to affect the public agenda. Some of the techniques outlined above for advocacy about an issue can be used to lobby parliamentarians, where relevant. For instance, it is important to be well-informed and to argue your case clearly, and to back this up with solid evidence.

Encouraging other people to lobby members of parliament, and to keep at it by regularly contacting them, will increase the chances of success. Face-to-face contact is more effective than telephone contact. Ask for an appointment time, and go well prepared, with documentation to reinforce the main points you wish to make. Explain why the issue should matter to them, but attempt to understand and acknowledge their perspective. Consider using stories from the field to illustrate and add impact to the argument. Legislators like to be treated with respect. Always be polite and take time to thank them for their time. You may need their support on another issue in the future.

The mass media is also a very useful tool in lobbying members of parliament and other key decision-makers, who are increasingly reliant on the mass media for their understanding of important policy issues. The role of the media in social marketing is discussed in more detail in Chapter 7.

Responding to calls for public comment

Departments of health, and other government sectors, place advertisements in all the major metropolitan newspapers, usually on a Saturday, when they wish to advise of the availability of a new report for public discussion, canvass public opinion on an issue, invite public involvement in an activity or advertise the availability of funding for health-promotion activities or research. Other bodies, for example, the National Health and Medical Research Council in Australia, do the same. It is therefore extremely valuable to examine the major newspapers regularly in order to identify these calls for public comment. They provide a valuable opportunity to influence government policy on issues affecting health.

Unfortunately, many health workers miss out on opportunities to respond to these calls because they assume that they will gain access to any relevant discussion papers through their workplace. In fact, in many instances these discussion papers do not trickle down through the bureaucracy to health workers.

More often than not, calls for public discussion are responded to by more skilled and articulate members of the community, and many other people do not feel confident about writing to government departments with their opinion. Regrettably, this may mean that the final reports of government do not accurately reflect a broad range of public opinion, and so it is vital that as many people as possible put forward their views. It is most worthwhile to respond to these calls for submissions, and to encourage as many people as possible around you to do so.

It may be a good idea to arrange for a group of people to get together to discuss these draft documents, and perhaps to put together a group response. This can be very useful if the people who may be affected by the proposal are unlikely to respond individually because they do not have enough time, confidence or skills.

Responding to parliamentary inquiries

In situations where a government may need to explore an issue in some depth, a parliamentary committee may be established, to investigate the issue and make recommendations to parliament. When a parliamentary committee conducts an inquiry, submissions are called for in the press and all members of the public are invited to respond.

Some of the people who make submissions are then invited to appear at a public hearing to answer questions. These hearings are usually open to the public, although it is possible to request to speak to the committee in private if necessary.

Using the mass media

As a key influence in placing issues on the policy agenda, the mass media are powerful tools to use in working for healthy public policy. Using the media in this way is known as 'media advocacy', which will be discussed further in Chapter 7. Letters to the editor and media releases can put forward an alternative view and help to reshape the public perception of an issue. In addition, they can widen discussion on draft documents open for public discussion by making other people aware of the documents and their implications. There is widespread acknowledgment that politicians rely on the mass media for most of their information about public issues, so the value of using the mass media to lobby for change should not be underestimated.

Ensuring community representation on committees

If public committees are to conduct work that reflects a broad view of community opinions, community members or consumers need to be adequately represented on them and have adequate decision-making power. Health workers have an important role to play in lobbying for community representation on, and effective participation in, committees whose work impacts on the life of the community. Working to achieve these two goals is an important way in which the work of these committees remains in touch with community perspectives.

Some people may wonder why community representatives are necessary if health workers are committed to presenting a community perspective. However, there will be times when the perspective of community members may clash with that of health workers, and health workers should not assume that they are always able to represent the community perspective in an unbiased way when representing their professional interests (Consumers' Health Forum 1999, p. 3). Furthermore, accepting community members as partners with health workers means according them partnership status, not simply speaking on their behalf. In situations in which community representatives are present, health workers can add support by adding their voice to those presenting the perspective of community members.

Representing consumer interests, whether as the community representative or as a health worker concerned to represent the consumer perspective, is not always a comfortable position to be in. The perspective of community members can be threatening to many professionals if they believe that it is their job to make decisions on behalf of the community and that they know what is best. This is especially so if the consumers or community members do not agree with these professionals' opinions. Recognising that the community perspective may challenge professionals on the committees may help those representing it to deal with any negative feedback they receive from committee members. Supporting members of the community in this position, or finding support for yourself if you are in this position, is vital if the community perspective is to be maintained on the committee for a length of time that enables things to be achieved.

The Consumers' Health Forum has produced a very useful booklet, *Guidelines for Consumer Representatives: Suggestions for Consumer or Community Representatives Working on Committees* (1999), which addresses many issues relevant to community members becoming involved with committees. It is worthwhile ensuring that agencies keep a copy of this booklet and make it available to any community members or budding community representatives, so as to help them increase their effectiveness on committees.

Advocacy and lobbying are the work of empowered individuals, groups and communities. In the following section, we discuss empowerment in the light of using policy in health promotion.

Using policy in health promotion

Power and empowerment

Definitions of power and empowerment were presented in Chapter 2, along with a brief discussion about the ways that power is exerted in society resulting in disempowerment of some people and groups. The term empowerment is widely used, and is found in a range of policy documents and strategic approaches.

The *process* of empowerment is central to community development work (Ife 2002, p. 53).

The process of empowerment is aimed at increasing the power of those who are disadvantaged. As the section in Chapter 2 outlined, people and groups can be disempowered because of the way existing structures in society maintain their powerless situation, such as being unemployed, or by virtue of their personal characteristics, such as their gender, sexual orientation or personal values.

In health-promotion activities across the continuum of approaches, the Primary Health Care philosophy directs us to focus on the most disadvantaged groups in terms of their equitable access to health care. A fundamental way to achieve sustained change is to strengthen community involvement in decision-making so there are more community-based structures in place. Empowerment may be a by-product of other community-based activities. For instance, policy that is already in place at various levels of administration including national, state and local government, and within organisations, can be a very useful tool of empowerment. In addition, individuals and groups who become active in influencing policy formulation or change gain a number of very useful skills along the way.

Working towards empowerment

Ife (2002, p. 208) describes the role of the community development worker seeking empowerment of a vulnerable group as one of providing people with the resources, opportunities, vocabulary, knowledge and skills to increase their capacity to determine their own future, and to participate in and affect the life of their community. Ife (2002) offers four perspectives on empowerment:

1. Various groups in society are competing for power (politicians, unionists, lobby groups, professions, media, etc).

   Empowerment is a process of helping disadvantaged groups to compete more effectively with other interests.

2. Elite groups have more than their share of power and exercise disproportionate influence over decision-making. They control the institutions, media, education, political parties, public policy, the bureaucracy, parliament, professions, etc.

   Empowerment is learning the ability to compete for political power, to seek alliances with elites, or to limit their power, such as service clubs, school networks, the Australian Medical Association and other professional associations.

3. Structural inequality and oppression are major forms of power (white, wealthy, men).

   Empowerment is achieved through challenging structural disadvantage through social change.

4. Power is expressed through the use of language (discourse) which is used as a mechanism of control.

   Empowerment is achieved through validating other voices than those currently dominating the discourse.

As set out in Chapter 2, working in partnership with communities is the key focus of community development work, as well as being the ultimate aim in a Primary Health Care approach to health promotion. Partnership as an outcome is most likely to bring about changes that are sustained over time because they represent the wishes of the community itself. Healthy public policy will most likely be developed and accepted in partnership with others.

Sustaining partnerships

The *hardware* and the *software* of health promotion

The metaphors 'hardware' and 'software' of health promotion were used by community project workers in Canada (Labonté 1997, p. 48). The terms are used as symbols for the 'things' that are necessary to make health-promotion activities successful in enabling people to work in partnership with health agencies to achieve equitable access to health opportunities. Across the spectrum of health-promotion activities, from community action or policy regulations to health education, the work of health promotion is to 'enable', 'mediate' and 'advocate' on behalf of the community members. The hardware and software provide metaphors for how we, as health workers, can think about our ways of working with our communities to achieve desired changes. A fundamental approach to health-promotion work is that of enabling community members to participate fully in all aspects or activities. Participation is essential if the community is to achieve equitable access to health opportunities, and to become empowered as part of the process. It is not possible to achieve equitable Primary Health Care unless people are able to take an active part in decisions that affect them. Empowerment of community members is a conscious process with deliberate steps, which does not necessarily mean a consequent loss of power to the health-promotion practitioner.

The hardware and the software relate to the tools that people can use to be active towards their own health gains, in ways that are most suitable to them. They set out the 'toolkit' for the formal structures and the ways of working with communities.

Labonté (1997, pp. 48–9) describes *hardware* approaches as being like the 'potential power of a computer hard drive'. These may be the formal lines of authority, such as policies that may already be in place at national, state, local or agency level. They may be procedures and structures that are enshrined in the goals, objectives and strategic plan of an authority or an agency. These formal structures may relate to equitable allocation of resources, decision-making and representation on management committees or existing partnership agreements between agencies or authorities. We can view them as tools to support us in attracting, maintaining and supporting community members to take part and to achieve what is desired. The policy and procedures guidelines can be a very strong ally for health-promotion workers when they need to advocate on behalf of disempowered or disadvantaged members of their communities.

Software approaches 'focus on the nature of relationships between people' (Labonté 1997, pp. 48–9). The software approaches can be likened to the programs the computer might run; the processes used to achieve an outcome. In health-promotion activities these might describe patterns of behaviour in workplaces or on committees, such as whether they are conducted in a respectful, inclusive and ethical manner, whether the processes are congruent with guiding principles of the agency, whether some participants are allowed to dominate discussion or decision-making and others feel excluded or disempowered. Successful software approaches are largely in the hands of professionals who are often in positions of power, and have the capacity to set appropriate processes in place, or not.

Both approaches are necessary and interdependent. Positive and supportive software approaches require clearly articulated and strongly enshrined hardware to be successful; 'good hardware without any software is merely potential, but not actual, "empowerment"' (Labonté 1997, p. 49).

Developing networks for inter-sectoral action

Community participation

Participation is a concept that attempts to bring different stakeholders together around problem-posing, problem-solving and decision-making. Participation is difficult to describe because the purposes that bring different interested parties together will be diverse and, in addition, the course and outcomes of the coming together will be just as varied. The process of participation constantly changes. So there can be no predetermined set of steps to guide practitioners. Community participation is best described by the values enshrined in the process. It is defined by the *Macquarie Dictionary* as 'a taking part, as in some action or attempt, with others'. Without participation there can be no partnerships.

It is important to recognise that merely because various stakeholders come together around an issue does not mean that true participation is achieved (Labonté 1997, Ch. 4). Labonte (1997, p. 45) argues that true partnership is the most desirable outcome, because it is neither desirable nor possible to achieve citizen control; it is the ability of community groups involved in partnerships to negotiate their own terms of relationship with agencies and achieve mutually satisfactory outcomes.

Community participation benefits

For the individual
- Self-esteem, new skills.
- It is empowering — it gives people a sense of power over the forces that determine their own lives.
- 'Connectedness' is positively related to health in both morbidity and mortality data.

For the community
- More educated public, more cohesive community.

- Identification and mobilisation of untapped resources of community members, use of citizens' knowledge.
- Improved planning and decision-making by the proponents.

For the health-promotion program
- More relevant program action, better programs.
- Improved service delivery, greater public acceptance.
- Increased accountability.

For healthy public policy
- Gaining professional entry into social justice issues.
- Demonstration of government commitment.

Community participation limitations

Local decision-making is actually limited in scope. The decisions that people have made may be strictly limited to the local context, whereas policies and financial decisions are usually made at higher levels. This may mean that they are not aligned, and local initiatives are deprived of funds because they fail to demonstrate relevance to, for example, nationally funded priorities. Local agencies' decisions are always constrained by the amount and criteria set on funding and the policies that apply to everyone.

A second difficulty affecting local community participation initiatives is that the programs and strategies that are developed in one setting are not able to be generalised to other settings, meaning inefficiency in re-planning. A third limitation is that activities that are locally driven may still be 'captured' by powerful interest groups. The activities may continue to support the existing power inequalities and not have power to intervene in wider social decisions.

Health workers need to be cautious in accepting the rhetoric about the benefits of community capacity building and community participation. Strategies to encourage local decision-making are being introduced at the same time as social service cutbacks in line with the neo-liberal philosophy discussed earlier. If communities take responsibility for community development approaches, but are not supported with adequate infrastructure provision, they are setting themselves up for failure. And in this scenario, it is the community that can be blamed for failures in health improvement, rather than the weaknesses of the social welfare philosophy of the government (see Rose 1996 for a wider discussion of this point).

Moving from participation to partnerships

The process of establishing and maintaining effective partnerships is as important as the outcome. In the partnerships approach there is recognition that community members have a great deal of expertise regarding their own lives. Community members are directly involved in decision-making and implementation and there is negotiation and agreement between community members and service agencies. Achieving partnerships begins with considerations of two important concepts that have already been discussed in this text: power and participation. Community participation involves *sharing* power, rather than achieving power *over*.

Partnership is not a matter of replacing one authority for another; for instance, by the health care agency making decisions on behalf of a disempowered community. Power is often vested in those who are seen to have the 'expert' knowledge, such as health workers. Their position of authority may have to be gradually diminished. It is often a new and complex role for the health professional to relinquish control to community members.

Working to overcome powerlessness is the essential first step in mobilising community action to make structural social, political and economic change. It brings immediate benefits to the individual because they gain a sense of control, hope and purpose (Syme 1998). The partnerships and collaborative approaches outlined below are together aimed at addressing the social determinants through social change.

Inter-sectoral collaboration

Reorienting the health system to focus on health determinants demands that sectors collaborate around an issue, rather than acting in a separate 'silo' of action about a singular behaviour. This process is described as 'inter-sectoral collaboration'. Collaboration occurs between sectors which might have some involvement in health care in its widest definition through agencies that have some role to play in addressing the social determinants of health. Collaboration is aimed at reducing the barriers between sectors. It could be seen as a 'top down' approach. Inter-sectoral collaboration can be defined as a:

> recognised relationship between a part or parts of the health sector and part or parts of another sector, that has been formed to take action on an issue to achieve health outcomes in a more efficient, effective or sustainable way.

> (Harris et al 1995)

Collaboration is a process through which parties who have different perspectives about an issue, or who can address different aspects of it, can constructively search for solutions together. The solutions will go beyond one partner's own limited vision of what is possible, and intervene more than their own scope of practice.

The inter-sectoral collaborative approach is now recognised in international, national and local health policies, such as in the Primary Care Partnerships (PCP) strategy in Victoria.

When arguing for the need to 'reorient health services' the Ottawa Charter for Health Promotion outlines the responsibility for health promotion that 'is shared among individuals, community groups, health professionals, health service institutions and governments' (WHO 1986). Sustained health enhancement can be achieved when health strategies across the full range of sectors move their attention 'upstream' to the determinants of health.

This approach is the basis of the settings approach to health promotion and illness prevention, where sectors that have a role in settings such as schools, workplaces, health care facilities, and cultural and recreational venues, come together to work on a health issue of concern. The approach aims to draw on what works best in each setting and use the skills and strengths of the collaborating agencies to achieve a broad approach.

Collaborations may be between:

- organisations from areas of interest, such as education, childcare or agriculture;
- large organisational structures such as local, state or national government;
- community-based structures such as neighbourhood centres, service clubs and other non-government agencies.

Collaborative action can take many forms; for example:

- health promotion;
- community development;
- advocacy; or
- service delivery models, such as shared management.

Collaborative action can use a wide range of strategies, such as:

- an agreement between managers;
- a joint approach to a common problem;
- collaboration of workers in a specific case; or
- a change in legislation — for example, Municipal Health Plans.

Guidelines for putting inter-sectoral collaboration into practice.

1. The collaboration has a purpose. The collaboration may arise out of a formal or informal needs-assessment process. The key issue to be addressed (the prioritised need) becomes the purpose for bringing stakeholders together. Some of the agencies or groups represented may already be working on the issue.

2. All relevant stakeholders are involved. Thinking broadly considers all those who may have a role to play in the approach to the issue. In the early stages of development a 'reference group' could be formed, representing some of the groups. This group could then identify strategic approaches, and the relevant sectors to be approached. As the action evolves, different sectors may need to be co-opted.

3. Stakeholders' interests and concerns are considered. By its collaborative nature, the processes action will need to be described in detail to make sure that no stakeholder is later confused about expectations.

4. Each sector or organisation outlines its level of support for a proposed action. Small and large organisations will be able to commit different levels of contribution, financial, staff or in-kind. In the same way different agencies will be inclined to commit different support according to how closely the issue aligns with the core business or strategic plan of the agency.

5. Effective action must engage all major stakeholders. Invite stakeholders because they consider they have a role to play, not because they 'should' be invited. Make sure each has a role that is congruent with their core business. Even when they refuse to participate, their views should be considered. It may mean that they are more willing to participate at a later date.

6. Organisations need to recognise their interdependence in achieving a common end.

(Primary Care Partnerships 2004)

Inter-sectoral action is effective for a number of reasons. Firstly, it enables broad multi-focused approaches to addressing the determinants of health that would not be possible by smaller agencies acting alone. The factors that affect health are beyond the control of only the health sector. For instance, there are a number of approaches to reducing road accident deaths, including car design, public transport approaches, road design, school education, driver training, pedestrian awareness, safe use of alcohol and others.

Secondly, the availability of support services is not the business of any one sector. If we consider the needs of disabled older people living in the community, many sectors collaborate in order to support their health needs. For instance, allied health professionals, district nursing, public transport services, local government, home help and mobility support, federal and state legislation may provide pension and pharmacy assistance and local service clubs may collaborate to provide specifically local needs, such as provision of firewood.

Thirdly, if inter-sectoral collaboration allows those most affected to take part in decision-making and action about an issue then the information used and strategies developed are acceptable to the group (for example HIV strategies).

Fourthly, it promotes efficient use of resources. Collaboration makes best use of resources without duplication. Specialists are able to do what they do best, and this results in improved quality, and greater continuity of activity. Scarce resources are efficiently allocated, based on mutually agreed need. The process ensures partners must negotiate with other service providers in the settings.

The fifth reason is that inter-sectoral collaboration is effective because the process multiplies the impact because of its breadth of interventions. In turn this extends the capacity to influence policies elsewhere and increases the likelihood that the partnership is able to demonstrate a sustained improvement in the health determinant.

Finally, inter-sectoral collaboration is effective because it gives credibility and legitimacy to the issues and those involved in the process because, as suggested above, it encourages long-term commitment to an issue.

Agencies will not commit to a process unless they believe there is a chance of success and they have a part to play in it. The process allows a network of relationships between individuals and organisations to be developed, that are reinforced over time. It is not dependent on having the expert from outside to keep the action going; the activity is owned by the community and stakeholders work with the community to achieve a common goal. Even when community members or collaborative partners do not necessarily agree with the community decision that was made, they are more likely to abide by the decision if they were a part of the process and a range of sectors are involved in the activity. During the process partners will develop new skills and capabilities and these will enhance their commitment to the outcome, as well as being transferable to other settings.

Conclusion

The World Health Organization encourages the building of healthy public policy because it creates supportive environments. This in turn, provides people with an opportunity to live a healthy life. Policies for health are developed at the global, national and local level.

This chapter has reviewed some of the ways in which we can work for healthier communities. It is in this area more than in any other area of health promotion that change and development are occurring, as health workers develop more innovative ways to work with communities. It is in working with communities that we are working to change the environment rather than the individual. This is done by lobbying, advocacy and working in partnership with communities to develop healthy public policy. These policies include regulatory activities, such as laws, position statements, regulations and informal rules.

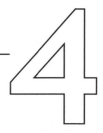

Community action for social and environmental change

In Chapter 1 you were introduced to the continuum of health-promotion approaches. In this chapter we will move along the continuum from 'healthy public policy' to 'community action for social and environmental change' and we examine the potential of community development as a way of working with communities, on issues they identify with, to achieve changes to the environment and enable community empowerment.

In community-level work, the environment, rather than the individual, is defined as the target for change (Labonté 1986, p. 347). Work at this level has the potential to address some of the structural issues, specifically at the local level, that lead to poor health. In addressing those issues, 'community action for social and environmental change' is obviously political since it means working for change to create social justice. While any form of health work can be political in nature, by using a community development approach the political nature of the health worker's action is usually more explicit.

Working at the level of the community, and community development in particular, has become popular in the health field since the Declaration of Alma-Ata highlighted community development and community participation as important strategies for health promotion. Before that, many health workers were unfamiliar with the concept of community development, although it had been used in other fields and by health workers in majority countries for some time.

An essential component of the Primary Health Care approach to health promotion is the recognition that it is necessary to change the structures that influence people's lives in order to improve their health. There is also recognition that the people who are affected most, need to be integral to that process. A key challenge in health-promotion work is to put these ideas into practice by encouraging and supporting community-led and community-controlled activities, rather than only those activities that are led and controlled by health workers or the health system.

Community involvement in change

The philosophical belief that underpins community development work centres on people's entitlement to have control over issues that affect their lives, and the worker's role is to support these rights, on the basis of equity and social justice principles.

Defining community development

Community development aims to increase people's participation in the life of their community and the interdependence of community members. It has been defined as a process of 'working with people as they define their own goals, mobilise resources, and develop action plans for addressing problems they collectively have identified' (Minkler 1991, p. 261).

While Minkler's definition (1991) refers to community organisation, it actually describes community development. The terms 'community development' and 'community organisation' are both defined variously, and often overlap in their definition. Rothman and Tropman (1987) describe community development as one form of community organisation. Egger et al (1999, p. 87) have described the difference between the two terms as one of 'directiveness', because they regard community organisation as being a process more directed by workers, while community development is more directed by members of the community.

At this point it is valuable to review the definitions of 'community' outlined in Chapter 2. We noted that community can mean a variety of things. In community development, emphasis is placed on community as a social system, bounded by geographical location or common interest, recognising that community is 'a "living" organism with interactive webs of ties among organisations, neighbourhoods, families, and friends' (Eng et al 1992, p. 1). It could also be said to be 'people who live within a geographically defined area and who have social and psychological ties with each other and with the place where they live' (Mattessich & Monsey 1997). We also noted in Chapter 2 that communities often include groups with conflicting interests, and that this fact is often hidden behind the romantic connotations of the term 'community'.

The notion of a 'sense of community' was also discussed. This is an ideal state in which everyone affected by the life of the community participates in community life. The community as a whole takes responsibility for its members and respect for the individuality of the members is maintained (Daly & Cobb 1989, p. 172). It is described by Clark (1973, p. 409) as a 'sense of solidarity and a sense of significance'. This sense of community can be an important component of people feeling as though they belong to a community, and it also has implications for the process of community development. However, two points are worth making here. Firstly, we need to take care not to oversimplify the consequences of human beings living in communities. Secondly, we must be careful not to assume that this sense of community is an ideal state for everyone, because some people may not choose living in a community as their ideal. As we have said, there are romantic descriptions of community life. These issues are of particular importance in considering community development, as these aspects of community may really come to the fore in the community development process. Indeed, workers using the community development process may have to regularly consider the implications of these issues in their work. Box 4.1, however, provides some ideals to work toward.

Box 4.1 Some principles of community
• A community is a group of people who share equal responsibility for and commitment to maintaining its spirit.
• A community is a highly effective working group.
• A community is the ideal consensual decision-making body.
• In community, a wide range of gifts and talents is celebrated.
• Community is inclusive.
• Individual differences are celebrated.
• Community facilitates healing.
• Community is reflective, contemplative and introspective.

(Source: Johnson, K. in Hoff, M. D. 1998 *Sustainable community development: studies in economic, environmental, and cultural revitalization.* Lewis Publishers, Boca Raton, Fla, pp. 175–6)

Community development is the process by which health workers are most able to work *with* communities. The aim in community development is for communities to be in control of decisions that affect them and gain control over the determinants of their health. The task for the health-promotion worker is to involve the community or group in each aspect of the decision-making process, so that the group is then able to take on the task, rather than just being the participants in a program that the workers conduct. The role is complex because it involves stepping back from the actual intervention, and facilitating community members' access to the conditions and resources that will enable them to exercise control and set their own directions. When health-promotion workers work in this way, their work is defined as community development.

Community development can be used in ways that manipulate people, through co-opting them to take a predetermined action, or in ways that do not encourage true community control. However, this thoughtless or manipulative use of power is likely to create distrust among community members.

A continuum of community development activities

Community development is not one form of health promotion, or one style of activity. The tasks involved in community development can be diverse, depending on the existing strengths, vulnerabilities and desires of the community of interest. What is consistent, and is set out in the definition of community development provided above, is the way of working; community development is a 'bottom-up' approach, that always involves working with a community, as they 'steer' the activity in their community. The worker must choose the way of working that best suits the needs and realities of the community they are working with. The range of community development approaches could also be expressed as a continuum, depending on community need at the time. The range of parallel skills a worker may use might extend from social action to one-to-one case work. These various community development 'tools' will be presented in more detail in this chapter.

At this point, it will be valuable to examine some key principles of community development. Together, these help construct a picture of what community development practice is about. Perhaps the two most important principles are:

1. the community's identification of its own needs; and

2. the importance of the process as well as the outcome of the participation by community members in the community development process.

Other important concepts are empowerment, creating critical consciousness, the development of community competence, and the careful selection of issues to be dealt with (Minkler 1991, pp. 267–74).

Community developers are particularly concerned with the needs of those who have little power. It is these people who are most likely to be suffering ill health as a result of their lack of access to, and influence over, the structures that are impacting negatively on their health. If people are not skilled in articulating their needs, or do not believe they are likely to have them met, then they are not likely to express them. Finding out what they believe they need may be a slow (but important) part of the community development process.

Unless we start from where people are at, we are unlikely to succeed, as people will not be committed to act on issues they do not see as relevant to them. Therefore, community members must identify with the needs being addressed if they are to involve themselves in working for change. However, communities may act on locally identified needs without knowledge of the 'big picture'. Acting on the combined knowledge of the community and experts is most likely to be successful. For example, if a community is working for increased public housing in its area, evidence of a low rate of public housing or a high rate of people on low incomes (expert knowledge) will provide valuable support for increased housing, and will be a stronger argument than if residents' demand for more housing was the only rationale.

Community development — process and outcome

In Chapters 2 and 3, we discussed a range of approaches to participation. In examining the importance of participation by community members in community development, it is apparent that approaches to participation that are appropriate in Primary Health Care are generally also the approaches to participation necessary in community development. In other words, for the process of participation to be empowering, it must be one of true participation in which decision-making power is shared by community members. Control over decision-making by community members is encouraged and supported by health workers with a community development philosophy. Participation that fits into the upper rungs of Arnstein's Ladder of Citizen Participation, discussed in Chapter 2, in which power is shared between workers and community members, or even completely handed over to community members, is a fundamental part of community development.

As mentioned above, the process of participation in change is often considered to be just as important as the outcome. This is particularly so in community development. By participating in community development, people gain skills in such things as negotiation, submission writing, organisation, working with the mass media and working as part of a group. These skills, the networks people establish with others in the community, and their sense of being able to negotiate the system and achieve something, are regarded as valuable, and sometimes as more valuable, than any outcome of the group's activity.

Although the process elements of community development are extremely important, giving more importance to them than to the outcome elements has some limitations. There is a real danger of this being paternalistic towards community members, for it effectively says that, even though they worked long and hard and lost, it was good for them. Community members themselves may not define this as success, but rather may be quite horrified by the suggestion (although they may acknowledge that they learnt from the process). Certainly the process of involvement may be very important for community members, but they may regard it as such only if they are successful in achieving what they set out to achieve.

The particular process and outcome (or objective) elements of community development have been described by Butler and Cass (1993, p. 10) and are outlined in the text that follows.

Process elements

- **Control of decision-making** — community members participate to control the project and particularly to control the identification and definition of the issue.
- **Development of community competence** — the project enables the community to recognise and address its problems.
- **Involvement in action** — the project involves the people concerned with the issue in action for change.
- **Development of community culture** — the project contributes to a culture of groups of individuals taking responsibility for improving and protecting their area and services.
- **Learning** — the participants are acquiring new skills, information and/or new perspectives on themselves, their community and their concerns.
- **Organisational development** — the project builds a new organisation or improves an existing one.

Process elements will be discussed in more detail later in this chapter.

Principles underpinning community development processes

The *process* elements of community development refer to the ways of working with communities. Two important concepts presented earlier in the text provide theoretical guidance for health workers' actions with their communities. These key concepts are:

1. Social justice
2. Empowerment

The challenge for health workers is to incorporate these concepts into each of their activities. Principles of social justice and empowerment need to become the personal philosophy of health workers; the lens through which the quality of their activities is judged.

Principles underpinning community development outcomes

Butler and Cass (1993) set outcome or objective elements of the community development process. These observable elements relate to the benefits that a community might see as a result of their taking part in the community activities. These are discussed below.

Objective elements

- **New power relationships** — the project changes the social landscape of the community so that new and more equitable power relations are formed (this is also a process aspect).
- **Concrete benefit** — the project sees the achievement of some new or improved service or facility, or the protection of something valued by the community.

It is clear that the objective or outcome elements relate to qualitative and quantitative differences that come about as a result of the activity or project. These are the lasting effects, not what happens along the way.

The *qualitative outcome elements* relate to the less tangible benefits for individuals and communities being actively involved in each aspect of an activity or project. As the framework from Butler and Cass (1993) indicates, being actively involved in community activities and actions will bring about changes in personal skills and competencies, which will in turn influence the capacity of a community or group to advocate for themselves. Power relationships will change within the community, and in the relationships between a community and wider society. For instance, there may be denser and stronger networks of association in the community creating the potential for future health-enhancing activities. These processes could be seen as *creating social capital*.

The *quantitative outcome* of community development is the tangible and lasting change that occurs as a result of the efforts the community put into an activity or project. The key concept that sums up the observable outcomes of community development activities is *sustainability*.

The process and objective (outcome) elements of community development provide workers with the 'toolkit' of activities for working with their communities. These elements will be expanded in more detail in the following two sections.

Goals of community development

Community development builds people's skills for current issues and for the future. In the process it enhances their feelings of competence and personal self-esteem. It means their community is competent to adapt to future changes and that legislators will be more likely to consider their perspective in the future, and more accountable for their actions in the future.

Successful community-based movements of radical activists and local concerned citizens have ensured legal rights and brought about changes in legislation. Outcomes might range from a change in the decision to dam a pristine river and lake, to local government by-laws relating to the disposal of mine tailings.

> Through community development people learn that their problems have social causes and that fighting back is a more reasonable, dignified approach than passive acceptance and personal alienation . . . Community organizing is a search for social power and an effort to combat perceived helplessness through learning that what appears personal is often political.
>
> (Rubin & Rubin 1992, p. iii)

The concept of community development is complex, perhaps because the skills and activities that are required vary with the situation, and also because the outcome will be defined by the community and known only after the activity has commenced. It is difficult to bring ideal global visions of capable communities deciding their own courses of action down to practical, day-to-day achievable goals. However, it is important to have visions broader than meeting local objectives if real empowerment of the community is to be achieved and sustained.

The following themes offered by Rubin and Rubin provide a very useful framework for working with communities at goal-setting.

1. *Improvement of the quality of life through the resolution of shared problems.* This may sound far too grand for a small community activity, but it may be as seemingly simple as having a local by-law changed that tip-trucks are prevented from carrying their uncovered loads of dusty mine tailings contaminated with arsenic, through residential areas. The potential for health enhancement by this action is clear.

2. *Reduction in the level of social inequities caused by the social determinants of illness such as poverty.* Actions may entail provision of transport for local people to attend community health activities, but in order to make sustained change for a community, provision of access to services needs to be enshrined in the operational plans of service providers, rather than being provided on an ad hoc basis.

3. *Exercise and enhance democratic principles, through peoples' shared roles in decisions that affect them in their communities.* Maintaining democratic principles, when it is easier and quicker to get on and do it oneself, is one of the biggest challenges to community workers. The processes and skills outlined in the next sections provide more specific guidance for this goal.

4. *Enabling people to achieve their potential as individuals.* The involvement in community activity brings its own personal and non-tangible rewards, as well as the development of new knowledge and skills. At the outset of a program,

these gains need to be acknowledged and documented in the objectives of the activity or project.

5. *Creation of a sense of community*. A strong cohesive and successful organisation or community will be powerful in creating the sense of belonging and ownership for its members. It is a means for people to achieve their vision.

(Rubin & Rubin 1992, pp. 10–16)

Community development process elements

A number of other sections presented so far have emphasised how important it is for the health of individuals and communities to be able to make decisions about issues that affect their lives, property, environment and community. The process elements of community development work, introduced in the previous section, are now presented in more detail to provide guidance for action.

Control of decision-making

Alinsky (1972, p. 105), has provided theoretical and personal leadership in community development strategies from his remarkable work with residents in ghettos in American industrial cities such as Chicago. In *Rules for Radicals* Alinsky argues one of the challenges in working with disempowered communities is that 'if people feel they don't have the power to change a bad situation, then they do not think about it'. Key theoretical approaches that enhance opportunities for community control include using social justice principles to underpin all activities, encouraging community participation using 'hardware' and 'software' approaches (Labonté 1997), and forming equitable partnerships with communities to enable their individual and collective empowerment. If a community learns to better solve its own problems, then it is being empowered and becoming a more competent community. Community control of decision-making allows a community to illustrate that it is the expert in its own affairs; that people 'on the ground' know best what they need and how this should be achieved.

> It is local community members who have this knowledge, wisdom and expertise, and the role of the community worker is to listen and learn from the community, not to tell the community about its problems and its needs.

(Holland & Blackburn 1998 cited in Ife 2002, p. 102)

This is a significant challenge to planners, policy-makers, health workers and the community members, because it challenges the traditions of outside 'experts' making decisions on behalf of communities (Ife 2002, p. 101).

Community control of decision-making occurs on two fronts:

1. decision-making within the affected community, to ensure that decisions reflect the aspirations of the whole community; and

2. decision-making between the community and relevant agencies of authority, to make sure the issue comes onto the authority's agenda for discussion, and that the community voice is heard.

Communities can be in control of decision-making when they are assisted to identify the issues and structures that prevent them from meeting their needs. After a community identifies its strengths and vulnerabilities it must then decide what actions and changes it can make to become healthier. The emphasis here is on community identification, rather than expert 'diagnosis'. The process of needs identification and solution generation in communities is called a 'needs assessment'. The process is set out in detail in the next chapter. For a community worker to be effective in facilitating community control of decision-making, she/he must get to know the community members, listen to, 'hear' and learn from the local people, and validate with community members that the information provided is correctly interpreted. Effective communication between community and decision-makers demands honesty, clarity and responsiveness by those running the participation process. A number of factors may get in the way of community members being 'heard', such as a professional being unable or unwilling to set aside their 'specialist' knowledge of how things should be, or the kinds of information provided by a community may not fit within the expected paradigms of what constitutes 'evidence' of need. An issue that has been a particular barrier to Aboriginal and other minority community groups in Australia taking control of decisions that affect their communities has been that local knowledge and local solutions derive from different forms of 'knowledge', or ways of understanding the world. Another barrier to communities being heard is their inability to influence the wider public agenda, to influence social values and policy or legal decisions. It takes a great deal of effort to raise an issue in public profile sufficient to move it from a local concern onto the public agenda. Many of the strategies of advocacy set out in the previous chapter are relevant to increasing community control of decision-making.

Development of community competence

The concept of community competence is very much linked to community empowerment (Minkler 1991, p. 268). A competent community is one that is able to recognise and address its problems. People and communities can feel powerless because their problems are complex and solutions often require knowledge and skills that they lack. Some feel powerless because they are left to deal with problems that they did not cause, such as unemployment or environmental degradation. They have been socialised to believe that authorities act in the best interests of the population and there is little they can do to challenge the decisions of authority. In some cases, a lack of action is also motivated by the fear that voicing or acting on concerns will worsen the risk or will have negative implications.

Hawe et al (1990, p. 114) suggest that an increase in a community's competence can be examined by considering 'changes in the community itself, its networks, its structures, the way in which people perceive the community, ownership of community issues, [and] perceived and actual "empowerment" in health and social issues'. Being aware of the existing community resources is the first part of that process. Community resources can be knowledge and skills of community members, tangible things such as buildings and spaces, or they can include non-tangible resources; for example, aesthetics, or positive values such as trust and reciprocity; that is, the 'glue' of social capital (Putnam 1993). It is important for the community health workers to gain an understanding of these resources and existing social processes, such as communication patterns, social commercial and economic networks, key informants and decision-making traditions, so the way they work in the community do not exclude some people from participation, or in another way act as a barrier which discourages people from getting involved.

Involvement in action

If we want and expect community members to be active in local decision-making they need to believe that the action is worthwhile, and likely to bring about change. Several writers suggest that the choice of issues used in community development is important. Minkler (1991, p. 272) suggests that if an issue is to be a good one for community development, the community must feel strongly about it, and it must be 'winnable, simple and specific'. She argues that this is particularly the case early in the community development process. Once people have started to develop a sense of their ability to effect change, they may be less easily swamped by resistance from others, or by lack of success on a particular issue. In the early stages, however, failure or resistance may lead the group to give up, so starting with winnable issues while people develop some skills can be productive. Other more difficult issues can then be tackled, with people building on the skills that they have already developed through these experiences.

The main aim of getting community members involved in the action is that they will become self-reliant in managing the issue in their community, or in solving the problem; that their processes and outcomes are sustainable. 'Change comes from power, and power comes from organisation. In order to act people must get together' (Alinsky, 1972, p. 113). At the start of a community development activity or project it is usual for external funding and/or an outside 'expert' facilitator to get the project or activity started. The project must develop in such a way that when these resources are reduced to a bare minimum, or are removed altogether, that the activity continues in a form that the community is satisfied with. The value of community involvement is that the project develops in a form that uniquely matches the local resources and setting.

Development of community culture

Development of a community culture gives collective recognition of an issue that a number of individuals may have believed affected only themselves. It allows them to move towards action for change (Ife 2002, p. 126). There is recognition that communities acting together are far more effective in bringing about desired and sustained change when they act in unity, rather than pulling in different directions.

An essential element in building a culture of strength and unity in the community (or building on it if it already exists), is establishing mutually respectful dialogue between all parties involved in any activity or project. This relates particularly to agencies and personnel in authority, who are in positions of power because of their authority, and for this reason, they are at particular risk of perpetuating feelings of powerlessness or incompetence. Effective communication with a community demands honesty, clarity and responsiveness. Refer again to the discussion of community participation 'software' (Labonté 1997) presented in the previous chapter.

Community development work, especially in the early stages, frequently involves 'consciousness raising', where the community members are assisted to recognise that existing values, structures and ways of viewing the world, are keeping them feeling oppressed, perhaps believing there is little they can do to improve their situation. Feelings of powerlessness, felt, for instance, by many unemployed people, can be reinforced by social structures such as all forms of media, the health and education systems, and religious institutions. Such seemingly simple issues, as the use of jargon, or wearing certain clothing, or terms of communication or greeting, can be oppressive and exclusionary.

Consciousness raising involves 'sharing experiences to learn that what appears personal is really political' (Rubin & Rubin 1992, p. 7). Communities can gain collective strength by learning from the development journeys and the wisdom of experience of other communities in similar situations. A groundswell of opinion or reaction to an issue can create a culture of unity in the need for action. The collective culture can make the issue public and political. It enables members to portray and publicise their life experiences in the context of existing inequitable policy frameworks, or give wider recognition to an issue; it can be a means of advocating for policy change.

Development of a community culture happens gradually from within the community, but community development workers can be powerful catalysts in enhancing the culture when they link or re-frame personal experiences of individuals with the wider political dimensions.

When one issue is resolved successfully, the empowered community will have no difficulty in finding another problem (Alinsky 1972).

In short, there are not specific activities involved in creating a community culture but it involves ways of working with communities 'that seeks any opportunity to engage in dialogue and to explore paths toward collective understanding, shared experience and action' (Ife 2002, p. 126). The core public health values that we have presented earlier, including equity and social justice and human rights, can provide tools for community development workers to illustrate where injustices are occurring. In this way an issue can be framed as structurally inequitable, rather than being viewed as a personal complaint.

Learning

Community members who become engaged in the processes and decisions that concern them need to be open to the learning and dynamic changes that this entails. Communities of all descriptions constantly change and evolve, and as they become empowered to act on their own behalf, the process of change demands new skills and creates new opportunities for learning. Whilst people learn as individuals, their additional knowledge is added to the community 'toolkit' of resources, to be used on other occasions in different settings. People may learn to work with media agencies, for instance to write a press release, or they may learn to read budgets and financial statements or a piece of legislation. People learn in a great deal of ways when they decide to challenge legal authority formally in the courts, or informally when they use disruptions as a means of gaining attention for their issue. People may feel they don't have the professional skills of many in formal organisations, however, the sheer weight of numbers with enthusiasm and determination can be sufficient to raise the profile of an issue across the social spectrum, and to bring about acceptance for their agenda.

Organisational development

The key process in community development, reflected in the definition presented earlier, is that citizens increase their abilities to control decisions that affect their community. Whatever the reason that has brought community members together, and no matter how disempowered they have felt, the challenge is to enable their progress along the continuum towards greater community control. The wisdom and experiences of local people is the starting point on which all other processes are built. Ife (2002, p. 109) has a salutary message for those workers who want to impart their own expertise, or speed the community processes along:

> Barging in as the person with the expertise, intent on 'intervening' and bringing about change from a position of 'superior' knowledge and skills, is to guarantee failure, and will simply perpetuate structures and discourses of disadvantage and disempowerment.

For a start, the community development worker must earn the trust and support of the community, who are likely to be distrustful, on the basis of their prior experiences with 'professionals'. To be an advocate for a disempowered community may mean the worker is seen as the enemy of the mainstream (Alinsky 1972). It can be a solitary, isolated role initially, until there is wider acceptance from the community.

It is also easy when working with communities for the 'outside expert' community development worker to transfer control over community decisions, and therefore to transfer power to the 'elites' within the community. These people may be the most vocal, articulate, active or politically or economically powerful community members. Processes that enshrine shared and collaborative and consultative processes in the routine activities of the community are needed from the beginning. Constant attention to democratic and participatory principles is required. The community development worker models these processes in the way she or he works with the community. The community needs to make early decisions about how information is to be collated, distributed and acted on so that all members can be informed and be as active as they wish to be.

The community development worker, therefore, is not independent of the community, but joins the community team, and the skills that they bring become part of the 'toolkit' of skills the community can call upon when needed. The specific roles of the worker are addressed in more detail later in the chapter.

Development and strengthening within the organisation, group or community happens gradually and incrementally. As people become aware that they share problems and can bring about collective solutions, strength will be gained to tackle other issues, and additional individuals will join. The more that people take part, the greater their future capacity to solve community problems through political action. As Rubin and Rubin have said, 'Participation in community organisations helps make people more politically sensitive and more effective political actors' (1992, p. 9).

Community development workers may consider applying the following DARE criteria (Rubin & Rubin 1992, p. 77) as a means of ensuring that decision-making continues to reflect the needs and concerns of the communities they work with. These criteria are:

Who **D**etermines the goal?

Who **A**cts to achieve the goal?

Who **R**eceives the benefits from the actions?

Who **E**valuates the actions?

The process indicators presented here are more likely to be successful and to be sustained when communities work in partnership or collaboration with government and non-government agencies which have similar philosophies or areas of interest, or are sympathetic to their cause. Working to achieve these criteria does not mean that another agency loses power, or that there needs to be a power struggle. The criteria provides a basis for negotiation and shared decision-making to reach mutually satisfactory outcomes. Box 4.2 provides another schema to assess process indicators for effective participation. Consider these with Arnstein's ladder (presented in Chapter 2), and the DARE criteria presented above.

Box 4.2 Principles of effective community participation

Transparency
All aspects of the process must be clearly stated and easily accessible.

Inclusiveness
Everyone must be given that opportunity and assistance to participate.

Information
Information must be timely and presented in a way that is easily understood. Access to further information must be facilitated.

Communication
Effective communication demands sensitivity, honesty and reciprocity.

Respect
Mutual respect for the multiple perspectives that are inevitable is essential.

Evaluation
The nature, extent and success of the participation processes must be known to improve the processes following.

(Source: derived from the State Government of Victoria Department of Human Services 2003. *Health Promotion Short Course Facilitators Guide. Module 1.* Victorian Government, Melbourne)

Objective elements

While the goals of developing and strengthening an organisation, group or community are admirable, people tend to come together and give their energy voluntarily when they are trying to achieve a specific outcome or change. The following objective elements provide the reasons for coming together and provide people with the satisfaction and energy to tackle a new issue concerning their community.

Concrete benefit

The key factor that makes all the processes of community development desirable and worthwhile is the burning issue that brings the community together in the first place. As set out in the earlier section, headed 'involvement in action', careful selection of the issues used in community development is important, and Minkler (1991, p. 272) suggests the criteria should be 'winnable, simple and specific' to ensure participants develop skills, are productive and have some early success. However, the issue must be chosen by the community and it will attract the most community engagement if it is an issue that many people are impassioned about. In practice, the idea of starting with winnable issues may not be possible, as it may well be a difficult, even almost un-winnable, issue that brings a community to the point of wanting to act. In that case, the idea of starting with winnable issues goes out the door. This is more likely to be so where the community development process begins spontaneously, as a result of people responding to an issue crucial to their lives, where change will bring a concrete benefit.

New power relationships

Sustainable changes in communities will arise when members have acquired new skills and recognised their existing talents during the process. Being involved in a project changes the social landscape of the community so that new and more equitable power relations are formed. People reflect on and acknowledge the value of the process elements. For instance, through the processes of community development former adversaries may now be able to work together, and relationships with government agencies may be less confrontational than they were previously (Johnson in Hoff 1998, Ch 9).

The role of the health worker in community development

Insight 4.1 The role of the health worker in community development
Go to the people Live among them Love them Start with what they know Build on what they have But of the best leaders When their task is accomplished Their work is done The people all remark We have done it ourselves

(Source: Chabot 1976 in Ashton 1990, p. 8)

The approach described by the poem in Insight 4.1 is the approach taken by a health worker using a community development approach. However, the community development process may also begin without the assistance of employed health workers. Local people and community leaders are often committed to using that process and may work away quietly in their own areas or groups, attempting to build consensus and initiate collective action to address people's needs.

Health workers have an important role to play in supporting the people involved in community development, whether the community development process began through the efforts of strong local leaders or was instigated by health workers themselves. There are a number of reasons for this. Firstly, it is quite clear that the Ottawa Charter for Health Promotion urges health workers to take up community development strategies if they are to promote the health of the people they are working with. This may mean that their work becomes uncomfortable because it has political implications, but it is not sufficient reason to ignore this way of working. Secondly, health workers are well placed to work for community development because they come into contact with members of marginalised groups as part of their everyday work. Indeed, because of the special relationship that develops between many health workers and members of the community, the context in which they work and the 'crisis' situations in which they often meet the community member, health workers are often already in a position of trust with regard to these community members. In addition, their close involvement with people in crisis situations means that they see quite clearly the health implications of poverty and disempowerment. However, health workers may still need to break free from some community perceptions that they should be dealing directly with ill health through clinical services only. Health workers need to join in the life of the community, making the most of opportunities to listen to the community and develop relationships with community members, if they are to identify opportunities for community development.

Integrated community development work requires health workers to be generalists. It is not appropriate to be confined to some roles more than others. There are some skills that are constantly required, others less so. There are five interdependent roles: *facilitative*, *educational* and *representational* roles, *technical* skills and being a *catalyst* is also a role. You can see once again how well these fit in with the particular roles of advocate, enabler and mediator which the Ottawa Charter for Health Promotion highlighted as important roles for health workers in health-promotion action.

Working in the role of a *catalyst*, the health worker is an instrument of change by assisting others to take action. In the *educational* role, the health worker facilitates learning to increase the capacity of people through enhanced knowledge and problem-solving skills. *Facilitating* the process of turning decisions into actions by providing administrative or technical skills for small groups may also be required of a health worker. The *representational* role in this context is an advocate or champion. A health worker may also be required to be a linking person between individuals, groups, organisations, or between the community and the government. This may mean knowing where to go to link the different areas of expertise, bringing the parties together and being a translator for groups with different 'languages'. *Technical skills* may be required; for example, in research.

Reading textbooks about the process of working in a community may make it appear that the process can be ordered and linear. In fact, working in communities is rarely like that. Ife (2002, pp. 226–8) provides a critique of the 'cookbook approach' to working in communities. This critique is useful for health workers who work in any setting. It is important to recognise while there are many roles that health workers play, each setting is different and so each approach needs to be different. The culture, the resources and the reason for the community's existence needs to be considered. Furthermore, each health worker is different.

The community development continuum

Jackson et al (1989) outlined a community development continuum as a way of conceptualising the various practice modes or 'ways of working' in community development. They emphasise that community development is a 'philosophical belief' which underpins the way a worker engages with the community, whether it be working to support an individual at a time of crisis, or being active in a social movement across a wider community. The philosophical belief is centred on people's entitlement to have control over issues that affect their lives, and the worker's role is to support these rights, on the basis of equity and social justice principles. Jackson et al argue that (1989, p. 67):

> the choice of practice mode should be made in response to the needs and realities of the communities with whom one works, and that techniques from social action and locality development models, and from one-to-one case work, can be adapted to achieve community development goals.

People in times of crisis will have different needs for support than those who feel strong enough to take on policy-makers to bring about social change; therefore the role of the worker will differ accordingly. The continuum in Figure 4.1 gives some guidance to the role most suitable at the time.

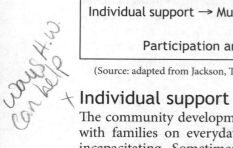

> ### Figure 4.1 The community development continuum
>
> Individual support → Mutual support → Issues identification and campaigns →
>
> Participation and control of services → Social movements

(Source: adapted from Jackson, T., Mitchell, S. and Wright, M. 1989. *Community Health Studies.* 13(1): 66–73)

Individual support

The community development practice mode in crisis situations involves working with families on everyday survival issues, because suffering is paralysing and incapacitating. Sometimes people are not in the position to think any more broadly than their day-to-day survival needs, and it would be unethical not to address these as a first priority. However, community development workers need to nurture people's abilities to make informed decisions rather than fostering their dependence on welfare provision and health worker power.

Mutual support

The role here is to link vulnerable people into existing social networks of support because of the recognition that socially integrated people have greater senses of empowerment and wellbeing. Social isolation of individuals is reduced through group discussion with others in similar situations, formation of self-help activities and facilitation of programs that enhance community integration. The worker supports activities which enable people to 'shift their safety net from dependence in unequal power relationships of worker/client to a more equal base amongst peers' (Jackson et al 1989, p. 69).

Issue identification and campaigns

This is an important part of the community development workers' role because it marks the transition of community members' capacity and strength to take part in community-wide issues that directly affect their lives in order to bring about wider change, rather than as a means for their personal survival. This emphasises the importance of careful selection of issues, discussed earlier. The role of the worker is to have a 'repertoire of strategies' that 'foster confidence that joint action will achieve the desired change' (Jackson et al 1989, p. 70).

Participation and control of services

The key role at this stage on the continuum is one of empowerment of community members. Refer back to earlier discussions of empowerment and participation and to the discussion of Arnstein's Ladder of Citizen Participation which emphasises the importance of true participation in decision-making and control of services, rather than degrees of tokenism. At the beginning people tend to become involved in decision-making at a localised level to ensure that service provision meets their needs in activities such as neighbourhood houses or school councils. Community members are encouraged to view this local participation as a means of getting involved in wider social issues, not as an end in itself.

Social movements

At this point on the continuum the worker is facilitating the activities of social activists who are engaged in far-reaching campaigns. These people now have the strength and capacity to 'see an important part of their lives to be ongoing commitment to social change' (Jackson et al 1989, p. 71).

From this summary of the community development continuum it is apparent that when the worker is working within the practice modes on the left of the continuum the emphasis must be on the process elements presented (described earlier), whereas when working to the right of the continuum, the worker facilitates actions towards the objective elements outlined above.

Everyday tasks

In playing the roles outlined above, there are many practical resources that health workers can provide to effectively resource and support a community if they are to take up their responsibility for community development and health promotion. These can be valuable, whether the community development activity in progress began spontaneously or as a result of worker encouragement. Greater support will be needed if the activity did not begin spontaneously, as it is possible that the community involved is less prepared to act.

Providing resources

Workers can support the community by providing necessary resources in their campaign. These might include access to photocopying and typing facilities and the use of meeting rooms if this is necessary. Negotiating to find accessible, neutral meeting places that are comfortable for group members will be an important component of this process. Assisting with applications for funding for some projects may be necessary also.

Assisting with skills development

Community members may need assistance with developing skills in such things as communicating with the media, writing press releases and writing letters to members of parliament, the public service or local companies involved in a particular issue. Health workers can be active in assisting people to learn how to carry out these tasks effectively in order to get the message across.

Assisting with research

Health workers may have better skills than community members in researching information, and better access to databases holding useful information. They can therefore assist communities in developing their research skills where appropriate and can themselves conduct research through information systems to which members of the public may not have easy access.

Planning action

If health workers have a better knowledge than community members of the bureaucratic process and other useful channels to follow and approaches to take, they can provide valuable information that will help the community group to plan an effective campaign. This can save much worry and uncertainty, as well as a great deal of valuable energy that might have been wasted if the group had acted inappropriately owing to lack of knowledge.

Supporting localism

While not all communities are locality-based, many of them are. Health workers can assist opportunities for community development through actions that support the local community. For example, encouraging the establishment of local credit cooperatives will help keep local money in the local area and will make more money available for financial support of local endeavours (Williams 1986). Local employment initiatives, too, present valuable opportunities to support local economic development (Sindal & Dixon 1990, p. 246).

Supporting community members

Unless support is provided when necessary, community members involved in the process can end up burnt out, unable to continue and feeling disempowered. Community development is hard work and can be exhausting, physically and emotionally, for those involved. Health workers therefore have a key role to play in supporting and encouraging community members involved in community development.

Community development work may also be a tiring process for health workers, and so it is valuable for health workers using this approach to support each other. This can be particularly so when progress seems slow, and when community development is not endorsed enthusiastically by some health decision-makers.

Everyday skills

To perform the required roles and undertake the necessary tasks as discussed above, there are some fundamental skills that health workers need. Communication skills, consensus building, collaboration and conflict management skills are constantly required.

Communication skills

Authentic, effective communication is probably one of the most important skills a health worker can work on to improve their practice. Health workers need to be able to communicate information and viewpoints effectively. To do this they need to be fluent in the language of different groups to translate the various constructs to others who have different languages, perspectives and understandings.

Effective verbal and non-verbal communication requires highly developed interpersonal skills as well as knowledge about communication patterns in and between communities. Being aware of your own perspectives, including prejudices, expectations, ideologies, judgments and the need to control, is the first step. The personal skills required include the ability to:

- ensure that the conversation is one of genuine dialogue and not a game of power and control;
- create and maintain an atmosphere of mutual trust and acceptance;
- be aware of cultural differences and sensitivities in communication;
- listen carefully;
- allow the other to speak before formulating your answer;
- state one's message clearly using language that is readily understood;
- use 'I' statements when speaking;
- keep a conversation focused and directed where necessary;
- understand the value of silence in communication;
- be aware of the other person's time constraints and priorities;
- be aware of the importance of the physical environment;
- encourage the other to reflect on the implications of what is being discussed; and
- be prepared to share vulnerability and brokenness as well as courage (Hoff 1998, p. 175; Ife 2002, p. 240).

Consensus

In some cultures consensus in decision-making is the norm; in others it is not. To reach a consensus, groups need to agree on a course of action that best meets the needs of the whole group. The decision may not be the preferred option of some, but diversity is respected and commitments are made to the action. The process of talking the issues through may take some time and skill and so health workers need skills in listening, empathising, re-framing and communicating (Ife 2002, pp. 235–6).

125

Collaboration

Health workers need to be able to develop cooperative strategies to assist communities to develop shared visions about the future. Some of the strategies include building trust, building teams and building community competence. There can be no community without some level of commitment to cooperation. Health workers may need to seek to challenge the dominance of the competitive ethic which is so entrenched in many cultures (Verrinder et al 2005). Thoughtful networking sets up fruitful collaborations. It is necessary to network with a wide variety of people and groups in and outside one's usual context. Networks need to remain open and to involve people from the grassroots. This prevents the possibility of unofficial network elites forming.

Conflict management

We all need to be able to work toward negotiated resolution of conflict, so it is advisable to explore causes of conflict and forms of conflict resolution. At various times in community work, there may be tension due to unclear expectations, broken agreements, irrational outbursts, conflicting agendas and so on.

Classic conflict resolution techniques include controlled discussion, role reversal, hidden agenda counselling and cooperative problem-solving.

- Controlled discussion — designed to get combatants listening to each other. The health worker mediates an exchange of views. There are two rules: each person makes only one point at a time, and each person restates the point to the other's satisfaction before replying.
- Role reversal — the health worker mediates an exchange of views with each person taking the other person's position.
- Hidden agenda counselling — each person is asked to state what he or she needs from the other by addressing an empty chair: this can uncover a hidden agenda that has nothing to do with the current situation.
- Cooperative problem-solving — the health worker takes people through the diagnosis, treatment and follow-up problem-solving cycle. Each person must state clearly what the problem is, to what degree each is responsible, and if there are any other causes. Possible solutions are identified and an appropriate action plan, including an evaluation of the plan, is agreed on (Heron 1999 in Verrinder et al 2005).

Critical reflection

Critical reflection is acknowledged as an important part of practice. The Marxist tradition uses 'praxis' to describe a cycle of doing, learning and critically reflecting. Through this process we achieve a deeper understanding from which we can inform practice and build theory; this in turn creates further understanding of practice, community and social change. 'Reflective practice includes both reflection-*on*-action and reflection-*in*-action' (Lehmann 2003, p. 83). It is a skill we can learn and in this context, is an empowering experience. Some health workers put time aside to reflect on their practice, others keep a diary or talk things through with colleagues or friends. To contextualise your practice you may find reading widely is helpful. Ife (2002) suggests that community values on particular issues will be reflected in policies, social commentaries and through the media. We can also learn a great deal about society, social change and our own values by reflecting on the work of painters, film-makers, writers and artists of all descriptions (Verrinder et al 2005).

Insights 4.2 and 4.3provide two 'snapshots' of community-based programs that have been successful, but which illustrate differing forms of community development. In Insight 4.3 an inspirational 'community champion' supported individual empowerment, which had a ripple effect through the community. In Insight 4.4, the Torrens Valley project was to provide a supportive environment of structures and agencies which gradually built empowerment of vulnerable youths. These brief stories illustrate that community development can be supported using a range of skills and approaches.

Insight 4.2 Putting people before structures

Healthy Living Centre in Bromley-by-Bow

Bromley-by-Bow is a 'healthy living centre', set up in 1997. The aim is to put 'people before structures' by listening to people's interests and passions, and unearthing their talents and investing in their skill development. This empowers the individual and strengthens the community.

As a young clergyman, Rev Andrew Mawson arrived at the Bromley-by-Bow parish, where church was attended by '12 old people' on Sundays. He did notice that in the parish there were also people from many parts of the world, who among them spoke 50 different languages, and lived in run-down estates. From where the Rev Mawson was sitting in those early days, it looked as though there were many disempowered people.

The idea to rip the interstices of the church out, leaving only the shell, and turn it from a place of worship used once a week by the regular church goers, into a church, a nursery and an art gallery, used every day by many people came from the Reverend, some artists, some nursery workers, and a person running dance classes. Initially, there was a great deal of opposition from public service workers, but one worker was interested and backed the idea.

People share their skills in this place to a point where they now run several nurseries, have an artist cluster that produced a 200-piece art exhibition, and church is still conducted on Sundays. The Rev Mawson describes the action at Bromley-by-Bow as social entrepreneurship and suggests that people really 'learn by doing'. He suggests that this approach fosters a 'social democracy that empowers individuals to act rather than representative committees to talk' (p. 21).

Social entrepreneurship is the way that the volunteer sector can provide public services. Those services are developed by becoming interested in the passions of individuals. In Bromley-by-Bow there are now 125 choices in health and education services and the so-called disempowered have many skills that they are now sharing. The Rev Mawson firmly believes that 'you become a citizen not by what you talk about but what you practically do in the community'.

(Source: Mawson, A. 2004 *Putting People Before Structures*. VicHealth Letter, Special Issue, Issue No. 22, Summer, pp. 20–1)

Insight 4.3 Community partnership

Torrens Valley Youth Program

This is the story of a partnership that developed between the Torrens Valley Community Centre, Lutheran Community Care and the community, to develop a youth program in a group of isolated towns in South Australia. 'The Torrens Valley Youth Program aimed to promote the spirit and vision of young people and address priorities by working in partnership with 8 to 18 year olds in the Torrens Valley' (Packer, Spence & Beare 2002, p. 319). This program addressed issues facing many young people in small rural towns in Australia; namely: geographical isolation; loss of population to the city; decline in employment opportunities; a reduction of many services, including youth services and activities; and lack of anonymity.

> The financial and social capital sustainability of the program is attributed to project management based on community development principles and positive peace processes. The partnership approach, values empowerment and inclusion of all young people, and builds the capacity of rural communities to find local solutions to local needs.

(Packer et al 2002, p. 319)

Objectives were developed in consultation with local young people. These objectives were developed despite the temptation to shift the focus to specific funding opportunities such as drug and alcohol, mental health or suicide. They included:

- to promote a positive image and respect for young people;
- to provide opportunities for young people to have a voice and participate in their community;
- to increase recreational opportunities for young people;
- to increase community involvement and support for young people;
- to advocate on behalf of young people for equitable access to youth information, resources and services;
- to facilitate sustainability of the project through life-skills development by young people, and funding support from the community sponsorship and grant bodies.

A considerable amount of goodwill and a Partnership Agreement assisted the partners to overcome issues of power, and facilitated the building of trusting relationships where concerns could be voiced, listened to respectfully and responded to collectively. This in turn ensured that the objectives were able to be met.

(Source: Packer, J., Spence, R. and Beare, E. 2002 Building community partnerships: an Australian case study of sustainable community-based rural programmes. *Community Development Journal*. 37(4): 316–26

Theories of change in communities

At the beginning of the chapter we talked about how the terms community development and community organisation are defined. These are two of three theories that are commonly discussed in health promotion: identifying key approaches by organisations and workers to bring about change in local communities (community organisation); and making communities more central in decisions about their futures (community building) (Nutbeam & Harris 2004). There are a number of other theories that have been developed to help health workers understand how the social environment impacts on health and assist them to develop skills in working with communities; introducing new ideas into communities (diffusion of innovation) is another. There are many similarities within these approaches and we have drawn primarily from the first two in this chapter; however, it might be useful to outline the *diffusion of innovation* theory given the expectation that one of the roles of the community development worker is that of change agent.

Diffusion of innovation

The diffusion of innovation theory provides us with a way of understanding how new ideas are taken up (or not); that is, how change takes place in a community (Rogers 1995 in Verrinder 2005). Diffusion is defined as the process by which an innovation is communicated through certain channels over time among members of a social system. An innovation is defined as an idea, practice, or object perceived as new by an individual or other unit of adoption (Rogers 1995 in Verrinder 2005, pp. 10–11). The process works in a group as clarity to a few, then gradual and later rapid uptake by the rest of the group. Five general factors that influence the speed and success with which new ideas are taken up have been identified: relative advantage, compatibility, complexity, trialability and observability (Rogers 1995 in Verrinder 2005).

There are several kinds of adopters: innovators, change agents, transformers, mainstreamers, unwilling laggards, reactionaries; there are also iconoclasts, spiritual recluses and curmudgeons (Rogers 1995; AtKisson 1999 in Verrinder 2005). Innovators are the progenitors of new ideas; they may be considered 'fringe', eccentric or unpredictable by the rest of the community and so may not be trusted. Change agents are the 'ideas brokers' for the innovator. Transformers or early adopters in the mainstream are open to new ideas and want to promote change. Mainstreamers can be persuaded that the innovation is a good idea and will change when they see the majority changing, but unwilling laggards (who are the late majority and who constitute about the same number as the mainstreamers) are the sceptics who need to be convinced of the benefits before they adopt a change. Reactionaries have a vested interest in keeping things as they are. Iconoclasts highlight problems but do not generate ideas; they are often silent partners of innovators. Spiritual recluses may proffer the philosophical underpinning and influence the atmosphere for change, while curmudgeons see change efforts as useless (Rogers 1995; AtKisson 1999 in Verrinder 2005). As we have said, we propose that community development workers are agents of change for community-led ideas.

In theory the success or otherwise of innovation depends on how it is seen by various groups — whether the innovation is seen as compatible with the established culture, for example, or the perceived relative advantage of the innovation. The simplicity and flexibility of innovation together with its reversibility and the perceived risk of its adoption will affect the extent to which innovation is taken up by the community. Finally, the observability of results will influence whether others take up the change (Rogers 1995 in Verrinder 2005). An in-depth study of these factors and other theories may provide useful information for agents of change.

The important thing is to know the community and what is likely to influence its response.

If we are to work with community development realistically and optimistically, we need to recognise its limits as well as its potential. There has been a tendency to expect a great deal from community development processes. It is important to recognise that while community development processes can have some impact on power relationships and equity at a local level, these processes will not shift power relationships on a broad scale without a vision and a plan to create a social movement. Even with the best intentions in the world, these processes at the local level will not change widespread social, economic and political conditions that are creating inequality and ill health.

Global challenges to community development

There are three major challenges operating at the global level that have local implications. The first is that, in recent times the rhetoric of many governments around the world and large organisations, such as The World Bank, has been that 'community' and community development are valued processes that advance the wellbeing of the most marginalised groups. However, challenges to participation in civil society and to social capital have come from globally dominant neo-liberal ideologies advocating values such as individualism, competitiveness and meritocracy, and governments have hijacked the language of community development while in reality offering simplistic and contradictory solutions to meeting the needs of the least powerful (Craig 1998 in Craig et al 2000, p. 329).

> The structural violence inherent in economic and political hierarchies privilege the few at the expense of the many and in doing so deny them access to channels of power, resources, communication, and participation.
>
> (Packer et al 2002, p. 317)

The co-option of the language on to the agendas of governments and powerful international organisations has often meant that instead of working with communities to address the structural issues that determine their ill health, communities have been encouraged to solve the problems without the resources or power to do so.

The second and related challenge with local implications is that the demands that local communities face participating without resources are enormous. The government discourse of empowerment through participation ignores the reality that communities are not homogenous. Forming partnerships takes time and skill and conflict arises within and between communities for the scant resources made available. There is often 'burnout' for the committed few (Craig et al 2000).

A third challenge, that is related to the first two, is that the language of governments masks not only the conflicts within communities but also the inequalities in community development processes. Large non-government organisations (NGOs) and professional organisations may be at odds with small community-based organisations, social movements and self-help collectives. They have the greatest opportunity to participate because of their resources.

The rhetoric of the powerful few about empowerment through community development processes often masks and creates these challenges. All of these challenges have implications for the worker, operating at the interface between the community and the state.

Encouraging community development: in whose interests?

Community development workers are involved in a process by which members of a community are enabled to work together to solve a problem they face and, through their participation, develop skills and greater power over some of the issues that impact on their lives. However, as we have said, community development is not always used to empower communities and increase their access to a range of choices. In many instances, some of its principles may be used to increase the compliance of community members with a program being imposed on the community, as a means of increasing the success of that program.

Tones and Tilford (1994, p. 271) suggest that there is a continuum of approaches to the use of community development strategies, ranging from community development as empowerment at one end through to the use of community development strategies to impose the beliefs of workers, professional groups or politicians at the other end. In between these extremes lie a number of variations. Werner (1981) describes the two extremes of this continuum as the difference between community-supportive programs and community-oppressive programs:

> *Community-supportive programs* or functions are those that favourably influence the long-range welfare of the community, that help it stand on its own feet, that genuinely encourage responsibility, initiative, decision-making and self-reliance at the community level, that build upon human dignity.

> *Community-oppressive programs* or functions are those which, while invariably giving lip-service to the above aspects of community input, are fundamentally authoritarian, paternalistic or are structured and carried out in such a way that they effectively encourage greater dependency, servility and unquestioning acceptance of outside regulations and decisions, and in the long run cripple the dynamics of the community.

> (Werner 1981, p. 47)

In terms of community development, this difference can be described as the difference between community development *as* health promotion and the use (or abuse) of community development *in* health promotion. When a more limited form of community development is used, it is worth asking whose interests are being served. To what extent is this type of community development likely to serve the needs of the disempowered in the community? As Werner's (1981) definition of community-oppressive programs suggests, some uses of community development may serve the needs more of the workers or bureaucracies whose decisions are being imposed than the needs of the people they are meant to assist. There may be times when the community may benefit from the imposition of good ideas, but this may be the case only in the short term. In the longer term, the community may have become more, rather than less, dependent on the health workers, and so the principles of Primary Health Care may not be operating. It is only when the principles of Primary Health Care underpin community development processes that community development can live up to its reputation for addressing the structural causes of ill health. While it may be argued that some of the projects that use the more limited form of community development are useful, they will not result in structural change or change in the power relationships between health workers and community members, and so they cannot rightly be regarded as community development.

Walker (1986) has described the aim of community development as being to 'establish a dialogue between people and the system, so that people can demand things from the system, and the system can be responsive to their needs'. If community development activities result in people being more obedient to health workers, rather than making the system more aware of and responsive to the needs of the community, then we have a fair indication that the aims of community development and the principles of Primary Health Care are not being addressed.

Critical evaluation of community development practice is therefore vital. It often needs to include critical evaluation of the way in which the employing agency or funding body sees community development being applied. If they have unrealistic or manipulative uses of community development in mind, you may need to provide some clarification, because administrators and bureaucrats, like others, do not always understand the intention of the approach to community development endorsed in the Primary Health Care approach.

Community development places emphasis on people working together as a group to achieve things for themselves, and changing the structures that influence their lives at the local level. Governments might therefore support community development because it takes the focus of responsibility away from government, public policy and broad social change. Community development also provides a cheap option for government. In supporting community development for those reasons, governments may have little regard for its goals of empowerment and increased community competence. This may mean that they support community development in theory, but in practice support only those limited forms (Cox 1995). Further, governments may reject community development as an approach to community health work because of their recognition that it emphasises drawing people together to work for common problems. Governments may be nervous of an approach that encourages people to work for social change, as it is possible that people may start demanding increased accountability from government. McArdle (1999, p. 4) argues that the growth of economic rationalism and move away from nation-building by government actually makes the need for community development even greater. Health workers with a commitment to the Primary Health Care approach cannot afford to lose their focus on community development.

Conclusion

With the endorsement of community development as a health-promotion strategy in the Ottawa Charter for Health Promotion, and recognition that it reflects the Primary Health Care approach due to its focus on working with people, health workers need to make it a central part of their practice philosophy. Creating empowering conditions at the local level enables communities to work on the social and environmental determinants of their health. We also need to develop skills in those forms of action that may help bring about social change on a broader level.

5

Program development and evaluation

The continuum of health-promotion approaches outlined in Chapter 1 continues to guide health-promotion action in this chapter. We continue to work within the socio-environmental approach which fosters community action for social and environmental change to develop and evaluate programs for health enhancement.

In this chapter we examine the continuous cycle of program development, from needs assessment through to evaluation. Research skills form the basis of the process and we outline the steps necessary to develop an effective program. Using these skills facilitates the development of a research base for health promotion in a way that both strengthens the relevance of health-promotion work and enables health workers to be accountable for their practice. A broad range of approaches can be used which are grounded in Primary Health Care and there are clear relationships between the philosophical approaches and the methods used. Community engagement in the process is fundamental to the success of program development and evaluation.

Why do we need to plan?

The purpose of program-planning is to devise a program that addresses the health issues of concern for the community within the available resources. The Primary Health Care approach ensures that the process and outcome of the planning are acceptable to the community and mindful of social justice, while ensuring the efficiency and effectiveness of the organisation or agency. The fundamental propositions to program development and evaluation are that health and health risks are caused by multiple factors. Efforts to effect environmental and social change must be multidimensional and/or multi-sectoral.

Successful programs do not happen by chance. The process elements of planning in program development and evaluation are:

- focusing attention on and clarifying what the stakeholders are attempting to do;

- allowing for quality and participatory decision-making and better collaboration;

- knowing what types of interventions are most acceptable and feasible for specific populations and circumstances;

- taking a multidimensional approach;

- assisting in identifying the resources and activities required;

- assigning responsibility to specific stakeholders to meet program objectives;

- reducing uncertainty within the program environment;

- informing everyone involved with the program as to the:
    — implementation requirements
    — desired outcomes; and
- reviewing existing practice to assess whether the intervention is meeting a justifiable need.

(Talbot et al in State Government of Victoria, Department of Human Services 2003)

The outcome elements of program development are:

- understanding the determinants of an issue or problem;
- designing an intervention;
- ownership of problems and solutions; and
- relevant theory, data and local experience informs the development of the program.

What is the program development and evaluation planning cycle?

The program development cycle is a continuous cycle or spiral of planning which includes identifying, analysing, prioritising, implementing and evaluating. That is, we need to define the issue, work out what to do about it, act, and then evaluate what impact this has had. The steps in program development and evaluation are:

1. Identifying a specific issue, community and focus for a program:

> The needs assessment — identify and analyse the health issue
> > Conducting consultations
> > Gathering information about the issue
> > Examining characteristics of the community
> > Analysing the information and making a judgment

2. Designing the program:

> Specifying the broad purpose of the program
> — the program aim
> Converting the analysis of the issue into a draft plan
> — identifying the program objectives
> — stating the expected outcomes

      Developing roles with key people
      Reviewing available resources
      Ensuring the program is realistic and achievable

3. Developing an action plan:

      Planning for the organisation of tasks
      — selecting and sequencing activities
      Selecting the program strategies
      Preparing materials, resources, activities
      Training staff

4. Implementing the program

5. Evaluability assessment

6. Evaluating the program

      Process evaluation
      Impact evaluation
      Outcome evaluation

This chapter deals with step 1, identifying a specific issue, step 5, evaluability assessment, and step 6, evaluating the program from the cycle. Designing the program, developing an action plan and implementing the program will be dealt with in other chapters according to the activities the community decides upon. The steps in program planning and evaluation are best thought of as a continuing cycle (as illustrated in Figure 5.1) rather than as a linear sequence of events. The cyclical process indicates that the process is never 'finished'; when one round of interventions is complete, one reflects on the evaluation findings and plans relevant new interventions.

Theoretical frameworks that guide program development and evaluation

Research in Primary Health Care

The research process has an important role to play as an ongoing, integrated part of practice. When participatory research is integral to practice, practice is strengthened in a number of ways. Firstly, health-promotion practice will be built around the needs of the people for whom it is designed. It will be responsive to those needs and based on recognition that needs are dynamic rather than static, and therefore change over time. Secondly, with grounding in community needs, health workers are less likely to implement programs that do not meet these needs, thus preventing expensive mistakes. Thirdly, when research is integral to practice, health promotion and other activities of health workers are routinely evaluated, and the findings used to improve the quality of health-promotion work.

The inextricable relationship between research and practice means that the additional resources required to carry out research may not be as great as expected. When research is an integral part of practice, it is as much a state of mind and

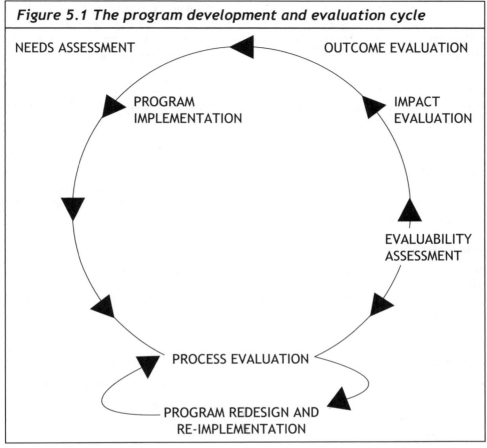

Figure 5.1 The program development and evaluation cycle

NEEDS ASSESSMENT   OUTCOME EVALUATION

PROGRAM
IMPLEMENTATION   IMPACT
                                   EVALUATION

                                   EVALUABILITY
                                   ASSESSMENT

PROCESS EVALUATION

PROGRAM REDESIGN AND
RE-IMPLEMENTATION

(Source: Hawe, P., Degeling, D. and Hall, J. 1990 *Evaluating Health Promotion: a Health Workers' Guide*. MacLennan and Petty, Sydney, p. 78)

an approach to working as anything else. Certainly there are times, for example, when a major community assessment may be required, and this may necessitate an additional commitment of time and resources and the active involvement of people with expertise in community assessment. However, not researching and improving practice may result in wasting the limited resources that are being allocated to health promotion.

Participatory research: the Primary Health Care approach in action

A Primary Health Care approach to health promotion emphasises the importance of health-promotion work being socially relevant and conducted *with* people, rather than working *on* people. Research conducted as part of health promotion needs to meet this criterion also. If research is to reflect a Primary Health Care approach, the emphasis must be on working with people as equal partners, involving them in the research process and acknowledging their expertise. This will ensure that the research conducted is relevant to their needs and therefore useful.

This approach to research, known as 'participatory research', is growing in recognition. The participatory approach to research is an approach to working collaboratively with consumers or community members while drawing on a wide range of research methods of direct relevance to the problem at hand.

In such situations, planning committees comprised of researchers, health workers and community members can work together to design, implement and evaluate research projects. Contributions of community members in defining the parameters of the research and reviewing issues that arise, from their perspectives as community members, add much to the value of the research.

Some research methods are of particular value in Primary Health Care because they actually have this participatory approach embedded in the research process. Of note here are *participatory action research* and *feminist research*. It is worthwhile examining them briefly in order to understand how these methods can be utilised in health promotion.

Participatory action research

Participatory action research is a dynamic process built on a foundation of working with people, enabling them to be the key developers of problem-solving and change. Participatory action research has developed simultaneously in a number of fields, with slightly different styles, taking account of the different circumstances, but following similar general principles (Selener 1997). Of particular relevance for our purposes is participatory action research as it has developed in community development, and action research as it has developed in organisations.

Participatory action research in community development has been defined as

a process through which members of an oppressed group or community identify a problem, collect and analyse information, and act upon the problem in order to find solutions and to promote social and political transformation.

(Selener 1997, p. 17)

Participatory action research is based on a strong set of values relating to social justice and empowerment of oppressed groups, through working to change those things that constrain their lives, including dominating social structures (Selener 1997, p. 18). There are several characteristics of participatory action research:

- The problem originates in the community itself and is defined, analysed and solved by the community.

- The ultimate goal of research is the radical transformation of social reality and improvement in the lives of the people involved. The primary beneficiaries of the research are the community members themselves.

- Participatory research involves the full and active participation of the community in the entire research process.

- Participatory research involves a whole range of powerless groups of people — the exploited, the poor, the oppressed, the marginalised.

- The process of participatory research can create a greater awareness in people of their own resources and can mobilise them for self-reliant development.

- Participatory research is a more scientific method, in that community participation in the research process facilitates a more accurate and authentic analysis of social reality.

- The researcher is a committed participant, facilitator, and learner in the research process, and this leads to militancy, rather than detachment.

(Selener 1997, pp. 18–21)

Participatory action research in community development clearly has many applications within health promotion, as it provides a process by which community members can identify and address problems by dealing with some of their root causes.

Two streams of action research have developed in an organisational context, based on the work of Lewin (1946). These approaches, action research in organisations and action research in education, are very similar. What they offer health promotion is a framework for using an action research approach within an organisational context, which can be quite different to working at community level. These organisational approaches may be particularly valuable when working for health-promoting settings.

Organisational action research is a continuing cyclical approach to work that involves an ever-developing 'self-reflective spiral of cycles of planning, acting, observing and reflecting' (Carr & Kemmis 1986, p. 162). It is likely to be a more consensual process than participatory action research in community development, because it is conducted within an organisational context to address problems at this level. Like participatory action research in community development, organisational action research is a participatory process, although it may be instigated and led by an outside researcher. Its focus is on solving practical problems through organisational change and development (Selener 1997, pp. 65–8). It is therefore regarded as a learning process, both for the individuals involved in the action research process and for the organisation itself.

Because organisational action research is built on recognition of the inextricable links between research and practice (Carr & Kemmis 1986), it has a great deal to offer health workers. It is ideal as an approach to working with community members, enabling them to reflect on their own experiences, plan how they can act to change their situation, act and then evaluate the impact of the changes in order to then re-plan, re-act and re-evaluate in a continuing cycle of change, development and learning. It can also be used to provide a framework for health workers to continually analyse and develop their own practice. That is, it provides a framework for good reflective practice.

Feminist research

While feminist research developed originally for work with women as an oppressed group, it has potential as a set of principles of use when working with any marginalised groups. Feminist research has been defined as:

... research that relates to an understanding of women's position as that of an oppressed social group, and which adopts a critical perspective towards intellectual traditions rendering women either invisible and/or subject to a priori categorisations of one form or another.

(Oakley 1990, pp. 169–70)

139

Feminist research is therefore conducted in a way that is not oppressive to those involved in it and care is taken to ensure that the research findings can be used by the research participants (Roberts 1981, cited by Oakley 1990, pp. 169–70).

Feminist methodology is built on recognition of the expertise of the people affected by a particular issue. Mies (1983, pp. 124–7) suggests several key issues to guide feminist research. These are:

1. There is a recognition that research is not value-free. Therefore, rather than attempting to remain totally distant from and uninvolved with research participants, feminist researchers identify with them sufficiently to see the problem from their perspective as well as their own.
2. The relationship between researcher and research participants is an equal partnership, not one where researchers are the 'experts' and the people being researched are mere subjects. This is reflected in the use of the term research 'participant', rather than 'subject'. Without this partnership approach to research, researchers contribute to the oppression of people they are attempting to help.
3. Research is inseparable from the wider actions for improvement of women's position in society. Therefore, researchers are also engaged in 'active participation in actions, movements and struggles for women's emancipation' (p. 124).
4. The interrelationship between action and research indicates that an inherent part of feminist methodology is 'change of the status quo' (p. 125). In particular, feminist methodology is built around changes to women's position in society and the fight for emancipation.
5. 'The research process must become a process of "conscientisation", or critical consciousness raising, for both researchers and research participants' (p. 127). That is, through the research process, people are enabled to see the social, political and economic constraints on their lives and therefore recognise the context in which their lives are lived. This process also results in recognition of the experiences individual women share with each other; consequently, the power of the group becomes recognised and can be used for collective action (p. 127).

Towards a Primary Health Care approach to research

It is quite apparent that there are links between feminist research, participatory action research and the process of 'conscientisation', or critical consciousness raising developed by Freire (1973). Together these form a powerful basis for dynamic relevant research that has the potential to promote the health of the people for whom it is designed. This Primary Health Care approach to research can be described by the following elements:

- Research is a dynamic cyclical process, inextricably intertwined with action. Its aim is to improve the conditions under which people live.
- The research process is guided by critical self-reflection on the part of the 'researcher' and the research participants. The values of researcher and research participants are acknowledged up front and are the subject of critical self-reflection as part of the research process. Conscientisation is a key feature of this process.

X • The relationship between researcher and research participants is a partnership that itself acts to change the status quo by breaking down the traditionally 'top-down' approach of researchers. Thus, all people involved in the research process are best described as research partners.

Developing participatory research in a way that is both rigorous and accepted by professional colleagues and funding bodies on the one hand, and meaningful and acceptable to community members participating in the process on the other, is a challenge that has been identified by several researchers committed to working in this way (Boutilier et al 1997).

Involving community members as partners in the process means that the process may become unpredictable and uncontrollable, which may create difficulties for people if the framework in which they are working doesn't allow for that kind of flexibility, or if the community members want to take the process in a direction that is against the principles of Primary Health Care. This is by no means a simple issue. How do you balance the need to be flexible in your approach and to ensure community members are true partners in the process, with the need to remain committed to certain principles, which may mean being inflexible if those principles are transgressed? However, these are challenges worth grappling with if we are to see the Primary Health Care approach to research reach its potential.

Ethical considerations in program development and evaluation

There are international and national rules governing how research is conducted. In Australia, the National Health and Medical Research Council (NH&MRC) governs the conduct of research and Human Research Ethics Committees (HREC) oversee research on this organisation's behalf and are guided by the NH&MRC rules. These committees are found in large organisations such as universities, education departments, health departments and large hospitals.

It is not proposed that we deal comprehensively with ethical issues here. The guidelines are easily found on websites, such as the NH&MRC website.

There is some debate about whether HREC approval is needed for community-based needs assessments and evaluations. HRECs are charged with supervising research with publication of the results in mind (Posavac & Carey 2003, p. 110). Some believe that much can be gained by seeking approval in any circumstance, others believe that if the community is involved in identifying their own needs, planning the implementation of the program designed to address the need, and evaluating the program, seeking approval from an outside HREC is unnecessary. Further, reflective practice is a form of evaluation and that does not need HREC approval. Awareness of power-relationships is probably the most important consideration in gathering information. Power imbalances may emerge in the research procedures in needs assessments and evaluation.

The principles of Primary Health Care provide a solid foundation for conducting needs assessments and evaluation within the program-planning cycle. However, research procedures form the basis of these processes and therefore further discussion is needed concerning some of the ethical issues that health workers need to consider, whether they seek HREC approval or not.

Five categories of ethical issues have been identified:

1. treating people ethically;

2. recognising role conflicts;

3. using valid methods;

4. serving the needs of the program participants; and

5. avoiding the negative effects of the research.

(Posavac & Carey 2003, p. 97)

Treating people ethically

Health workers need to consider whether any harm will be done during the research process. One way of protecting people is to obtain informed consent prior to the research. The emphasis here is on *informed*, which means that the information sheet explaining the research and the participants' role must be written in a way that they can understand, therefore enabling them to truly make an informed decision about whether they participate or not.

Another way of protecting people is through a confidentiality agreement. It is often not necessary to identify the participants, because usually it is their opinion that is needed, not a record or the need to keep a record of their name and contact details. However, if it is necessary, utmost care must be taken to protect the participant's details, and if confidentiality is promised, it must be preserved (Posavac & Carey 2003).

Recognising role conflicts

Ethical dilemmas sometimes arise from the conflicting interests of the stakeholders. How the stakeholders could be affected by the findings is a significant issue to be considered before the research takes place.

- Why is the research being done?
- Who is conducting the research?
- Who will have access to the findings? and
- How will the findings be used?

These are important questions which, when addressed, prevent conflict and compromised research procedures (Posavac & Carey 2003).

Using valid methods

When it is clear that the participants can come to no harm and that the potential for conflict is minimised, then it is important to focus on the validity of the project. Research design must fit the needs of those who will utilise the information. Conducting research that is not suitable for the purposes for which it was commissioned is unethical. Experienced data collectors and analysts need to be involved in research. If quantitative methods are to be used, then a standardised test appropriate to the setting will minimise the risk of invalid results (Posavac & Carey 2003). If interviews form part of the process then experienced interviewers are required, if the time of the interviewee is not to be wasted or the money of tl research program because of meaningless or inadequate interviewing. Interviewing requires tremendous skill.

Serving the needs of the program participants

People will not benefit from the findings if they are not published (Posavac & Carey 2003) and as we have said, working with participants in program development and evaluation maximises the chances of serving the needs of the participants. Collecting data that does not serve the needs of the participants is unethical.

Avoiding the negative effects of the research

People can be hurt by inaccurate findings. False negatives and false positives can be minimised by clean research design (Posavac & Carey 2003).

Planning in Primary Health Care

Conceptual models or health promotion planning models are the means by which structure and organisation are given to the programming process. They provide health workers with direction by supplying a framework on which to build. There are no perfect planning models. The important thing to remember is that health workers must fit the needs of the planning situation with the characteristics of the group/community/issue/setting.

PRECEDE-PROCEED

The PRECEDE–PROCEED planning model 'grew out of . . . combined and cumulative experience in practice, research, teaching, consultation and government service, all guided and enriched by significant teachers, colleagues and students' (Green & Kreuter 1999, p. xxix). It is not offered here as the exclusive road to quality health planning. There are many models for health promotion for planning. It is, however, a theoretically robust model. It can be applied to health promotion in a variety of situations and is acknowledged as *the model that addresses planning comprehensively*. It takes into account the multiple factors that determine health. It helps planners arrive at a highly focused subset of factors for intervention. In this section we provide an overview of the model before expanding on the steps of program development and evaluation.

- PRECEDE — an acronym for predisposing, reinforcing and enabling constructs in educational diagnosis and evaluation.
- PROCEED — an acronym for policy, regulatory and organisational constructs in educational and environmental development.

There are nine phases in this model for program development and evaluation. The information gathered is often referred to as *primary* and *secondary* data. Phases one and two are primary sources and phases three, four and five can be either primary or secondary sources.

Phases one to five (PRECEDE) are addressed here. Phases six through nine (PROCEED) relate to the development of appropriate strategies using organisational, regulatory and policy approaches and are encompassed in the subsequent chapters of this book. For a detailed discussion on PROCEED, refer to Green and Kreuter (1999).

The first phase is social assessment, which refers to the needs that are defined by a community in terms of the dimensions of their quality of life. This means asking the community to identify and discuss their needs and aspirations (Green & Kreuter 1999). The kinds of social problems a community experiences are a practical and accurate barometer of its quality of life and include such things as discrimination, poverty, isolation, self-esteem or poor nutrition.

The second phase is the epidemiological assessment. These needs are defined by health professionals in terms of morbidity and mortality. This builds on phase one, although it can and often is done in isolation. The task of the second phase is to identify the specific health issues that may contribute to the social issues identified in phase one. In this phase we begin to analyse and prioritise the health issues. Combining existing epidemiological data and the social diagnosis you have made, health issues can then be prioritised. Prioritising is necessary because there will always be too many issues to deal with (Green & Kreuter 1999).

Phase three consists of identifying the specific health-related behavioural and environmental factors that could be linked to the health issues chosen as most deserving of attention in phase two. Because they are the risk factors that the intervention is tailored to effect, they must be specifically identified and carefully ranked. Environmental factors are those external to the individual, often beyond his or her control, that can be modified to support the behaviour, health or quality of life of that person or the community through organisational or administrative action. Being aware of these factors reminds health workers of the limitations of health-promotion programs consisting of health education directed only at personal behaviour and of the multidimensional nature of health issues and of the need often for multi-sectoral approaches (Green & Kreuter 1999).

Phase four consists of sorting and categorising the factors that seem to have direct impact on the behaviour or the environment. Interventions that are planned within these categories will depend on their relative importance and the resources available. The PRECEDE model groups them according to the educational and organisational strategies likely to be employed in a health-promotion program to bring about environmental and behavioural change. The three broad groupings are *predisposing*, *enabling* and *reinforcing* factors. These are described as (Green & Kreuter 1999):

- Predisposing factors — a person's or population's knowledge, attitudes, beliefs, values and perceptions that facilitate or hinder the capacity for change.
- Enabling factors — can be viewed as the skills and resources necessary for change. The vehicles or barriers, created mainly by societal forces can enhance or hinder change. Facilities or community resources may be ample or inadequate; laws may be supportive or restrictive. Enabling factors thus include all the factors that make possible a desired change in behaviour or in the environment.

- Reinforcing factors — the feedback received from others following adoption of the changed situation may encourage or discourage continuation of the changed situation.

Phase five is the administrative assessment. This is the assessment of organisational capabilities and resources for the development and implementation of a program.

Limitations of resources, policies and abilities and time constraints are assessed. Some of these limitations and constraints can be offset by cooperative arrangements with other local agencies or larger organisations at state or national levels or through the development of alliances at the local level. All that remains is the selection of the right combination of strategies. The program is then implemented and evaluated. This is PROCEED and we will be discussing evaluation later in the chapter. However, listing evaluation last is misleading. Evaluation is an integral and continuous part of working with the entire model from the beginning.

Needs assessment

The PRECEDE–PROCEED model can guide health workers in program development and evaluation. Phases one through to four are the phases where we identify, analyse and prioritise the needs. However, before expanding on the steps in a needs assessment we need to reconsider who the 'community' is. Is it local, state/territory, or national? Is it a community of interest or a geographical community? How homogenous is it? Can you assume that all the views of community members will be represented? These are important initial questions for health workers.

Community assessments

Community assessment can be defined as a process that results in:

> . . . a comprehensive description of the needs of a population that is defined, or defines itself, as a community, and the resources that exist within that community, carried out with the active involvement of the community itself, for the purpose of developing an action plan or other means of improving the quality of life in the community.

> (Hawtin et al 1994, p. 13)

This definition highlights several issues that are central to meaningful community assessment.

- Community assessment is a process of determining both the needs and the resources of a community. While considerable attention tends to be focused on the needs of communities, and these certainly are important, a focus on needs alone tends to paint a 'deficit' picture of communities. This itself can be a negative disempowering experience for communities and can ignore the positive characteristics and resources of that community. These community strengths can be a source of pride for the community, and may hold a key to successfully addressing the needs that arise.
- Community assessment should be carried out with the active participation of community members. As discussion in each chapter so far has noted,

community members have the right and ability to be meaningfully engaged in determining what their needs and strengths are. Good community assessment is a participatory process.

- Community assessments are carried out for the specific purpose of achieving change that improves the quality of life of those living as part of that community. A community assessment is not an end in itself, but a guide to action. Unless community assessments are acted on, they are a waste of time and energy (Hawe 1996; Feuerstein 1986, p. 153). Community assessments that leave you with few resources for acting on what you find, or for which there is no real commitment to act on after their completion, are likely to do little to help those for whom the community assessment is purportedly being carried out and are likely to result in significant community frustration (Hawe 1996; Rissel 1991, p. 30).

Need — what is it?

While comprehensive community assessment examines both the resources and needs of a community, it is true that the notion of needs has a central place in community assessment. This is especially so when there is a focus on social justice and working to achieve equity for those who are disadvantaged. Any examination of community assessment should start, therefore, with an examination of just what need is, and a review of some of the issues surrounding the definition of something as a need. Need has been defined as 'the condition marked by the lack of something requisite' (*Macquarie Dictionary* 2001). This definition highlights the fact that the very concept of need itself is value-based and socially constructed. Whether something is identified as a need will depend on the perspectives and values of those involved. In addition, it is through the way in which issues are defined at a social and political level that individuals, groups and societies come to decide which issues are of concern to them and which things they need. Which issues are constructed as needs depends on the particular values in place in the society or group. Given the value-laden nature of need, it is important to be clear about which values should be driving the needs-identification process in the Primary Health Care approach.

There are several different ways in which needs can be classified, according to the perspective used to identify need. Bradshaw (1972) has identified four types of need: felt need, expressed need, normative need and comparative need. The categories of felt and expressed need include need determined by people themselves, while the category of normative need represents need determined by experts, and comparative need represents need determined by past responses to similar problems. These needs are expressed in the PRECEDE model in steps one through to five discussed earlier in the chapter. With an emphasis on equal partnership between professionals and community members in a Primary Health Care approach to health promotion, all these types of need have something useful to contribute to an assessment of need.

Felt need

Felt need is most easily described as what people say they need. For example, if a local community is surveyed regarding its highest priorities for health-promotion action, people may say that they want more intensive-care beds, safer streets in which their children can play or less youth unemployment in the local area. This is closest to the social assessment in the PRECEDE model or the predisposing and reinforcing factors of phase three.

Felt need is important because it involves asking people themselves what their needs are. However, on its own it may not give a complete picture of need for a number of reasons. Firstly, people may limit what they tell you they need to what they think they can have (Walker & Dixon 1984, pp. 16–17). If they believe that meeting some of their needs is beyond their reach, they may not ask for them.

Secondly, people may only voice needs that they believe you are interested in. For example, if a health worker asks someone about their health needs, that person may interpret the question as referring to his or her illness problems alone, and may not think of health in its broad context.

Thirdly, powerful groups in the community can have a strong influence in determining how people see their needs. Community members' beliefs about what they need can, in fact, be socially constructed by interest groups, opinion leaders and the mass media. Groups and communities may 'adopt' certain needs as their own because these have been sold to them through the mass media. In many instances it is not the need alone but also one potential response to the need that is presented as the 'solution'. One example of this process can be seen in the establishment of the need for national mammography services. A concerted media campaign, 'sold' the importance of mammography screening rather than providing a balanced discussion about the issues. The problems of false negatives and false positives and whether it actually makes a difference to people's lives were not discussed (Browning 1992; Wass 1990). Through the impact of the medical profession and medical insurance companies, which have advertised mammography as 'the only safe way to detect breast cancer', the need for appropriate breast cancer screening has been redefined for many people as the need for mammography.

Fourthly, the perspective of a small group of community members may not reflect the perspective of the whole community. Careful consideration needs to be made of whom a group of community informants represent — a section of the community, a small subsection or only themselves (Hawe et al 1990, p. 19).

If we are to take the principles of Primary Health Care seriously, we need to work to promote health based on people's own assessment of their need — that is, felt need must be among the types of need present. However, because of the all-pervading forces that influence people's felt need, most particularly through the media, people may not have had a real opportunity to decide for themselves. In health promotion, as in any other area of health, workers need to ensure that people are able to make informed decisions and that they have access to the information they need to make those decisions. Of course, this process may require more than giving people information; it may require them to examine the forces that influence their decisions. That is, this process of helping people clarify their felt need may well involve the process of conscientisation.

The presence of felt or expressed need alone, without the presence also of normative or comparative need, raises some questions. What if a group or community wants something but there is no evidence to demonstrate the need for it? In such a situation, more information may be needed. Does the group or community know that it is comparatively well off in the area concerned? This may change the priorities that the group sets. Conversely, is it the case that there is a lack of formal evidence in this area because of the shortcomings of information collection, rather than that there is no objective need?

Another issue worth mentioning is that the felt need may be expressed in the form of a solution. This can be very limiting. It is always worth digging deeper. It is worth asking what is the issue or problem rather than what the solution to a problem is. There may be many creative solutions to identified issues.

Furthermore, currently, health-promotion funding is made available for specific projects, often aimed at particular diseases or risk factors. Frequently, funding may be granted and the project begun without any prior systematic assessment of the community's felt needs. The particular project being funded may be a long way down the community's list of priorities, and people may not be motivated to participate in the project. It is then imposed on the community, at 'best' with the community being educated about why they should want it. This approach to funding presents some very real dangers, as it encourages health workers and bureaucrats to ignore communities' own assessments of their needs or regard them as a simple 'add on' rather than an integral part of the project.

Expressed need

Expressed need is need that is demonstrated by people's use of services or demand for new or more services. That is, expressed need can be described as 'felt need turned into action' (Bradshaw 1972, p. 641). Examples of expressed need include waiting lists for services such as childcare, housing or public dental services. In PRECEDE, this could be the environmental or behavioural assessment in phase three, or the enabling factors of phase four. Needless to say, this expressed need has even more limitations on it than felt need, as people can only add their names to waiting lists for services that already exist or are about to come into existence. Indeed, waiting lists are limited to issues of service provision: it is not possible to join a waiting list for a new public policy, for example, although the number of letters written to a politician on a particular issue may be regarded as another form of expressed need.

The constraints on people's choices here are even greater than in felt need, since the specific service they are demanding must already be there. Moreover, expressed need can easily be misinterpreted. For example, a waiting list at the local dentist might be interpreted as the need for more dental treatment services, when in fact it could reflect inadequate oral health promotion or lack of awareness of school dental therapy services, to give just two examples. Another problem with expressed need is that in many situations people may add their names to all available waiting lists for a particular service, although in reality they would accept only one place (for example a nursing home placement). In such a situation, adding up the numbers of names on waiting lists is likely to give an inaccurate impression. In other situations, people may refrain from placing their names on waiting lists if they believe the waiting lists are already long and their chances of success low. In addition, people's beliefs about whether they have a right to particular services, or deserve to have access to them, will influence whether they act to formally express a need.

Normative need

Normative need is need determined by 'experts' on the basis of research and professional opinion. Examples of normative need include safe levels of water pollution, recommended daily allowances of different food groups and unsafe levels of lead ingestion. The epidemiological assessment described in the PRECEDE model would form part of this assessment. Normatively determined need is often regarded as objective and unbiased because it has been determined by experts. It often carries the assumption that it is value-free and beyond reproach, but this assumption needs to be called into question. In addition, professional opinion often changes over time, leaving the public confused (Bradshaw 1972, p. 641). For example, Becker (1986) cites the example of professionals' changing views of the dangers of cholesterol, and the consequent confusion among the public. As a result, the public is beginning to develop some healthy scepticism about professional opinion. Normative need may reflect some level of paternalism, and it certainly can provide conflicting information, depending on the values of the experts themselves (Bradshaw 1972, p. 641).

One crucial issue that influences normative need and that requires examination is the fact that many professional groups act, often unconsciously, as gatekeepers in society. They may be unable or unwilling to acknowledge publicly that something is occurring at an unsafe level if their judgment in this case has political implications. This, then, represents another possible limitation of normatively determined need. Finally, an over-reliance on epidemiological data to provide evidence of normative need is increasingly being called into question, as the limitations of only relying on one type of data are recognised.

Comparative need

Comparative need is need that is determined by comparing the services available in one geographical area with those available in other geographical areas. Therefore, it may be argued that a particular area requires a certain service because other areas with similar demographic characteristics have one. In PRECEDE, this could be the result of a social assessment, but it could also be part of phase five, the administrative assessment. Comparative need can be useful in highlighting relative deficiencies in some communities. However, it can also be problematic because it is based on the assumption that the service provided in the place of comparison was the most appropriate response to the problem (Bradshaw 1972, p. 641), and that the needs of the two areas are in fact the same.

All of these needs tell us different things. As we discussed earlier in the chapter, a combination of social, epidemiological, environmental, behavioural and administrative assessments provide us with a comprehensive base from which to plan programs.

In preparing to assess the needs of any individual, group or community, it is vital to know why the particular assessment needs to be done. What needs to be known, and to what end? This will help determine how the assessment should be conducted. Adequate resources need to be available. As discussed above, uncovering needs, creating the expectation that something will be done about them, then not acting, is unlikely to develop confidence in those whose time has been wasted. Box 5.1 outlines the principles that underpin a Primary Health Care approach to community assessments and Box 5.2 outlines the steps.

Box 5.1 Principles of community assessment

1. Community assessment should be an integral part of health-promotion work.
2. Community assessment should reflect the social view of health, which is so much a part of health promotion and Primary Health Care (Baum 1992, p. 83).
3. Community assessment should involve both formal and informal assessment of needs and resources.
4. Community assessment should recognise the partnership between people themselves and health workers in determining their needs and resources, planning action and evaluating any outcomes. Part of this process may involve negotiation between community members and health workers.
5. Needs assessment should involve a combination of felt, expressed, normative and comparative need.

Box 5.2 The steps in community assessment

1. Identify the purpose of the community assessment.
2. Identify available resources.
3. Establish a project team and steering committee.
4. Develop a research plan and time frame.
5. Collect and analyse available information.
6. Complete community research.
7. Analyse results.
8. Report back to community.
9. Set priorities.
10. Determine responses to the needs identified.

(Source: South Australian Community Health Research Unit 1991 *Planning Healthy Communities: a Guide to Doing Community Needs Assessment*. South Australian Community Health Research Unit, Adelaide)

Gathering information for a community needs assessment

Program-planners need to make themselves aware of what information is already known. There are a number of sources and collation services to assist this process. Planners need to consider all the sources of available information before committing new funds to needs assessment. As we have said, health workers' information about a community is only as good as the techniques used to collect it. A lot of precious time and money can be wasted collecting information that is unusable, or in planning and implementing activities based on information that does not reflect community needs. Three 'groups' of data need to be gathered to inform a community needs assessment, which fall into the two sources outlined earlier.

Primary data sources:

    1. data from the community members; and

Secondary data sources:

    2. statistical and epidemiological information; and

    3. information from the literature.

In a community needs assessment, primary data consists of information gathered from community members, specifically for the purposes of the needs assessment. Secondary data are information that may be collated from existing sources, that have been gathered for other purposes, but which may be relevant to the needs-assessment process.

Because it is important to establish what is already known about the community before setting out to gather even more information, the secondary sources of data will be discussed first.

Secondary data sources

Secondary data are those data that already exist that can be accessed relatively easily. These data are essential to provide a strong rationale for a new incentive, or to argue the case for 'comparative need' (Bradshaw 1972). Good examples are Australian Bureau of Statistics (ABS) population data, and state-wide mortality and morbidity data, such as regional 'Burden of Disease' reports.

Social and economic indicators

Social and economic indicators include a range of statistical information that helps to construct a picture of the community. Information such as proportions of people in each age group, income levels, number of people on each type of pension, number of single-parent families, number of single-income families and level of home ownership is useful in helping to construct a picture of the issues likely to be affecting a particular community. This information is available from ABS data, which are often held by each local council or health department for its own area and should be available for public viewing. In addition, information on such things as amount of land available for recreation, shopping facilities and availability of public transport may also be useful to access. It should be available from your local council.

Epidemiological data

Epidemiology has been defined as 'the study of the distribution and determinants of disease in human populations' (Christie et al 1987, p. 1). Epidemiological data provide information about the levels of death (mortality) and disease (morbidity) in the community and their distribution according to such criteria as gender, age and place of residence. They come from a number of sources (Christie et al 1987, p. 8):

- death rates;
- cancer mortality and morbidity rates from state cancer registers;
- health surveys and studies, for example those conducted by the Australian Institute of Health and Welfare;
- hospital discharge records; and
- reports of notifiable infectious diseases.

By providing information at a population level, epidemiology provides a useful tool against which to confirm or question the hunches of health workers or community members regarding health problems in an area. This can be valuable because assumptions about problems in an area may not always be correct. The reports produced by the Australian Institute of Health and Welfare, for example, are of particular value in providing and analysing up-to-date epidemiological data. These include biennial reports, such as *Australia's Health 2004* (Australian Institute of Health and Welfare 2004). Also, local public health units or health-promotion units may prepare epidemiological data relevant to their own areas. Many libraries and municipalities may keep some of this material if it is relevant to the surrounding area. In addition, a growing range of this data is available on the worldwide web, especially in the validated reports of government agencies, such as reports on women's health, domestic violence, injury surveillance, mental health and wellbeing, and others.

It is important to note that epidemiological data are not equally available for all health problems. Some health problems have well-developed databases (for example, cardiovascular disease) while others, such as depression or family violence, do not (Hawe 1996, p. 474). Similarly, until relatively recently the seriousness of Aboriginal health problems in Australia was ignored because data on Aboriginal health were not collected. Relying on pre-existing epidemiological data risks focusing further attention on conditions that are already well identified, at the expense of those that may be serious but that have been ignored in the past.

Beyond epidemiology: the need for a broader approach to health assessment

If we were solely interested in preventing disease, rather than being interested in health promotion and a social view of health, we might be happy with the information we can gather from morbidity and mortality data. However, from a social health perspective, morbidity and mortality data are simply not sufficient to enable us to see the problems we are concerned about. In addition, epidemiological data are of limited use in situations where no simple cause-and-effect relationship exists or where delayed onset of symptoms occurs (Auer 1988, p. 41; Public Interest Advocacy Centre, cited by Brennan 1992, p. 18). This may particularly be the case, for example, with environmental health issues. Epidemiology also requires a fairly long time frame before there is 'evidence' of a problem, by which time a number of people will have already experienced illness or even death. Nor is epidemiology sufficient to measure the extent of wellness of a community and of individuals in that community. Using a conceptual model, such as the PRECEDE–PROCEED model outlined earlier, when planning a community needs assessment, guides the researcher to think more broadly about health and wellbeing. It provides a framework for planners and practitioners to consider multidimensional strategies for addressing health needs. The same process also enables identification of existing community strengths and capacities and provides a means of valuing these in future projects.

National and state policy documents

National and state policy or strategy documents often provide material from a combination of sources, particularly epidemiological data, social and economic indicators and the views of professionals. They will also have been developed with varying degrees of community consultation, depending on political will and the 'need' for expediency. It is important to note that national and state policy documents are often reflective more of political priorities and processes than of the needs of the community. The politically determined nature of these documents must be acknowledged. They will also need to be compared with local evidence of need rather than be assumed to reflect the local picture. With recognition of these issues in mind, such documents can be useful sources of information and should be used wherever possible as one component of identifying needs. Further information about the policy documents relevant to your state or region should be available from your state's health department or a regional public health unit, and are often available to view or download from the web. In addition to national and state documents, some regions or areas may have their own policy and strategy documents. These may be even more useful because they are one step nearer to your community and so may reflect its needs more closely. However, it is worthwhile finding out about the process by which these documents were developed. Were they simply summarised from state and national documents, or were regional needs assessments carried out? They may have been prepared without consulting the community members in the region. Their value may therefore be limited.

Reviewing the literature

A literature review sets the current activity into the context of wider public health practice. Skills in accessing and reviewing literature are essential to inform different phases of a needs assessment as will be illustrated throughout this chapter. Literature review skills are frequently used in other aspects of public health practice, such as preparing an application for funding or reporting on a research project or community program. This section does not provide a comprehensive overview of the literature searching and reviewing process. For that, consult a core text in public health research. The following provides a brief overview of the main steps in the process and some practical guidelines.

A literature review is defined as '. . . an extensive, exhaustive, systematic and critical examination of publications relevant to a chosen topic' (Seaman & Verhonick 1982 in LoBiondo-Wood & Haber 2002, p. 78). It has two main purposes: (1) to critically evaluate published research material; and (2) to place current information and activities in the context of previous research. Conducting a literature review before commencing a program not only allows health workers to draw wisdom from the experts, but also prevents wasting time, or making the same mistakes that others have made. A later review of the literature may allow extension of existing knowledge, identification of methods that could be used, or to guide modification of previously tried approaches in order to enhance their effectiveness locally.

Searching the literature

A literature review, which fits with the definition above, requires good knowledge of data sources and skills in using them effectively. These days, much of the information which is accessed is available from the internet using a search engine or browser (such as 'Google' or 'Yahoo') and computer bibliographic literature data bases (such as 'Proquest' or 'Cinahl'), rather than in 'hard copy' journals or books. Primary research, reported in refereed journals, should be the key criteria used for selecting literature. Be wary of using the easily accessible, but completely non-validated, writings and opinions contained in many internet addresses that turn up from a 'key word' search.

Books provide a foundation, particularly in historical, theoretical and conceptual areas, including definitions. However, they contain material assembled from other sources, so they are not so up-to-date, they may not provide in-depth details of the topic, and they do not usually provide data-based research literature.

Primary sources are first-hand accounts; research reports written by the researcher.

Secondary sources are at least once removed from the primary author. These could include summaries of research studies (for example an annotated bibliography) and textbooks. Primary sources are preferred because anything interpreted by a second author has potential to be biased by the views of the second author (LoBiondo-Wood & Haber 2002, p. 83).

Critical evaluation of the literature

It is essential to critically evaluate published material in order to determine the quality of the research that is being reported and the 'trustworthiness' of the information that is retrieved. The review must identify the strengths, weaknesses, conflicts and gaps in the literature. A literature review is not simply a matter of just reading large amounts of literature and providing a narration. It should provide some critique to the reader, as to the usefulness of the findings for the current purpose.

Use the following questions as a guide to reflecting on each piece of literature:

- Is each piece relevant to the community/group/topic?
- Are the research processes and outcomes credible and sound?
- Are there flaws in the research design?
- Are reasonable conclusions drawn?
- Is the information *vital* to this review?

Be systematic in collecting the material. After deciding that an item is relevant and useful for the purpose, keep a copy of the article on file or in hard copy so it can be reread, and quoted from if required. Be sure to have all the citation requirements at the time. However, random printing of something that may be peripherally relevant is a waste of paper and time. How broad the review needs to be depends on its purpose. A review to inform data gathering for a major research process or higher degree will necessarily be very comprehensive. A short review for a small funding grant may be limited to literature that relates to the local context.

Making a literature review grid

Making a grid in the reviewing process is a useful activity, which will assist those who are less experienced with writing literature reviews to collate relevant material and to structure their review well. Use a large sheet of paper or a whiteboard that will not be erased. Most people find it easier to have a hard copy of key articles, so they can highlight main points, but this can also be done within computer files. Read all the material first time without marking them, to get an idea of what the key themes are. In this way new key words can be generated and specific sub-topics identified and explored.

In the second reading, highlight aspects of the paper, according to the key themes that are emerging, using the series of questions mentioned in the previous section to critically evaluate each piece. As you do this, collate the grid — add new themes into new columns as they arise. Use a new row for each article. In the cell, write very brief prompts to enable easy identification of the section of the paper

Journal details	Theme 1	Theme 2	Theme 3	Theme 4
Figure 5.2 The literature review grid				
Article 1 *Author* *Title summary* *Location*				
Article 2 *Author* *Title summary* *Location*				
Article 3 *Author* *Title summary* *Location*				

when writing the review (see Figure 5.2). (You may also use a series of different coloured highlighters, according to the different theme in each paper — one colour per column.)

Organisation of the literature review

A good review should answer the following questions:

- What is known about the topic?
- Why is it an important topic?
- What is unknown about the topic?
- Why is it important that the knowledge gap is filled?
- What activities or processes might fill the existing gaps?

The organisation of a literature review needs to tell a logical 'story' to the reader. The process is the same, irrespective of the size of the review. It is useful to conceptualise a literature review as a funnel, which takes the reader from the broad general topic or problem at the start, and narrows through the exploration of key themes to the specific focus of the research or program which emerges at the end of the review.

This conceptual diagram (see Figure 5.3) is useful and draws directly on the grid that was constructed during the reading phase.

Commence with an introduction which sets out the purpose of the review and provides a rationale as to why it is a worthy topic. Introduce any key terms and definitions that are necessary for the reader. Outline any limitations in the breadth of the topic being explored or the search parameters. Next, provide a summary of current knowledge of the problem and introduce the key themes that the review will address (that is, list off the column headings from the grid, in an order that will tell a logical 'story'). Then, depending on the size of the review, a separate section is composed for each of the themes. Use a series of headings as 'signposts' to ensure that everything that is included in the section directly relates to that theme (take the headings out at the end). Each theme becomes a 'mini-essay' in itself; it needs a

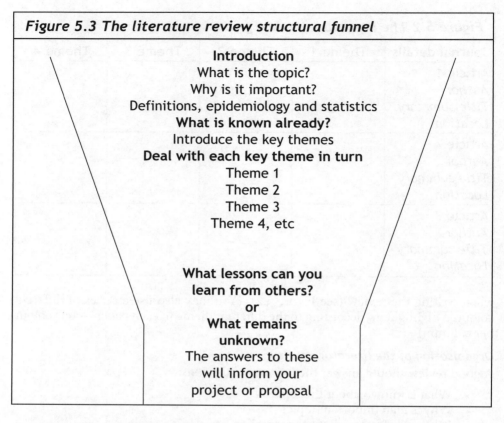

Figure 5.3 The literature review structural funnel

Introduction
What is the topic?
Why is it important?
Definitions, epidemiology and statistics
What is known already?
Introduce the key themes
Deal with each key theme in turn
Theme 1
Theme 2
Theme 3
Theme 4, etc

**What lessons can you
learn from others?
or
What remains
unknown?**
The answers to these
will inform your
project or proposal

strong introduction. This is followed by a 'discussion' of the literature relating to that theme. Include the critique, what was useful, relevant, reliable about the research, what other research concurs or contradicts the findings. Also, highlight gaps in the knowledge. After each theme is dealt with, the conclusion should highlight what has been the purpose of the review. For instance, if it has a research purpose, the conclusion should highlight the topic 'demanding' further exploration; if the review has been to inform health-promotion planning or practice, the conclusion should highlight key action areas or wisdom from the field.

Community profile

Every service that has responsibility to a community will need to have access to a relatively up-to-date profile of that community. This is necessary to have a sense of what needs there may be and what demographic and social issues are likely to be shaping the lives of people in the community. Community health workers may be part of the team that sets about preparing or updating a community profile. It is worthwhile to examine what sort of information will be needed to include in a community profile and some of the general principles involved in preparing it. Henderson and Thomas (1987, pp. 57–68) suggest that a community profile can be considered under six interrelated categories. However, these are meant as a guide to adapt to the profile of each community. Taken together, the information in these categories will provide a picture of the community. However, communities are dynamic and changing and so information will need to be added along the way. A community profile is not something that can be completed and then filed away.

History

An understanding of the history of an area may help health workers understand a great deal about dominant values in the community and may help explain some of the current attitudes towards contemporary events.

Environment

The environment in which people live strongly influences the way in which they can interact with each other. It also may be the source of some health problems for the community (Henderson & Thomas 1987, p. 58). For example, a town that includes a number of dirty industries and is sited in a hollow may face serious environmental pollution; a community may have little recreational space within its boundaries; or a suburb may be designed around the needs of cars, often resulting in lack of access to services for those who do not own cars.

Residents

The information you collect here will include information about demography, housing occupation, employment levels, numbers of people receiving single-parent benefits and pensions, residents' perceptions of the area, community networks, and the values and traditions that guide life in the area (many of these may take some time to discover). This will also include epidemiological data and any other information already available about health problems.

Organisations

Several organisations may operate in, and influence, an area. Their presence and the role they play in the community could provide very useful information. Organisations can be classified under a number of categories, including local and state government bodies, industrial and commercial organisations, religious bodies and voluntary organisations. It is worthwhile finding out about the roles played by each of these organisations in the community. For example, is there a particular company that is the main employer? Is there a religious organisation that involves itself in a lot of community work?

Communication

Knowing which mass communication methods are used in the community will help you to keep in contact with many goings-on. For example, what radio and television stations are received in the area, and which stations seem to be listened to or viewed by which groups of people? Which newspapers are available locally? Is there a local newspaper? A number of other effective communication options may also be operating. For example, are there community noticeboards that are well used?

Power and leadership

Power and leadership can be both formal and informal, and an understanding of both is needed if you are to work in a community. Information of value here includes information about leaders of local political parties, local government and community groups as well as key influential people within those organisations. It may also include information about people who seem to have a strong voice in influencing public debate or a particular organisation but who may not necessarily hold a current position of formal power.

Community survey

Few communities are small enough for it to be possible to ask everyone to define their needs. Therefore, more often than not, a community survey will be conducted with a sample of people. Determining which people to ask in order to obtain an appropriate sample is a key component of planning a needs survey, and may require the involvement of people with expertise in survey development.

Primary data sources

Over the years a great deal of time and money has been spent, and an enormous amount of information has been gathered from communities' members, by researchers doing 'data raids'; that is, gathering information willy-nilly, without a clearly defined purpose in mind. Such processes are clearly unethical. Box 5.3 provides some guidance to screen data-gathering plans before they enter the process.

Qualitative and quantitative data-gathering options

Preliminary consultations

Qualitative and quantitative options are ways of collecting data. The community may inform health workers of issues of concern to them, which may trigger informal information gathering to clarify the felt need. Conversations with other people such as concerned community members, police, teachers, medical practitioners, community workers and others may occur. These health workers and other professionals working in areas related to the health of the community may contribute a great deal to the assessment of needs. In particular, other health workers may themselves have listened to community members or may have conducted formal needs assessments in the past. Furthermore, several different health workers may discuss an issue and each brings to it a slightly different perspective, based on individual experience and professional background. Similarly, they may each notice slightly different issues in the same community. This can all be useful in gaining an understanding of problems and issues facing the community. Combining the assessments is valuable and time and effort can be saved.

It is worthwhile briefly examining the relationship between health workers and their communities. Sometimes health workers suggest that, because they are a part of their community, there is little need to canvass community needs: what they themselves see as problems is an adequate reflection of community needs. However, although health workers may be members of the community, they cannot represent all groups in it. Indeed, as a result of their professional education and socialisation, they bring a particular perspective to health issues. Certainly this perspective is a valuable one that contributes much to the debate about health and health promotion. Nevertheless, it is but one perspective, and it can not be substituted for the opinions of other community members. Therefore, while professional opinion offers a great

---

> **Box 5.3 Why are we doing this needs assessment?**
>
> *Whose concerns are driving it?*
>   How can collaboration between health workers and community members be strengthened in the first instance?
> *Why do we need to know it?*
>   Is all of the information sought in the data-gathering procedures useful? Will it be essential for comprehensive planning?
> *What do we want or need to know?*
>   Use a conceptual framework such as the Ottawa Charter or PRECEDE to assist broad thinking about an issue.
> *How will the information be used?*
>   Gather information about community strengths and social determinants of health to avoid 'victim blaming'.
> *Have all the possible sources of information that will answer the questions been considered?*
>   What useful information sources already exist at local, regional, state or federal levels?
> *Does the plan encompass the best ways for all community members to be engaged in data gathering?*
>   What data-gathering options best suit the characteristics of community members?
>   How will those who are least likely to be involved be reached?
>   Do the funds allow for the preferred approaches?
> *How can the information be organised, analysed and presented?*
>   Participants in a potential program need to 'engage' with the process and understand the outcomes. Does data presentation create a 'living picture' of the data?
>   How can you make sure they know what you have discovered?
> *Have the existing strengths and capabilities of community members been used as a resource in data gathering?*
>   Successful outcomes and sustainability depend on community participation from the beginning. Community members have many under-utilised and under-valued skills.
> *What people and organisations should be involved in gathering the information? Why? How?*
>   Answers to these questions may assist you to answer some of the earlier questions.

deal, it cannot be assumed to reflect the views of the whole community or remove the need for listening to the community or checking external assessments of need. Consider different data-gathering techniques within the program-planning conceptual framework to answer the following questions:

1. What is the community like? What are the characteristics of people, types of organisations, values, beliefs, goals, concerns, problems? Who are the key stakeholders?

2. How does it compare with other communities?

3. What is unique about the community? What are its strengths?

Qualitative approaches

Qualitative approaches are useful for exploring the 'how' and 'why' questions in the community, rather than the 'how many' style of questions used in surveys, which can often be answered readily from national and local census data, and do not usually provide sufficient details to be a basis for planning a community program. Qualitative approaches usually involve face-to-face approaches as distinct from survey methods that are conducted most often using a questionnaire format by mail, telephone and sometimes in person.

There are a number of possible advantages of using qualitative data-gathering approaches in community needs assessments (the list is not exhaustive):

- people have a greater chance of defining and describing what is important to their health and why;
- it gives the researcher the opportunity to follow up on cues and explore issues in detail;
- people are not forced to choose one way or their other — they are able to take a middle ground, or to put up options that have not been previously determined; and
- people can begin to contribute to solutions and strategies.

At the same time qualitative approaches have some disadvantages:

- they are time-consuming and require a skilled interviewer;
- some people are unable to share personal or private information with others;
- anonymity cannot always be guaranteed;
- the process may generate more questions than answers, or problems that cannot be managed by a proposed program, and therefore generate further community frustration; and
- vocal participants can dominate.

Qualitative data-gathering options

- Community forum

A community forum is based on one or more public meetings to which residents are invited to express their opinions about community needs.

- Focus groups

A focus group is a group interview or discussion with a particular focus on an issue of concern. The group is also focused because it has people or characteristics in common.

- Interviews

Face-to-face interviews are conducted with members of the community. Participants may volunteer to take part or they may be identified because they have some particular relevance to the future wellbeing of the community, its services and its people.

In the qualitative data-gathering options mentioned here, it is advisable to use a broad schedule of open questions and themes to guide discussion, that prompt full responses, rather than narrow, closed questions that prompt monosyllabic responses and give no guidance for planning future strategies with the community. Consider using the WHO definition of health discussed in Chapter 1.

- What factors or issues make it easier or more difficult for you to achieve good physical health in your community?
- What factors or issues make it easier or more difficult for you to achieve good emotional health in your community?
- What factors or issues make it easier or more difficult for you to achieve good social wellbeing in your community?

General guidelines for gathering qualitative data in a community are provided in Box 5.4. However, this is a formal research process and it demands appropriate expertise.

Managing the data

Qualitative data are managed systematically using a four-step procedure.

1. *Organising* the data into a useable form, which may include collating notes and/or transcribing interviews.

2. *Shaping* the data, which means identifying key themes and categories. The interview schedule will be useful for this, but some data may fall outside what was anticipated by the questions.

3. *Summarising* the data by identifying the extremes of views or the range of opinion. All responses must be represented, but it is not appropriate to attempt to quantify the results.

4. *Explaining* what is meant by the data, consistent with the responses you have received.

Box 5.4 Guidelines for gathering qualitative data

- It will not be practical to talk to all of the chosen community, so the aim is to canvass a broad range of opinion from all of the sub-groups represented.
- Consider a data-gathering approach that will enable best access; take account of age, gender, ethnic or language background, employment status and area of residence.
- Informal networks as well as mass advertising may be the best way of recruiting participants from the various sub-groups.
- Choose an acceptable and convenient location for the interviews or meetings.
- Prepare a broad interview protocol in advance, which will take only about half an hour. Keep the questions specific to the general theme of health, but be flexible enough to follow strong responses from participants.
- Use a planning model or theoretical framework (such as PRECEDE) to develop the question framework. Pilot test the questions and then refine them.
- Have a research assistant to 'scribe' the responses or tape-record the session (with participants' permission). Allow plenty of time to prepare the seating and facilities.
- Focus groups and public forums need skilled facilitators to ensure that all potential participants have the chance to be heard.
- Journal and record overall impressions and reflections after each session.
- Consider using more than one form of data gathering.
- Involve local community people as researchers; provide training and support.

This is a very brief overview of a complex process requiring research expertise that is best gained through health workers gaining appropriate qualifications in research procedures.

Quantitative research approaches

Surveys

Surveys are particularly useful to study questions such as *how often*? or *how many*? about a particular condition or behaviour. A well-designed survey or questionnaire will enable the researcher to generate a large amount of accurate and reliable information at the least cost. It is important to structure the survey instrument in such a way as to encourage the participants to complete and return it, and also achieve reliable data that informs future planning. A variety of survey techniques can be used, which generally provide anonymity for participants. There are advantages and disadvantages of each approach.

Questionnaire design

Use previously validated questionnaires where possible. For instance the SF36 Short Form Health Survey provides a widely used and validated, quick indicator of health status. It has been developed to provide a general health survey that is 'comprehensive and psychometrically sound, yet short enough to be for practical use in large scale studies' (Stephenson 1996). It covers themes such as physical, social and emotional functioning, role limitations due to health problems, vitality and general health perceptions. As a means of validating the instrument for use in Australia, standard norms for the Australian population have been derived from ABS census data.

If the survey instrument has not been previously validated it is imperative to always pilot test the questionnaire to ensure the questions can be readily understood, that there is a logical sequence and that questions do not *lead* the respondent into a certain response.

Unless appropriate sampling techniques are used to recruit participants into the survey, the researcher must be cautious about making generalisations that apply to the whole community from the responses of a small number.

Reporting the findings to the community

An essential part of any needs assessment is reporting the findings to the people involved. This should be done as a matter of course, to ensure that the information obtained accurately reflects what people said. It will then enable community members to be involved in the priority-setting process discussed below. Responses should be presented in a succinct manner, with key findings in an 'Executive Summary'. The report should be made available through a range of venues/forums, so that all people who took part in the data gathering have an opportunity to know of, and discuss, the results, and to take part in priority setting. Use the media options that will provide the best access, according to the characteristics of the community. Present the information in a format that makes the findings clear and which can be easily understood by all who participated — use tables, graphs, colours, quotes.

Separating the problem from the solutions

In presenting and analysing the findings of a community assessment, it is possible that the need will be expressed in terms of a solution to the problem, rather than the problem itself. Indeed, often when this occurs, the assumption is that the solution presented is the only solution to the problem. This point has also been made elsewhere (Baum 1992, p. 81). It may be how the people interpret the questions about their needs that leads them straight to one well-known solution; for example, another service. You may need to 'peel the onion' and ask what the issue/problem is that leads them to this one solution. It is very important to develop a vision of the problem as separate as possible from any potential solutions, and so broaden the scope for solving the problem by coming up with a range of possible solutions. This process is one in which community members and health workers can think creatively together. It provides an excellent opportunity for consciousness-raising to occur. As people discuss the problems in their community, they may, layer-by-layer, be able to work their way through to alternative conceptualisations of them. This may broaden quite markedly the choices available to them in dealing with those problems.

Setting priorities for action

This step in the community assessment process corresponds with the fourth phase of the PRECEDE–PROCEED model, the educational and ecological assessment.

> Study of the predisposing, enabling, and reinforcing factors automatically helps the planner decide exactly which of the factors making up the three classes deserve the highest priority as the focus of the intervention.

> (Green & Kreuter 1999, p. 42)

It is rarely the case that a community assessment identifies only one need. Sometimes a number of needs may be able to be dealt with together if they all share a similar root cause and you have recognised this in your analysis, but this will not always be the case. It will, therefore, be necessary to set some priorities, as it is rare to have the time or other resources to be able to deal with all the needs at once.

So, how do you set priorities for action? Some people suggest that you deal with the easiest or most 'winnable' issues first (for example, Minkler 1991, p. 272), but there are some problems with this approach. The easiest issues to deal with may not be the ones that make the biggest difference in people's lives. Indeed, the most difficult ones may well have the biggest impact if they are acted on successfully. Priority setting, done in partnership with community members, is most likely to be the most successful approach because of the community support for, and action on, any decisions made. Planners need to be aware of complementary programs that already exist in the community, to avoid duplication, and at the same time they may 'piggy-back' strategies for added impact. Of course, there may be times when the health risks involved are great and time for community involvement may be limited. Even then, however, maximum possible involvement by community members should be built into the decision-making.

Priorities set by national health documents can be taken up if they are identified also as local health needs. The advantage here is that if they are national priorities, it is more likely that funding will be available to support health-promotion projects and health workers will be encouraged to take action in this area. Similarly, some areas may be included in the charter of the agency for which you work, and so these may need to be addressed first. Furthermore, some issues may be able to be dealt with first because the necessary expertise is available in the team with which you are working or because you have ready access to it (Henderson & Thomas 1987, p. 101). While it would be a mistake to build an agency's work around the interests of the staff rather than the needs of the community, acknowledging and working with the expertise of the staff and other available expertise is a valuable use of resources.

There are several questions worth asking about each identified need in order to help to set priorities for action. Those in the following list are based on Lund and McGechaen (1981 in Gilmore et al 1989, p. 22):

- What types of need are present? Does the individual, group or community consider this as a need? What programs are presently available?
- How many people are affected?
- What will the consequences be if this need is not met?
- Is this a critical need that should be met before other needs are addressed?
- How can this need best be met? Is it likely to be affected by health-promotion action?
- Does the need coincide with your department's or agency's mission statement or policies? If not, why not? Can you influence the agency's policies?
- With which community members and other agencies do you need to work in order to address the issue?
- Are resources (funds, staff) available?

Determining the most appropriate response to a need

Once you have determined which needs there are and which need (or needs) you are going to address, the next step is to determine what the best response to the latter will be, before you can plan any action. A very useful framework within which to consider this issue is the Ottawa Charter for Health Promotion. Should the need be dealt with by working for healthier public policy and so creating supportive environments; by working to strengthen community action; by working to further develop people's personal skills (through some form of health education); or by working to reorient the health system to a greater emphasis on health promotion? Or should it be dealt with by a combination of some or all of these approaches? You may decide that action will need to occur on some levels to address the problem in the short term, while you are attempting on other levels to address it over the longer term. For example, working for public policy change may take some time, and in the meantime you may need to help people to develop some of their own skills to deal with the situation they are in.

Working with the community, it is important to choose interventions that fit the purpose the community has chosen as its priority. The priorities for action could fit anywhere along the health-promotion continuum, presented in Chapter 1. Thus, details of strategies will be found in each of the remaining chapters. The final chapter provides more detailed guidance for using the Ottawa Charter for Health Promotion as a framework for health-promotion practice, including designing multifaceted interventions to address the needs of communities.

McKenzie, et al (2005, Chapter 8) provide a useful overview of the types of intervention strategies that a community may consider. They have been arranged here according to the action areas of the Ottawa Charter to indicate how the charter can be used to plan multifaceted approaches to a community issue.

Building healthy public policy

Environmental change activities are strategies that alter or control the legal, social, economic and physical environment. Changes in the things 'around' individuals that may influence their awareness, knowledge, attitudes, skills or behaviour.

Regulatory activities include executive orders, laws, ordinances, policies, position statements, regulations, and formal and informal rules.

Incentives and disincentives.

Creating supportive environments

Communication activities.

Social activities provide recognition that social activities and social support are good for health.

Behaviour-modification activities.

Strengthening community action

Community advocacy activities, such as those presented in Chapter 3, are used to influence social change.

Organisational culture activities.

Developing personal skills

Educational activities.

Technology-delivered activities.

Reorienting health services

Health status evaluation activities.

Funding programs

Before implementing the program, you may be required to write a submission for funding. Funding bodies usually provide guidelines and it is important to read them carefully. Successful applications are the result of systematic program-planning as described above, and careful budgeting. Part of the assessment is necessarily concerned with the organisational capabilities and resources for the development and implementation of the program.

The funding proposal

- **Project summary**
  This outlines who you will be working with, that is the people for whom the project is designed. It outlines the needs that have been identified, the aim, activities, partners and evaluation plan.

- **Background**
  The background describes how you determined the need. This means that you will describe the type of evidence you have collected from the assessments that you have made from both the primary and secondary data sources.
- **Determinants of health**
  How you propose to address the determinants of health for this particular issue is described.
- **Project aim and/or objectives**
  This is a clear outline of the changes you hope will occur as a result of the program.
- **Work plan and timetable**
  Outline the program objectives/strategies, who will be involved, what resources will be needed and a tentative timetable.
- **Evaluation plan**
  How you will evaluate the process is described and then, following an assessment of the process, if you intend to evaluate the impact of the program or the outcome of the intervention.

Evaluating health promotion

In practice, good health promotion is guided by a recurring process of assessing, planning, acting, implementing and evaluating, followed by re-assessing, re-planning, re-acting, re-implementing and re-evaluating, in a continuous cycle of reflection and action similar to action research. In such an approach, the lines between assessment, planning, action and evaluation become fine. Moreover, as this process continues and then recurs, the line between evaluation and assessment becomes particularly unclear. As a result, many of the issues discussed earlier in this chapter are extremely relevant to evaluation.

There is real value in health workers evaluating every aspect of their work, using appropriate methods and approaches. The daily practice of an individual health worker, the overall work of an agency or team, and specific health-promotion activities or projects will all benefit from regular evaluation, either formal or informal. Each health-promotion activity, whether it is community development, lobbying for public policy change or health education, will benefit from some form of evaluation.

This section will draw on needs assessment theoretical frameworks as they relate to evaluation in health promotion, and describe some of the important elements of evaluation applied to daily practice and the activities with which health workers are involved. It will also consider the importance of making evaluation itself a participatory, potentially empowering, experience for both health workers and community members.

What is evaluation?

Evaluation has been described as 'the process by which we judge the value or worth of something' (Suchman 1967, cited by Hawe et al 1990, p. 10). Evaluation is used to determine the strengths and weaknesses of an activity or intervention. The findings may be used as a basis for improving various areas within a program. Evaluation may be as specific as determining the effectiveness of a particular learning aid or activity, or as general as gauging the effectiveness of a community-driven social activity. Evaluation may also allow us to identify inconsistencies that may exist between program goals and implementation processes.

Who is the evaluation for?

Despite the impression we are often given that evaluation is an objective process that will inform us of the 'best' way to proceed, it is clearly a process of judgment, and this judgment can never be value-free. We may describe evaluation by using such terms as *measurement, appraisal, assessment* or *calculation*, but when we use terms such as these it is clear that the objects of interest are compared to some sort of standard or benchmark. Such baselines may be driven by competing values, such as cost control or prior political or organisational decisions to change services.

Evaluation is very much a value-driven process and in a Primary Health Care approach it is the values of Primary Health Care that drive the evaluation. That is, the needs of the people for whom the activity is carried out are foremost, as are issues of community control, social justice and equity. Bedworth and Bedworth (1992, p. 407) describe evaluation as a 'complex process of measurement and judgment which includes gathering and organising and interpreting information'. Judgments and interpretations can be based on different views of the world, by people or organisations holding contrasting values to those of the participants. The challenge is not to remove values from the evaluation process, but to ensure that the process reflects the values of the community *as well* as those of the health and/or funding agencies. Of course, community members or program participants are not the only people interested in the outcomes of health-promotion evaluation. Funding bodies, managers and other health workers may be keen to see health promotion evaluated, and their needs may be very different to those of community members participating in the program.

The ethical values in research, presented earlier in this chapter, are clearly as relevant to evaluation as they are to the needs-assessment process. Both are quality assurance measures using research processes.

Detailed evaluation of the effectiveness of different strategies is often beyond the scope of health workers in their everyday practice and more in the realm of special evaluation projects, conducted by either health workers or skilled researchers or a team of both (Hawe et al 1990, pp. 10–11). Several books examine in detail how to plan and implement evaluation. Although this chapter will examine some of the principles of evaluation, more in-depth examination of the issues and skills is available elsewhere (see, in particular, Wadsworth 1997; Hawe et al 1990).

Approaches to research in evaluation

Evaluation in health care has traditionally been grounded in the positivist approach to research, with a focus largely on quantitative measurement of outcomes. In this approach, experimental techniques, and particularly randomised controlled trials, have been regarded as the most acceptable approach to evaluation. However, this approach is not always appropriate for many health-promotion activities, such as working for policy change or community action, when outcomes may not be amenable to statistical analysis. Even in health education, focus on quantitatively measured outcomes may not always be appropriate because they cannot answer all the questions we need to ask and they are not appropriate for small local projects. There is growing recognition of the importance of both qualitative and quantitative approaches to evaluation, as well as recognition of the importance of a wide range of outcomes not directly related to morbidity or mortality, such as social wellbeing and community participation.

The limitations of a quantitative approach to evaluation have been recognised for some time (Guba & Lincoln 1989), although it seems that the primacy of the quantitative approach remains, particularly with many government decision-makers and funding agencies. Certainly quantitative approaches to evaluation can contribute significantly to evaluation processes when they are used appropriately and in balance with other approaches. However, by their very nature, they are often unable to provide the answers to questions regarded as important in health promotion, particularly to inform program refinement or redesign. Evaluating any activity needs to be built around evaluation methods appropriate to the program and enable it to maintain a level of flexibility sufficient to respond to the needs of the people for whom it is being implemented.

Participatory evaluation

One of the key features of working with a Primary Health Care approach is that the evaluation process actively involves the people for whom the project is running, building on their active involvement in the assessment, planning and implementation of health-promoting activities. It is for this reason that participatory evaluation fits most comfortably with a Primary Health Care approach — because it is built on this active involvement of community members in the evaluation process (Wadsworth 1997). Wadsworth points out that while non-participatory research may come up with useful outcomes, 'a non-participatory, non-democratic process of evaluation cannot *ensure* a user-appropriate outcome' (1997, p. 16). In addition to what is done to promote health, how it is done is very important and can have a positive or negative impact on the people with whom you are working. This is just as true for evaluation as for any other aspect of health promotion — the process of the evaluation activity can itself be a positive or negative experience for both community members and health workers. It is recognition of this fact, along with recognition of the expertise community members have on issues with which they are involved, that is behind support for participatory evaluation. Evaluation that makes conclusions about a health-promotion activity but does so in a way that is disempowering, will be of limited value for community members.

Why evaluate?

Guba and Lincoln (1989) argue that evaluation is the process of sharing accountability, not assigning accountability. On one hand, health workers have a responsibility to their employer to work in accordance with any reasonable demands made of them, while on the other hand they have a responsibility to the individuals and communities they are meant to serve. This dual responsibility has implications for each worker's practice, and the evaluation of the work of the agency. Whether working as a sole practitioner, in a team within a larger institution or as part of a small agency or centre, a health worker will need to find out if their work addresses the needs of those to whom they are accountable. This raises the issue of the dual accountabilities that health workers usually face.

If health bureaucracies and employers uphold a Primary Health Care approach, they are supportive of this primary responsibility and help health workers to respond to the needs of their own communities. Unfortunately, health bureaucracies in minority countries are not reoriented to a Primary Health Care approach, and health workers may often find themselves experiencing some difficulty as they attempt to grapple with their dual accountabilities to central planning agencies and their communities. Evaluating against the principles of Primary Health Care on the one hand, and the sometimes competing requirements of bureaucratic expectations on the other, may present some challenges. Box 5.5 outlines some of the different and competing perspectives that may underpin your decisions about evaluation of a program.

Box 5.5 Perspectives on program evaluation

Communities' or the public's perspective
- to learn about the value of planned change
- to increase community participation in a program or project
- to promote positive public relations
- to be accountable to the community, to enhance public relations

Project worker's perspective
- to be clear whether program activities occurred as planned
- to determine whether the program achieved its objectives, and if not, why not?
- to identify program elements that could be changed
- to inform planning of a new program or developing a comparable one
- to contribute to professional knowledge
- to identify areas for further research, or unmet community needs

The organisation's perspective
- for efficiency, to decide if resources were well spent
- to be accountable, to meet accreditation requirements
- to inform future planning and allocation of resources
- to secure future funding by fulfilling funding body's requirements

The funding body's perspective
- to demonstrate program effects for political purposes
- to provide evidence for more program support
- to contribute to the evidence base

(Source: Sarvela & Mc Dermott 1993, in State Government of Victoria, Department of Human Services 2003 *Health Promotion Short Course Facilitators Guide. Module 1*. Melbourne)

A 'culture' of evaluation

Evaluating practice can be a part of every working day. It can also be part of a more formal process in which health workers, either individually or as part of the team with which they are working, take time out every so often to formally review the activities with which they have been involved and the priorities to which they have been working. Building informal and formal evaluation into one's practice will add greatly to the relevance and the power of health-promotion work.

No amount of formal evaluation will be able to make up for the quality of evaluative work that is possible when informal evaluation is a part of your way of working or that of your team. As we have said earlier in the book, critical reflection is valuable. This process involves developing a 'culture of evaluation' (Wadsworth 1997, p. 57), and it is an essential part of Primary Health Care practice. Questions such as 'What went well there?', 'What would I like to do differently next time?' and 'What else would I like to experiment with next time?' are ones you can ask as a matter of course at the end of each activity. Such questions can easily be asked by every health worker on a regular basis throughout his or her working day as well as at various stages throughout health-promotion programs. Colin and Garrow (1996) describe this process as thinking, listening, looking, understanding and acting as you go along.

Planning for evaluation

It is essential to plan for evaluation at all stages of program-planning. Although the section dealing with evaluation is usually presented after the needs-assessment process has been discussed, as it does here, leaving evaluation planning until after the rest of the program has been planned (or implemented) sets one up for being unable to demonstrate the effectiveness of a program, or clarifying why it was not as effective as desired.

There are many perspectives that have to be incorporated at the planning stage. Evaluation from the point of view of whether or not the needs of the group for whom the service or activity is designed are being addressed should permit some common ground between evaluations from these various perspectives (Wadsworth 1997, pp. 15–16). It is important to note that evaluations cannot be expected to be all things to all people, and so evaluations conducted for different reasons can be conducted separately. Thinking through the implications of all these perspectives at the planning stage will mean that much of the information that is required by the different perspectives can be built into the implementation of the activity, making even formal evaluation for the managers or those funding a project easier than it might be if evaluation is regarded as an 'add-on' activity.

Evaluation challenges for health promotion

The Health Outcomes movement has been growing in momentum with the adoption of economic rationalism and managerialism. It is reflected in an increased expectation that strategies used in response to a health issue should be demonstrated to have a positive effect on health. This represents a serious challenge to much of medical and health care practice for, as the World Health Organization itself has identified, a significant proportion of medical technologies and treatments have not been evaluated for effectiveness. The consequences of this for acute medical care could be far-reaching if there was an increased expectation of health expenditure making an improvement in people's health. Indeed, it would be expected that this itself may result in the health system shifting to a greater balance between illness treatment and health promotion. However, it also raises some significant challenges for health promotion.

Many health-promotion activities are unevaluated, although in many situations there may be anecdotal reports from service users that they found the activity useful, or analyses by health workers that the environment seems to present less of a threat to health, for example. Also, because of the nature of much health-promotion work, which may be long term, developmental and complex, much health-promotion work is very difficult to evaluate, and attributing the cause of changes to specific activities almost impossible (see, for example, Chapman 1993). This by itself is a serious difficulty when decision-makers interpret this as a problem of the work itself rather than the realities of evaluation research. With the increasing evaluation requirements placed on health promoters, there is a great danger that the short-term simple (and potentially less useful) health-promotion activities will be encouraged over the more innovative, longer-term activities, which have the potential to make a real difference to the social determinants of health, primarily because they are more easy to evaluate and outcomes can be reported in a short time frame (Baum 1999, p. 38). That is, workers may be so driven to evaluate that programs are developed to match the evaluation methods available, rather than the other way round. 'Too often the evaluation tail wags the program dog as health workers choose objectives amenable to evaluation' (Freudenberg 1984, p. 46). This may also have the effect of discouraging health workers from taking up innovative health-promotion work — because it is difficult to evaluate.

It is not surprising that evaluation methods lag behind innovative strategies (Hawe et al 1990, p. 9), but it is vital that this should not prevent innovation and experimentation. Hawe and Shiell (1995) suggest that we need to think of health promotion as an investment package, balancing innovative but high-risk (because we can't yet make definitive statements about outcome) programs with the more straightforward low-risk programs in which evidence of effect is provided in the research literature. Indeed, such an approach is needed if we are to implement health promotion across the range of strategies of the Ottawa Charter for Health Promotion. For example, working to increase equity, to improve the health chances of the poor or Aboriginal and Torres Strait Islander people, would have to be regarded as the most important project of health promotion in Australia. Such goals require long-term commitment and resources and face many barriers, but the outcomes if successful could be great. However, if outcome criteria revolve around whether or not a project is easily measurable, specific and achievable within a short funding cycle, a great deal of 'evaluatable' activity may be achieved but it may do little in the long term to improve health.

However, some concern has been expressed recently that government and other funding bodies expect health promotion to be evaluated to a much greater extent than is expected of the rest of the health system. This is not to suggest that evaluation of health promotion is a useless enterprise — clearly, it is very useful. However, those who express concern about evaluation at a greater level than that expected of the mainstream illness management system are concerned that health promotion is being set up to fail by being required to demonstrate its impact on people's health over a short period of time and after relatively minor activities. Furthermore, evaluating activities beyond a reasonable level acts as a drain on the very limited resources available for health promotion. For those reasons, evaluation activities need to be critically reviewed and carefully considered so that inappropriate evaluation does not become part of the problem.

Cautions with evaluation

Thorough planning for evaluation can assist you to avoid a number of pitfalls associated with evaluation, which may fail to accurately indicate where the faults lie with a program. After all, it is a significant waste of resources if you cannot be sure exactly why a program works so well (or it doesn't). If a program is very successful, success really should be shared with others, to save valuable resources and time, or to prevent them from making costly mistakes. The key questions are: Why is the evaluation being done? and, What difference will it make? Two common pitfalls are:

1. Not sufficiently resourcing evaluation. It is better to do a thorough job of one form of evaluation, than to do a hasty, scant job of all forms. Inadequate resourcing, in terms of time, personnel and funds, can mean either that the valuable aspects of a good program are failed to be demonstrated, or you are unable to recognise where the faults lie in an ineffective program.

2. Ignoring the results of the evaluation because of evaluation faults. A poorly planned evaluation may not identify the causal link between goal, objectives and strategies. Therefore no matter how effective the strategies, the evaluation will never demonstrate achievement of an overly ambitious goal. Likewise, evaluation will fail to demonstrate that any form of intervention has been effective, if the program framework is based on an inadequate needs assessment.

Thus evaluation planning must always be done in partnership with program-planning. The following section provides guidelines for the skills involved. In Box 5.6 a series of questions are posed that may be discussed with program-planners and participants at the planning stage, to assist clarification of values and priorities in evaluation.

The question of how to collect the data forms part of the planning process. Questionnaires are often the first thing people think of; however, there are many ways to collect data including face-to-face interviews, telephone interviews, focus groups, stories, documentation, photos, artwork and process mapping.

Types of evaluation

Components of evaluation

There are three key components to evaluation — *process evaluation*, *impact evaluation* and *outcome evaluation*. Together, these components should paint a fairly comprehensive picture of your activity. Which elements fit into each of these categories will depend on just what your activity was aiming to do — something that forms the process of one activity may be part of the outcome of another. Two others, *program monitoring and accountability* and *economic evaluation* will only be covered briefly here.

Process evaluation

Process evaluation is about evaluating the way in which a health-promotion activity or strategies were implemented. Because of the centrality of process in the

---

> **Box 5.6 Foci of evaluation**
>
> *Why will you evaluate?*
>   Whose needs/agenda will be served?
> *Who will you evaluate?*
>   Participants? Wider community? Project workers?
> *What will you evaluate?*
>   Strategies? Objectives? Goal/Aim?
>   Are they able to be 'measured'?
> *Where will you evaluate?*
>   Location? Will your presence alter the outcome?
> *When will you evaluate?*
>   Before, during and/or after?
> *How will you evaluate?*
>   Is it a participatory process?
>   Qualitative approaches?
>   Quantitative approaches?
>   Observational approaches?
>   Is it ethical?
> *What are the expectations concerning the report?*
>   Do the stakeholders agree on these issues?

Primary Health Care approach to health promotion, examination of the process of the activity is particularly important. Several issues need to be examined:

- Is the program or activity reaching the people for whom it was designed?

- What do the participants think of the program or activity?

- Is the program or activity being implemented as planned?

- Are all aspects of the program of good quality?

(Hawe et al 1990, p. 61)

In addition, the particular process elements important in a Primary Health Care approach will include such things as how power was shared between health workers and participants — that is, what kind of participation occurred — and to what extent the direction of the project changed in response to the needs of the participants.

Impact evaluation

In impact evaluation, the immediate effects of the program are assessed. The questions relate to whether the objectives of the program have been met. The evaluation often relates to changes in knowledge, behaviour, attitudes at an individual level, or social support or community strength at the community level.

Outcome evaluation

Outcome evaluation is about assessing the long-term effects of the program and the questions in this type of evaluation relate to whether the program or project goal or aim has been achieved. The evaluation often relates to health indicators, health status or quality of life and so it is often the type of evaluation conducted beyond the organisational level. Health departments usually measure these things. However, it may also relate to community strength and this is within the realm of the organisation.

173

Aims and objectives that are clearly stated will be relatively easy to evaluate, while it will be difficult to evaluate those which are not clearly stated because it may not be possible to work out just what was intended by the person or people who wrote the objectives.

Both impact and outcome evaluation are known as goal-based evaluation because the goals set in the planning phase for the activity or project are evaluated (McKenzie & Jurs 1993, p. 204). Figure 5.4 shows the internal logic of goal-based program-planning and evaluation. The strategies need to be evaluated first. Without knowing whether the program reached the expected audience and what strategies worked we cannot proceed to assessing the objectives, and similarly, if the objectives are not evaluated we do not know what contributed to the success of the goal.

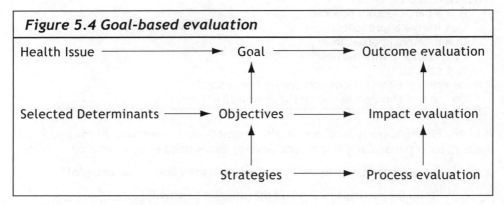

Figure 5.4 Goal-based evaluation

Health Issue ⟶ Goal ⟶ Outcome evaluation

Selected Determinants ⟶ Objectives ⟶ Impact evaluation

Strategies ⟶ Process evaluation

Evaluation carried out by comparing results with goals and objectives is not a complete evaluation of the outcome of a project because it does not provide an opportunity to note any outcomes that do not relate directly to the aims and objectives. These outcomes may either add greater benefit to the activity or undermine some of its other benefits. In either case, these unpredicted consequences are an important part of the program, and reliance solely on evaluation against aims and objectives would have caused them to be missed. For these reasons, some evaluation not directly linked to the aims and objectives is useful. This is described by some as 'goal-free evaluation' (McKenzie & Jurs 1993, p. 207). Wadsworth (1997, p. 39) describes this goal-free evaluation as open-ended inquiry. She highlights the importance of conducting it before starting any examination of whether specific aims and objectives have been met. This is because this process of measurement against objectives is itself fairly narrow and does not encourage creativity. Doing this evaluation first may mean that it is then very difficult for people to think broadly and creatively. Open-ended inquiry will not, however, make it difficult to examine later the extent to which aims and objectives have been met, and, indeed, may help health workers evaluate aims and objectives themselves.

Another limitation of evaluating against aims and objectives is that the value of the evaluation is dependent on the quality and appropriateness of the aims and objectives, and therefore on the quality of the research on which they were based and the process by which they were developed (Wadsworth 1997, p. 48). Relying solely on aims and objectives that may not have been drawn up under optimum conditions severely limits the potential value of any evaluation.

Wadsworth (1997, pp. 48–9) suggests that the philosophical values that guide the development of an organisation may provide better guidance for an evaluation than the specific aims and objectives. This is because aims and objectives may not reflect the value base and long-term goals of the organisation, and the extent to which this has been implemented may in fact be the most important thing for you to evaluate.

Basic program monitoring and accountability

This evaluation occurs at the organisational level and assesses management practices; for example, quality assurance processes such as regular review of planning processes. Evaluating the work of an agency or team is a vital process to prevent it wandering from its original goals or away from addressing the needs of the community. Informal evaluation can be incorporated into the normal work of the agency or team; for example, through discussion and reflection at weekly staff meetings. It will be necessary, however, for the agency or team to take time out to evaluate itself more formally and to involve the community in this process. This can be done by setting time aside specifically for evaluation and strategic planning. Although much of this can occur as a regular internal process, such as yearly evaluation and planning days, it can also be done by involving the agency or team in formal evaluation processes that include external evaluators. In these situations, however, care must be taken to ensure that the process is a supportive and useful one for the health workers and community members concerned.

Economic evaluation

This type of evaluation is based on a cost-benefit analysis. It assesses value for money and is assigned to the funding body. In this evaluation, the resources consumed, such as time and money, are assessed as being efficient relative to the population served.

Evaluating change at the community level

In Chapter 4 the discussion centred on citizens increasing their abilities to control decisions that affect their community and community development workers applying the DARE criteria (Rubin & Rubin 1992, p. 77) as a means of ensuring that decision-making continued to reflect the needs and concerns of the communities they work with.

Who **d**etermines the goals?

Who **a**cts to achieve the goal?

Who **r**eceives the benefits from the actions?

Who **e**valuates the actions?

The DARE criteria can be used to evaluate the success of an organisation that aims for community participation in program development.

There are other indicators that measure the extent of participation in activities such as:

175

- needs assessment;
- leadership;
- organisational focus and operation;
- style of resource mobilisation; and
- management and decision-making processes (Bjars et al 1991 in Baum 2002, p. 187).

The extent of participation and the different perceptions of the stakeholders about the degree of the participation can be mapped over time, by giving each indicator a score from one to five.

Evaluation reports

Having done the evaluation, it is then necessary to write the report. This helps health workers, organisations and funding bodies make decisions about the changes that need to be made to the program (if any). Reports also bring the issue to the attention of others and promotes greater understanding of issues. Individual, community or policy changes may take place as a result of disseminating this information. All stakeholders need to have access to the information, particularly those who designed the program or for whom the program was designed. In order that the evaluation report meets the needs of the widest possible audience, use the series of questions presented in Box 5.7 to guide evaluation and reporting planning.

Box 5.7 Evaluation reports
Who is the report for?
Do you need more than one report?
What is the appropriate format?
What is the appropriate length?
What is the appropriate language?
How should the report be disseminated?

(Source: State Government of Victoria, Department of Human Services 2003 *Health Promotion Short Course Facilitators Guide. Module 1*. Melbourne)

Conclusion

Research is an integral part of a Primary Health Care approach to health promotion. It has potential both to provide invaluable information for the understanding of major health issues and how best to address them, and to itself be a health-promoting activity when it is conducted using participatory research processes.

One of the key uses of research in health promotion is in the community assessment process. Community assessment incorporates assessment of both needs and resources and provides a firm foundation on which health-promotion priorities can be set and action undertaken. Community assessment may be both a formal and an informal process, but it is always a means to achieve health-promoting change for community members; it is never an end in itself.

The other key use of research is evaluation which should be an integral component of good health-promotion practice and therefore an integral component of the daily practice of health workers. It enables us to ensure the relevance and appropriateness of practice, enabling health-promotion practice to contribute to important long-term goals.

There are several challenges in evaluation for health workers aiming to work using a Primary Health Care approach. Firstly, the pressure to demonstrate success should not discourage innovation in health-promotion practice. Secondly, the accountability demands of those providing the funding should not prevent meaningful evaluation enabling the active participation of community members and should not prevent health workers from learning how activities may be improved. Thirdly, evaluation should not be regarded as an 'add-on' activity considered separately from other aspects of health-promotion planning. Finally, evaluations should rarely, if ever, be an end in themselves. The ultimate value of any evaluation will be determined by what improvement in health-promotion practice resulted.

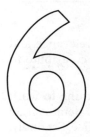

6

Education for health

In Chapter 6, we move along the continuum of health-promotion approaches outlined in Chapter 1 and begin to examine the behavioural approaches to health promotion. There is a range of strategies used in this approach, including education strategies, which will be the focus of this chapter. These strategies fit well with the Ottawa Charter for Health Promotion's action area of developing personal skills.

Education plays a central role in health promotion. Not only is education itself a common health-promotion strategy, but working for public policy change, community development, using the mass media, and working with individuals and groups, all involve education in some form or another — whether it be education of policy-makers, health workers or community members. Education is therefore inextricably linked with all other forms of health promotion. This chapter reviews some of the principles of education for health, and considers the particular approaches to education that sit most comfortably with the Primary Health Care approach.

Defining health education

Health education has been defined as '. . . any combination of learning experiences designed to facilitate voluntary adaptations of behaviour conducive to health' (Green 1980). There are two important elements in this definition. The first is that health education entails much more than the formal 'teaching' sessions that we may traditionally expect to undertake in this role. This point is emphasised by Bedworth and Bedworth (1992, p. 7) in their definition of health education.

> Health education includes all of those experiences — deliberate and planned, or incidental; direct or indirect — that affect the way people think, feel, and act in regard to their own health and that of the society in which they live.

The second important point in Green's (1980) definition (above) is that the focus of health education must be on skills enhancement to facilitate informed decision-making about health. Health education is not a matter of 'telling' people what they 'need to know'. Health education opportunities can arise on unexpected and serendipitous occasions, as well as in more planned and structured sessions. All health workers have an important role to play in enhancing knowledge and in assisting people to make informed decisions about their health-promoting

178

activities. It is essential that health workers have the ability to competently assess educational needs and to be able to enhance learning in the most appropriate manner for individuals, groups and communities.

The following chapter allows health workers to explore the teaching and learning role in a variety of health-related settings and campaigns. To enhance understanding, analysis and wider application of health education approaches, health workers should become familiar with core concepts and some selected educational models widely applicable in health education practice.

Rationale for health education

In recent times there has been criticism of the use of health education approaches, particularly when they are conducted instead of, or at the expense of, social and structural changes. These issues are dealt with briefly below. However, there are important reasons why health education still forms an essential component of the health-promotion workers' 'toolkit'. The first is that health knowledge is in itself empowering. Knowledge about health is a basic human right. People have the right to accurate information about issues that affect their health, in a form that is accessible and appropriate to their learning needs. Without knowledge people cannot make decisions about their own lifestyles or be equipped for political or social lobbying to change things for society generally. The second reason is that health education can enable people to make changes in their activities to reduce the risks to their health. In this way, some of the morbidity that is associated with chronic illnesses that affect many people later in life, such as heart and lung diseases, can be reduced. This has clear personal health benefits and economic benefits for the whole population in terms of reduced expenditure on medical care and pharmaceuticals.

Thus, the purposes of health education are to promote the presence of conditions that assist people in creating health-enhancing conditions for personal and community health.

Critique of health education behaviour change approaches

The first critical element relates to the concept of 'victim blaming'. When we place responsibility for managing the factors that make illnesses more likely with an individual — the so-called 'lifestyle' — there is potential to 'blame' those who are unable to make these changes for their 'failure'. The inference here is that because a person knows that a behaviour, such as smoking, is not good for their health, that they will be able to change this behaviour, and it is their own fault if they do not. The issue of victim blaming is also discussed in Chapter 2.

The second element of criticism is that expenditure on health education for behaviour change diverts attention from the structural causes of disease in social policy. Health education provides a political excuse for avoiding decisions about broad healthy public policies. Behaviour change approaches can be more expediently implemented during the course of one political term and they are more readily evaluated than the community building strategies that we outlined in Chapter 4.

Thus, it is useful to think of health education as a function of 'health literacy'. Being literate about one's health or the community's health is an enabling factor in health promotion. It enables one to make a whole range of choices and to take a whole range of actions at personal and community levels.

Values in health education

Chapter 2 reviewed several key values in health promotion, many of which have particular relevance to health education. In particular, the attitudes of health workers towards community members, the presence or absence of victim blaming or labelling, and whether health workers see education as an opportunity for encouraging compliance or empowerment, all have a major impact on both the way in which education occurs and the likely outcome of that education.

Health workers using a Primary Health Care approach work in partnership with community members, recognising the expertise that community members bring to the learning process. They are careful to avoid victim blaming, working with people to help change the environment as well as individual behaviours when people determine they need assistance to change these. As we have said, health workers using the Primary Health Care approach recognise education as an enabling strategy rather than one to encourage compliance with others' wishes. For this to occur the focus is on participation in which community members have decision-making power, not merely token involvement. Because of the central role of these values in health education, readers are encouraged to review Chapter 2 if you are not familiar with these issues.

Education approaches to address the social determinants of health

Education for critical consciousness

The concept of education for critical consciousness, critical consciousness-raising, or conscientisation was developed in its original form by Freire, although similar ways of working have also been developed by others. For example, the consciousness-raising techniques of the women's movement have much in common with Freire's education process. This approach to education offers a great deal to Primary Health Care because of the focus on working *with* people and because it provides a framework for action in dealing with the root causes of problems as recognised by people themselves. It provides an important link between the lives and experiences of individuals and change at a structural level.

Freire (1973, p. 13) criticised traditional notions of education for amounting to cultural invasion, as representatives of powerful groups impose their view of the 'facts' on less powerful members of society. He argued that education is never neutral because it in some way either confirms or challenges the status quo. On the basis of this premise, he argued for education that challenges the status quo and thus enables the empowerment of oppressed members of society and the development of a more just social system. Education for critical consciousness focuses on changing the environment rather than the individual alone, by working with people to examine the underlying issues behind their problems and to change the structures around them.

Freire (1968, cited by Minkler and Cox 1980, p. 312) argued that social change can be achieved only by the active participation of the people as a whole — it cannot be achieved by strong leaders alone. Therefore, action for change must be built on critical reflection and action by everyone concerned. This process of critical reflection and action is described by Freire as 'dialogue', a two-way process occurring between 'teachers' and 'learners', in which both are teacher–learners. Education for critical consciousness is a process of problem-posing that leads people through analysis of their personal situation, and then of the underlying social issues, to making a plan for action to address the issues they have discovered. The four steps involved in the process are:

1. reflecting upon aspects of their reality (e.g. problems of poor health, housing, etc.);

2. looking behind these immediate problems to their root causes;

3. examining the implications and consequences of these issues; and finally,

4. developing a plan of action to deal with the problems collectively identified.

(Minkler & Cox 1980, p. 312)

Before such a process can occur, however, health workers need to listen carefully to the needs articulated by community members and take the time to understand their problems as they see them (Wallerstein & Bernstein 1988, p. 382). They also need to observe the dynamics of the groups and individuals concerned to determine what sense of belonging or community exists. Some sense of community or group belonging seems to be important for the conscientisation process to work effectively (Minkler & Cox 1980, p. 320). It is for this reason that education for critical consciousness often goes hand in hand with community development.

Education for critical consciousness as described by Freire may not fit every learning situation that arises. However, the principles of problem-posing, two-way communication and sensitivity to people can be used in any learning situation, so that it becomes an enabling process for the people involved. The following general guidelines for more traditional health education give some indication of how this can occur.

Health education planning frameworks

By now you will be familiar with the continuum of health-promotion approaches, first presented in Chapter 1. The subsequent chapters in this text have presented approaches to health promotion, according to the particular focus of the activity. Community development approaches are most appropriate to address the social determinants of health, because they are most likely to lead to sustainable changes in the social context of people's lives. However, as we have argued above, there are times when a different focus is necessary and the aim of the health worker becomes one of enhancing the health literacy of individuals and groups. When planning health education strategies for individuals and groups it is useful to 'map' the activity, to ensure it meets the educational needs of the group, and that it enables them to make informed decisions affecting their health.

A clear understanding of the educational purpose is essential if we are to be effective in educating for health. A number of conceptual models have been used in order to understand the characteristics of the participants in an education program, and to enhance planning of activities that meet their educational needs. A conceptual model can be defined as 'a diagram of proposed causal linkages among a set of concepts believed to be related to a particular health problem (Earp and Ennett 1991, p. 164). In a model, the concepts or factors of influence are denoted by boxes, and the processes or relations between the concepts are delineated by arrows. In this way a model presents a visual image of the reasoned explanation of a hypothesis about a series of abstract principles — a theory. Models are based on theories.

The Health Belief Model is one health educational planning model (see Figure 6.1). Whilst the Health Belief Model has been presented in some detail here, because it is widely used and has been extensively validated, it is by no means the only useful model for health education planning. A number of other planning models are widely used in health behaviour approaches, such as the Transtheoretical (stages of change) Model and the Theory of Reasoned Action. Nutbeam and Harris (2004) and Naidoo and Wills (2000) both provide very useful overviews of a range of commonly used planning models.

The Health Belief Model is based on social learning theory, developed to provide a framework for explaining why some people take action to avoid a specific illness or condition, and others do not. The model can be used to suggest interventions that would make some individuals more likely to engage in health protective behaviours. The Health Belief Model is specifically useful when planning health protective activities for particular groups in relation to a specific condition. It is not designed for use in social change movements (Becker 1974).

The Health Belief Model predicts that an individual is likely to take the action based on the interaction between four conceptual areas.

1. Their perceptions about the seriousness of a given condition. *Perceived susceptibility* is a person's estimate of their probability of encountering the health condition. This estimate is dependent on their knowledge, and thus it is an important function of health education to provide accessible, reliable information as required.

2. Their perceptions about the severity of the condition. *Perceived seriousness* relates to the difficulties that individuals believe a given health condition would create. These difficulties may include the implications for work, family and social life, so the emotional response of an individual to a condition is significant here. It is only when the perceived seriousness is manageable — neither too low to be insignificant, nor too great to

contemplate — that a person can contemplate a change in behaviour. Thus, launching into a health education message, when a person is overwhelmed by other issues and needs support, is not only unethical, but also ineffective.

3. Their perceptions about the benefits of taking action to avoid or detect the condition. *Perceived benefits* of recommended preventive actions are important determinants of health protective behaviours. For example, women who believe Pap smears can detect cancer early, and this results in a good prognosis, are more likely to take part in screening.

4. People weigh up in their minds about the benefits of the action against their perceptions about the barriers to them taking action to avoid the condition. *Perceived barriers* may be personal — such as the embarrassment or unpleasantness of having the procedure — or they may be social — such as cost, inconvenience or the frequency of the desired behaviours that are required, and the extent of life changes. These barriers give important guidelines for health workers on planning their sessions according to the needs and characteristics of their audience. Perceived barriers may also provoke anxiety for the person, which prevents objective analysis of the choice of action. Hence, it is important to always provide an 'action-plan' when giving a health education message (Leventhal et al 1984).

The model predicts that people's perceptions in these four areas are influenced by a range of *modifying* factors; internal factors, such as personality, and external factors, especially socio-demographic and cultural factors. For example, women are predisposed to prevention more than men; peer groups can force conformity. Some factors such as age, sex, income and education have been correlated with health service use. To a lesser extent perceptions about particular health conditions, and undertaking the desired activity are also influenced by a number of internal and external cues. It may be that an internal cue, such as a physical discomfort, or a feeling of discomfort when a person thinks about a threat to their health, triggers them to act. It may also be that an external cue, such as mass media, advice from others or the illness of another person, triggers the activity. The cues to action make the person aware of their own feelings about the health behaviour. It is not clear how strong the trigger needs to be or the specific timing. A good example of the use of cues is the use of roadside billboards by the Transport Accident Commission (TAC) with graphic images of car accidents, used to prompt drivers to act safely. When all these influences on health action are taken into account and understood about the participant group, it is then possible to make assumptions about their likelihood of engaging in preventive action. Of course, health education alone may not be sufficient to overcome the barriers to change for some people. Issues such as addictions and social, economic, environmental and psychological barriers may be understood by using the model, but they may not be able to be altered to a sufficient degree to enable the person to change their behaviour.

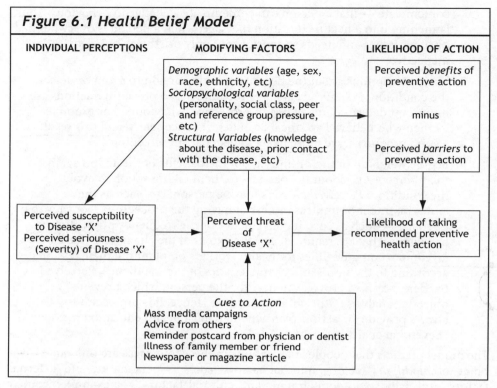

Figure 6.1 Health Belief Model

INDIVIDUAL PERCEPTIONS   MODIFYING FACTORS   LIKELIHOOD OF ACTION

Demographic variables (age, sex, race, ethnicity, etc)
Sociopsychological variables (personality, social class, peer and reference group pressure, etc)
Structural Variables (knowledge about the disease, prior contact with the disease, etc)

Perceived *benefits* of preventive action

minus

Perceived *barriers* to preventive action

Perceived susceptibility to Disease 'X'
Perceived seriousness (Severity) of Disease 'X'

Perceived threat of Disease 'X'

Likelihood of taking recommended preventive health action

Cues to Action
Mass media campaigns
Advice from others
Reminder postcard from physician or dentist
Illness of family member or friend
Newspaper or magazine article

Teaching and learning education theory

The role of the health worker has changed from the past where the role was to give people knowledge so they would be compliant people, to one now which is to generate competence and assist people apply their knowledge under changing conditions. These days, there is an added focus on what happens inside the 'learner', rather than what the 'teacher' does. Learners are no longer expected to be passive recipients of information delivered by experts. They have an active role in the teaching–learning process.

The teaching–learning process

Leddy and Pepper describe three key assumptions that should underpin effective teaching–learning (1989, pp. 317–33):

1. Teaching–learning is a process, not a product — that is, new information and skills are not the only goals. How that learning occurs is equally important and may contribute greatly to the learning process.

2. The teaching–learning process occurs between people who all bring their own expertise to the situation, whether it be the expertise of personal and collective experiences or the more theoretical expertise carried by health workers.

3. The teaching–learning process needs to be built on effective communication and mutual respect.

These principles demonstrate the importance of a partnership approach to working with community members. Both the community member (or members), and the health worker contribute to the discovery of potential solutions in a supportive atmosphere in which learners are allowed the dignity of risk and assume responsibility for decisions they make (Ewles & Simnett 1999, pp. 174–6). In such an approach, education is a guided problem-solving process in which both 'teacher' and 'learner' are open to learning from each other. It is worthwhile considering briefly the two major philosophical approaches to education that continue to underpin the way health education practitioners undertake their role.

Pedagogy

Pedagogy is the art and science of teaching children. The premise behind this approach is the transmission of knowledge. Using this approach fits within the traditional 'teaching' sessions where 'learners' are presented with information. Transmittal of knowledge as the main form of education was only appropriate when the time-span of major cultural change was greater than the lifespan of individuals. That is, what people learned in their youth would remain valid and useful for the rest of their lives. In some instances pedagogical strategies are appropriate regardless of the age of the learner, such as when someone is very dependent as a learner but needs to gain new skills. A key consideration is that the approach is not used by a 'teacher' who wants to keep the learners dependent (Knowles 1980, pp. 43–4). However, we must prepare individuals to face a variety of conditions in their lives, so this 'lecture' method is really only appropriate when:

- the basic purpose is to disseminate information;
- the material is not readily available elsewhere;
- it is necessary to arouse interest in the subject; or
- it is necessary to provide an introduction or reinforcement about a topic.

Andragogy

Andragogy has been defined as the art and science of helping adults to learn (Knowles 1980). In this situation an adult is one who behaves as an adult and whose self-concept is that of an adult; a person who can take responsibility for his or her own life. As people mature as learners their self-concept moves from dependency, such as we may observe in lower primary school education, towards increasing self-directedness, where the learner follows learning paths that interest them. Accumulated life experiences are an increasing resource for learning, and from this base more meaning is attained by learning from experience. Learning is problem-centred, therefore people become ready to learn when they need to solve a real-life task or problem. Learning is reinforced by immediate application of knowledge.

The andragogy/pedagogy models are not seen as dichotomous, but as two ends of a spectrum. Most realistic health education situations fall between the two ends where the facilitator makes use of a variety of teaching and learning approaches to create the context most conducive for the audience to learn. However, because most audience members for health education will have reached educational maturity, a number of adult learning principles should guide education strategies.

Facilitating the teaching–learning process

Adult learning principles

Several principles guide effective teaching–learning and build on the philosophical base of the teaching–learning process described above. They provide some general guidelines that can be applied to any teaching–learning situation:

- allow people to direct the learning process;
- get to know the people's perspective;
- be aware of the context of people's lives;
- build on what people already know;
- planned achievements need to be realistic;
- take account of all levels of learning; and
- present information in logical steps.

Each will be explored briefly in the following section.

Allow people to direct the learning process

Active participation of community members in the education process is paramount to successful education. Involve the learners in planning, carrying out and evaluating their own learning (Knowles 1980). Individual or community-controlled education is much more likely to address the issues of concern to people, when they are ready, and in the order that will help them to learn most effectively.

Participation to the point of control over the education process fits comfortably with the Primary Health Care approach. It is also supported by the principles of adult learning, which recognise the need for learners to direct the learning process and for learning to address the problems that learners themselves want to address. This principle was originally thought to apply only to adult learners, but there is growing recognition that it is just as relevant to child learners (Kalnins et al 1992).

Individual or group-controlled learning is most likely to occur if people themselves set the goals of learning. Helping people clarify just what it is they want to learn is therefore an important part of the education process. Active participation can also be encouraged by maximising interactive teaching techniques and activities, rather than taking an 'empty vessel' approach and 'filling' passive recipients with information. People need to be able to have their say, use their initiative, experiment and find out what works for them. Structuring education so that these things are possible is therefore another priority for health workers who are eager to facilitate learning. Which interactive techniques and activities are appropriate will vary depending on the situation, the people involved, and on whether you are involved in education for individual change or education for social change. Commonly used interactive activities include debating contentious issues, using structured group activities, planning action to address a problem and practising the action required (whether that be drafting a letter to a local councillor, role-playing the negotiation between work colleagues about smoking in the workplace, or preparing a low-fat meal). It is important to point out, though, that interactive techniques do not by themselves ensure interactive learning, nor is interactive learning precluded by the use of what are traditionally regarded as non-interactive techniques, such as lectures. Rather, it is how teaching techniques are used that ultimately determines the extent and success of interactive learning. Once again, emphasis should focus on how the health worker and learners use the teaching techniques, rather than solely on which techniques are used.

Get to know the people's perspective

Teaching–learning is effectively a communication process and as such is built on an understanding of the background and ideas of the other person or people. Build new knowledge on the base of the learners' past experience. This is often a long slow process and not necessarily one that can be completed before the teaching–learning begins. Rather, you need to be open to learning about the other person's perspective throughout the teaching–learning process, and to adapt your approach accordingly. A person's attitudes towards relevant issues, their cultural background, their life experience and topics currently of priority for them may all influence their approach to learning and their ability to act. To ensure that communication is effective, pay particular attention to the needs of people who have impaired sight or hearing, low literacy skills or any other communication problem.

Be aware of the context of people's lives

The active participation of people in directing the learning process will help to ensure that education does not occur out of the context of their lives. Centre learning experience on the real-life situations of the participants (Knowles 1980). This will again enable learning to be directed to the specific needs of the learners, taking account of such things as the particular barriers to action that they need to address and any other issues that may be more important to them than those identified by health workers. Being aware of the whole situation with which people are dealing will also help to identify other strategies that may be needed to address the issue at hand. Using conscientisation, this would then mean that these other strategies would become part of the education process. For example, letters may be written to members of parliament regarding the re-routing of a main road, while road safety education may be conducted to deal with the problem in the short term.

Build on what people already know

The active participation of community members in the learning process will help to ensure that education starts from the point where it is easiest for people to begin to learn. This builds on what people already know, providing new material in a format and at a pace that is appropriate to the learner or learners. Finding out what people know in a way that does not leave them feeling vulnerable is an important skill here. For example, 'Can you tell me what you have heard about osteoporosis?' provides people with more scope to express ideas they are unsure of than asking people what they 'know' about the topic. Treat mistakes as occasions for learning.

Planned achievements need to be realistic

Education is much more likely to be effective if realistic, achievable goals are set rather than expecting to achieve too much all at once. It will be useful, therefore, to spend some time with the people, finding out what they want to achieve and assisting them to adapt their plans if they seem unrealistically high or low. Helping people to plan what they want to achieve so that it is divided into a number of manageable pieces can also help them to keep track of their progress.

Take account of all levels of learning

Learning has traditionally been regarded as occurring on three levels — knowledge, attitudes and behaviour. While this schema has been criticised in recent years, it provides a useful guide. Consideration of whether knowledge development, attitudes and values clarification, or behaviour change and skill development are needed will help determine on what level or levels learning needs to occur. Several health education books describe teaching strategies and the level or levels of learning to which they are suited. In reality it is often impossible to separate knowledge, attitudes and behaviour, so attempting to separate them during the learning process is not always realistic. The following section on the domains of learning will assist in formulating broad educational objectives.

Present information in logical steps

If people are to learn effectively, new ideas need to be provided in a logical sequence in which more complex ideas are built on simpler ones. Some planning is therefore needed to structure ideas so that they are presented in an ordered fashion. Of course these plans may be let go, to some extent, as learners direct the process through their questions and other activities, but the plan remains a useful framework. The notion of learning having to start with simple ideas before moving on to more complex ones has been questioned in recent years. As with the notion of starting with achievable issues in community development, there is growing recognition that people may be quite able to deal with complex ideas when they relate to their own experiences or the problem to be solved, without needing to discuss the more simple ideas first. In these instances, people are likely to be motivated to learn about the complex issues, since they relate to the problem at hand.

Facilitating adult learning

When working with any audience, including adult learners, it is important to value and respect the wisdom that participants bring to the learning environment. In addition, we must recognise that many learners are challenged and unnerved by being placed in a learning setting, especially if they are made to feel inferior. The following points provide guidance as to how the facilitator can manage the environment positively.

- Be a good listener. 'Hear' the participants, value their contributions and make links between their contributions and the key themes around the topic.
- Communicate effectively with warmth, respect and encouragement. A superior attitude to participants will make them less likely to contribute.
- Be able to clarify points of difficulty or confusion. While a good knowledge of the topic is useful, the facilitator should not expect to know 'everything'. Knowledge gaps can be treated as opportunities for exploration, without losing the respect of participants. The participants will know very early if the facilitator is trying to make them believe they have more knowledge than them.
- Be flexible to adjust to the needs of the learners. The pace and detail in a theme will vary according to the prior learning, including life experiences of the participants, and their need for the information at the time.

- Don't 'own' the topic. This is a sign of a confident and mature facilitator. One of the key skills health workers need to learn is to relinquish 'control' of the group, and allow it to be led by the participants. A facilitator may need to 'steer' the discussion to ensure that topics the group decides are important, are covered.

Cognitive, affective and psychomotor domains of learning

During the process of learning, health education takes the learner through a series of stages. The Health Belief Model, presented earlier in the chapter, is one model that can be used to understand the learner's needs and to assist them to move through the different learning stages. The first stage is the acquisition of health facts. Accurate information is the basis on which a person develops their likelihood to take health-enhancing action. The second stage is the development of health attitudes and values about the health issue. The third stage may involve development of personal skills relevant to the health activity. Learning of facts does not necessarily alter behaviour. Personal attitudes and values about the health issue have the greatest influence on eventual health behaviour.

Domains of learning

Bloom (1964) developed a 'taxonomy of educational objectives'. A taxonomy is a system of classification. Bloom argued that learning can be classified into three domains (cognitive, affective and psychomotor) according to the type of learning that is taking place. Each domain is further categorised according to the level or complexity of behaviour that is being learned, progressing from the simple to the most complex. Classifying learning processes into these three domains serves to strengthen the understanding of the learning processes. The domains can be used as a framework for writing learning objectives, based on the adult learning principles presented earlier. As argued there, it is not appropriate to develop separate activities for learning knowledge (cognitive), attitudes (affective) and behaviour (psychomotor), because the concepts are interwoven. Each domain is related to a holistic process and to the individual needs and developmental tasks. It is clear that if one uses the Health Belief Model as a basis for planning health education activities, that each of the three domains is relevant to facilitating participant learning.

Cognitive domain

The cognitive domain describes learning which relates to the recall and recognition of knowledge and the development of intellectual abilities. This is a hierarchical domain, in that each level of learning becomes more complex and builds on the learning processes of the prior level (Bloom 1964). The hierarchical arrangement with illustrative examples is set out in Box 6.1.

Box 6.1 Taxonomy of cognitive learning domain		
Level 1	Knowledge	Recall of facts, methods and procedures
Level 2	Comprehension	Combining recall and understanding
Level 3	Application	Using information in new specific and concrete situations
Level 4	Analysis	Distinguishing components and understanding relationships between components
Level 5	Synthesis	Putting the information into a unified whole
Level 6	Evaluation	Judging the value of ideas, procedures and methods

(Source: derived from Bloom, B. S. 1964 *Taxonomy of Educational Objectives: the Classification of Educational Goals.* Longman Group, London)

Implications

The levels of the cognitive domain are useful for setting or clarifying expectations, planning objectives and assessment of cognitive abilities as the learning increases in complexity. The hierarchy demonstrates the way in which we put into practice what we know and value. This domain underlies concept development. Conceptual knowledge allows the learner to adapt readily to new learning situations.

Affective domain

The affective domain relates to changes in interest, attitudes, values, and appreciation, and also to the ability to make adequate adjustments. Attitudes and values are 'constructs' — terms that are used to explain things that cannot be observed directly. 'Values refer to the concept of what a person considers desirable, and so values have a large emotional component. A person's values might include sincerity, compassion and respect' (Quinn 1988, p. 242). Attitudes are positive or negative feelings about certain things. They consist of both cognitive and affective aspects; our attitudes are formed from our knowledge and our feelings about an issue. Attitudes affect what we see and how we see it.

Stages in affective learning

1. *Receiving* (attending). Willingness to receive information; giving selected attention.

2. *Responding*. Displaying acquaintance with and comprehension of the message.

3. *Valuing*. Acceptance and internalisation of values and attitudes in question, by demonstrating ability to apply the information personally.

4. *Organisation*. Conceptualisation of the value, and expressing a commitment and the ability to arrange the values in appropriate order.

5. *Characterisation*. The person gives a personal undertaking to adopt the behaviour that reinforces the attitude. The value becomes a philosophy of life. Practice reinforces the modified value system.

To enhance positive attitude formation the educational experience must provide the person with:

- intellectual stimulation, in that they understand the message and it engages their emotions;
- biological significance, in that they associate the message with themselves; and
- social significance in that the message is congruent with social values.

Psychomotor domain

The psychomotor domain is used in the observable performance of skills that require some degree of neuromuscular coordination. An individual uses the psychomotor domain when they apply accumulated knowledge and attitude to life situations. Three conditions are necessary:

1. the learner has the ability;

2. the learner has a sensory image of how to carry out the skill; and

3. the learner has the opportunity to practise.

The guided process of mentally preparing for a new skill, and the gradual development of competency through to creative adaptation of a behaviour is illustrated in Box 6.2. The box also suggests the close link between cognitive and psychomotor domains.

Box 6.2 Taxonomy of psychomotor learning domain		
Level 1	Perception	Perception of sensory cues that guide action
Level 2	Set	Readiness to act
Level 3	Guided response	Skills are performed with demonstration — may be incremental
Level 4	Mechanism	Performance is habitual. Movements are not complex
Level 5	Complex overt response	Skilled performance with economy of effort, smoothness of action, accuracy and efficiency
Level 6	Adaptation	Catering for special conditions
Level 7	Origination	Origination of new movement patterns to suit particular circumstances

(Source: derived from Quinn, F. M. 1988 *The Principles and Practice of Nurse Education*, 2nd edn. Chapman and Hall, London, Ch 10)

Teaching—learning strategies

By now it is probably quite apparent that all the health-promotion strategies described in this book so far are useful health education strategies. Community development, lobbying and advocacy, and group work often result in education of more than one group of people, and often at several different stages in the process as do mass media and social marketing campaigns. Which strategies are most appropriate depends on the issue at hand, the needs of the people, the context in which the learning is taking place and the particular skills that the teacher and the learner have. In addition, strategies can be adapted and new ones developed to better suit each situation. The following brief descriptions provide an introduction to some common education strategies.

Talks and lectures

Talks and lectures tend to be regarded as a relatively efficient way to pass on a lot of information to a group of people. They allow an audience to participate passively and learn in a relatively unthreatening way. However, they are largely a pedagogical approach to teaching and as such, their effectiveness can be limited in a number of ways. Firstly, people may attempt to provide too much information in a talk, swamping the audience in a way that tends to inhibit rather than foster learning. Secondly, unless combined with other strategies, talks tend to be one-way communication in which little interaction (and therefore little participative learning), occurs. However, it is also possible to combine talks and lectures with other interactive strategies, using a variety of approaches to get the message across.

Preparing and structuring a lecture

1. Introduce the lecture

   - Gain participant attention.
   - Establish rapport, perhaps with a warm-up exercise.
   - Provide motivational cues — explain why the ideas are important.
   - Set out the essential content.
   - Have only a few main points and summarise these with the use of objectives.
   - 'Pre-test' student knowledge to prompt awareness of relevant knowledge.

2. The body of the lecture

   - Cover the content according to the objectives.
   - Provide a logical organisation — use the levels in domains of learning as a guide.
   - Maintain participant attention by showing enthusiasm for the topic, using humour if it is appropriate and comes naturally, inserting questions for the audience, being physically active (but not with irritating mannerisms) or providing handout material.

3. Concluding the lecture

   - Recall the main ideas introduced earlier.
   - Specify what participants should now know.
   - Answer any questions.

Lecturing is less appropriate when:

- long-term retention is desired;
- the material is complex, detailed or abstract;
- learner participation is essential;
- higher cognitive objectives, such as analysis and synthesis, are being sought;
- learners are of average or below-average intelligence.

Buzz groups (quick discussion in pairs to discuss an issue) may be used during long presentations to help energise the group and keep the presentation interesting. In these situations, though, it is worth confirming whether such a long presentation is necessary.

Discussions and debates

Discussions and debates provide an opportunity for people to examine an issue by comparing a variety of views. They are useful to motivate intellectual and emotional exchange among learners. Engaging in debate helps learners develop respect for the ideas and opinions of others as well as to acquire insight into a particular health-related topic. Learners need to listen, communicate and analyse the issues of debate. Discussions and debates are a much more participative approach to learning than talks and lectures, although care still needs to be taken to ensure that they are effective. Firstly, discussion may need to be guided (perhaps through a series of questions) or provoked (such as through a challenging video or opinion). Secondly, if group discussion is to be a participative process for everyone, it may need to be facilitated so that everyone has a chance to participate.

Values clarification exercises

A number of activities can be designed to assist values clarification with participants. These processes are useful to assist learners to clarify their moral, ethical and social relationships, resulting in self-understanding. For example, the following strategies can be used for formulating one's value judgment:

- *Rank order* — the learner chooses among alternatives, or places alternatives in rank order.
- *Voting* on health issues then comparing and discussing responses with other learners.
- A *values continuum* where people identify and arrange values about issues on a continuum from one 'extreme' to the other.
- A *values whip*, which forces participants to state how they arrived at their decisions; use interview techniques that elicit the opinions of others.
- The use of *devils-advocate role-plays*, where participants are required to take a stance in a role-play that is opposite to their preferred values.
- *Autobiographical and biographical sketches* — the use of 'stories' (participants 'or others') can be powerful illustrators of the impacts social values (Labonté & Feather 1996; Lehmann 2003).

These methodologies are intended to help learners identify and clarify their thinking regarding health issues, and to understand their values. They are not intended to force the values of others on participants. Facilitators must not see these strategies as opportunities to indoctrinate participants.

Demonstration and practice of skills

Observing and then practising skills can be a valuable way to learn and may be vital when people are attempting to learn a new skill. If demonstration is to be effective, planning the demonstration as a series of logical steps, reserving explanation to the necessary key points, will help simplify the process for learners. A range of multimedia resources are available to assist learning psychomotor skills, from preparing an insulin injection to using a condom. Refer back to the learning hierarchy set out in the psychomotor domain of learning as a guide for when to introduce demonstration into a learning occasion, and following this, ensure that adequate opportunities are available for participants to practise the new skills.

Role-play

Role-playing often provides a useful opportunity for people to practise new or unfamiliar behaviour with others. It can also be used to provide an opportunity to explore values and feelings within a group. A word of warning about role-plays, though: they should be used to explore emotional or challenging issues only by health workers with the knowledge and skills to assist participants to debrief and de-role at the end of the process. Otherwise, role-playing may do more harm than good.

Games

There is a great variety of educational games or activities available to trigger learning. One example of these is the series of structured activities for group learning (Pfeiffer & Jones 1974–1985). However, if games and activities are to be effective learning tools, they need to be relevant to the issue at hand and well facilitated. Like other teaching–learning strategies, games and activities are not ends in themselves, and need to be integrated with other learning processes to be used to full effect. For example, a series of open-ended questions to guide discussion after a game may help draw out the key learning points, and link the message of the game to real life experience.

Self-contracting

Self-contracting provides a mechanism whereby people can contract with themselves to change their behaviour in some way and then support the behaviour change through rewarding the behaviour they wish to encourage. Despite the discomfort some people feel with its behaviour modification origins, self-contracting has often been found to be a useful tool in helping people change their behaviour. Very important in this process is that people themselves determine what they should change and how they should support their new behaviour.

Action

Enabling people to act on an issue of concern to them can provide an excellent opportunity for them to learn and make a difference at the same time. Writing a letter about an issue of concern, planning and conducting a health survey or media campaign, or developing educational materials for use with peers are just some examples of action for change that in itself may teach the protagonists a great deal. In these situations, health workers may play an important role as resource people, but otherwise allow people to act independently.

Learning organisations

A learning organisation is a health-promoting organisation. They foster inclusiveness and transparency in decision-making processes. There are many organisations, such as schools and workplaces, where health workers find themselves as a catalyst in promoting health, and in doing so, the learning process. This includes their own workplace.

There is a tendency to assume that learning is always positive and beneficial. This is not necessarily so. For example, employees learn that anger and cynicism is justified in situations where employers deny that risks have been taken with the employees' health.

The strategies needed for a health-promoting organisation fit well with the values of Primary Health Care described in Chapter 2 and the planning and evaluation process discussed in Chapter 5. That is, we work within a social justice framework and demonstrate respect for each other. We encourage participation of the workers in identifying the needs of the organisation and decision-making processes to address those needs and those processes are transparent. We emphasise teamwork; encourage innovative thinking; and celebrate achievements.

To avoid negative learning, organisations need a clearly articulated, shared and alive organisational purpose and formal planning and review structures based on a strong policy framework. Further, policies need to be in place that encourage critical reflection; support staff development; include the community in decision-making; and take a long-term perspective on issues within the context of the bigger picture (Legge et al 1996 in Baum 2002).

Community-level education

Education at the level of the community or population is a more complex process than education at the individual, group or organisational level — even more planning and teamwork is needed if it is to be successful. Nonetheless, the same general principles apply. The World Health Organization (1988, p. 175) suggests three points to keep in mind:

1. Get the support of influential people in the community — those who are called 'opinion leaders' or 'key people'.

2. Be sure that all the people of the community are informed about the problem and are kept up to date on plans and progress. All available channels of communication should be used for this purpose.

3. Get the maximum number of people involved so that the community will really strengthen its capacity to do things for its health. This can be done through community health committees, advisory or planning boards, etc.

Community-level education draws particularly on mass media and community development strategies. If it is to be effective, it needs to be built on the recognition of the nature of communities as being composed of a variety of groups, often with competing interests. This is likely to mean that a variety of different approaches are needed to work effectively with each of these different groups. Minkler (1994) has developed a set of ten principles or 'commitments' for community health education (see Box 6.3). In examining these it is apparent that they draw together the wide range of principles examined throughout this book, demonstrating the way in which these points all come together in community health education. This also serves to highlight the linkages and similarities between community health education and other strategies identified here.

Formulating goals and objectives

Being able to develop goals and objectives is an essential part of any health worker's 'toolkit'. In the previous chapter we talked about goals and objectives in program-planning and how they can provide a foundation that guides health workers through a program from planning through to implementation and on to evaluation. In education for health, they help health workers clarify the desired changes. Clear goals and objectives maximise the opportunity for change.

The use of the terms goals, aims and objectives differ in different disciplines. In this text we take goals to be statements about long-term outcomes and objectives to restate the goals in operational terms. Strategies are the activities that enable us to achieve the objectives. They are the actions or daily tasks. It may be useful at this point to review the model in Figure 5.4 in the previous chapter.

Goals usually express long-term changes. They express something about a desired change in the major issue that has been identified and this relates to the outcome evaluation. They may express desired changes in the social environment such as health indicators, health status, quality of life, social support or community participation.

Objectives state what must occur for the goal to be achieved. They address things that contribute to the major issue and so an analysis of the determinants of the major issue provides a guide for us to develop objectives. They are often expressed as either learning objectives or action/behavioural and environmental objectives.

Learning objectives address educational and organisational needs. If we use the PRECEDE–PROCEED model discussed in the last chapter to make our assessments, we would be addressing the predisposing, enabling and reinforcing factors identified in our needs assessment, which means that we would be addressing changes in knowledge, attitudes, beliefs or behaviour (McKenzie & Smeltzer 2001, p. 125). The domains of learning, discussed earlier in the chapter can be used as a framework for writing learning objectives, based on the adult learning principles, also discussed earlier in the chapter.

Action/behavioural and environmental objectives address the non-behavioural issues contributing to the goal. Using PRECEDE–PROCEED, they are derived from our behavioural and environmental assessments (McKenzie & Smeltzer 2001, p. 126). They may express changes in health indicators, social support, quality of life or community participation.

> ### Box 6.3 Minkler's ten commitments for community health education
>
> **Start where the people are**
>
> Respecting community members' own perspectives and priorities and working with them on the issues they identify is the basis for effective meaningful health education.
>
> **Recognise and build on community strengths**
>
> Paying as much attention to the strengths of communities as to their needs acknowledges the resources of the community and itself strengthens the community.
>
> **Honour thy community — but do not make it holy**
>
> While this focus on the community is vital, we need to ensure that we maintain our focus on social justice, or we run the risk of blindly committing ourselves to divisive community attitudes.
>
> **Foster high level community participation**
>
> True power sharing and control by the community should be the aim if people are to participate meaningfully in health education.
>
> **Laughter is good medicine — and good health education**
>
> Humour and light-heartedness themselves have health benefits, as well as improving the quality of good health education.
>
> **Health education is educational — but it is also political**
>
> Health education should not ignore the political aspects of health issues, but should instead recognise the social and political context in which health issues arise.
>
> **Thou shalt not tolerate the bad 'isms'**
>
> Health educators should ensure that they do not work in ways which encourage or ignore racism, sexism, ageism, homophobia or other attitudes which act to exclude people.
>
> **'Think globally, act locally'**
>
> Work at both the macro level and the micro level to address the immediate problem and the broader causal issues.
>
> **Foster individual and community empowerment**
>
> 'If we do start where people are; if we work with, rather than on, communities; if we believe in and work for high level community participation; and if we see our work in terms of its political and economic contexts, we will be doing empowering health education.'
>
> **Work for social justice**
>
> Work to advocate for social justice and improvements in public health, to help create an environment which is more 'conducive to individual and community empowerment'.

(Source: adapted from Minkler, M. 1994 Ten Commitments for Community Health Education. *Health Education Research*. 9(4): 527–34)

Objectives should be SMART; that is:

- specific; measurable; achievable; relevant; and timescale.

To be specific, you need to refer to the place and the people concerned. To be able to measure the change you need to refer to an amount. For example, you might refer to an increase in the percentage of local people on a board of management committee. Achievable and relevant refer to the scope of what is to be achieved. Timescale refers to when you think the change will have been achieved by. Working within a Primary Health Care approach means that it will be relevant to the people concerned and be able to be achieved by them.

It is important to note that one organisation's goal can be another organisation's objective. For example, the national government's goal may be to reduce the incidence of suicide in young people and plan to raise awareness of the signs and symptoms of depression through a social marketing campaign. There are many things that contribute to depression in young people and in your town you may have identified poor social support opportunities. Your goal might be to increase the social support opportunities for youth in your town. Your objectives may include engaging marginalised groups in particular, and your strategies may include identifying potential youth facilitators from the marginalised group for peer education programs in your town. All of these goals, objectives and activities contribute to addressing the nationally identified issue, but your goal may be a strategy for the national government.

Working with groups

Much health promotion, whether it is lobbying for political change, community development work or more formal health education, involves working with groups of people, both community members and work colleagues. These groups often have dynamics that are so much more than the sum of the individuals in them. It is possible to develop an understanding of group dynamics and skills in working with a group, so that the group works effectively for what it is trying to achieve, rather than allowing its dynamics to work against what it is trying to achieve. In the final section of this chapter, the important components of the group process will be outlined along with some practical strategies for working with groups.

Group theory

Group theory has been developing since the turn of the century, with several social psychologists researching the dynamics of group behaviour. After World War II, as concern for the future of democracy grew, there was a further increase in interest in group dynamics and the ways in which groups could be encouraged to operate democratically and collaboratively (Johnson & Johnson 1997, p. 40). It is from this base that group theory has developed, and so belief in the principles of democracy and collaboration underpins group theory and its application. Johnson and Johnson (1997, p. 12) define a small group as:

> two or more individuals in face-to-face interaction, each aware of their positive interdependence as they strive to achieve mutual goals, each aware of his or her membership in the group, and each aware of the others who belong to the group.

This focus means that the principles of group work are compatible with the Primary Health Care approach, and have much to contribute to the practice of health promotion. Clearly many groups that meet do not fit this definition. However, by recognising and working with the principles of group dynamics, health workers can help groups move toward this definition, enabling people to gain as much as possible from group membership.

Types of groups

Community groups will be created, sustained and facilitated in different ways, 'but all have to be conscious in the exercise of decision-making and finding a good balance between autonomy, cooperation and hierarchy' (Heron 1999, p. 329). Social change theory seminars, community action groups, occupational action groups, organisational action groups and new institutions are five approaches outlined below (Heron 1999 in Brown et al 2005).

Social change theory seminars

These study groups are consciousness-raising groups that explore issues of change. There is a critique of personal, transpersonal and social issues. The research, reflection and dialogue that occur during this process are more likely to produce more perceptive and effective action than if this had not been done. Relevant research data is collected to assist in the analysis of the current social structure and support the vision developed by the group.

Community action groups

These groups come together to engage in direct action for social change on issues of concern to them. The groups are communities of interest who perhaps share the same occupation, beliefs or concerns and who meet regularly to take action. These groups include: peer self-help, new society education and action, and community development groups.

Peer self-help groups

Peer self-help groups may work for social change or for personal change in their members, or a combination of both. Their roles include 'mutual support … education, advocacy, lobbying, research and information and service provision to both their members and other consumers of the health system' (Markos 1991, p. 4). Mutual support is given to group members with similar problems of a personal nature that affect them directly. The members share experiences and identify common needs and areas for social action for themselves or on behalf of others in similar situations. The problems may be anything from a particular disease affecting individuals, such as asthma, or to psychosocial issues, such as drug dependency, or life-stage issues, such as retirement and so on. These groups will be discussed in more detail below.

New society education and action groups

These are consciousness-raising groups where cultural and ecological issues for social action are identified. The issues may be global or local. But thinking globally/acting locally may be the thrust of their action. Heron (1999) sights many examples, such as green consumerism, pollution, renewable energy, work cooperatives and so on.

Community development groups

Community development groups are local groups that work at the local level on local issues with or without the support of local government. These will be discussed in more depth later.

Occupational action groups

Occupational ties alone connect the group who work collectively for the profession. Trade unions are the best example.

Organisational action groups

These groups work for organisational change. They may or may not have similar occupations but their aim is often for a better balance of hierarchy, cooperation and autonomy within an organisation.

New institutions

All of the previous activities converge upon the creation of new institutions; the social structures of a new society (Heron 1999 in Brown et al 2005).

Health workers may need to create, facilitate and help sustain any of these groups and so an understanding of group dynamics and facilitation skills is required.

Peer self-help groups in health

All of these approaches often develop as a challenge to the mainstream system, or find themselves challenging the system once they are established. Within the health system, peer self-help groups often form in response to inadequate services for their needs. Whether they actively challenge the system or not, health workers may feel threatened by people addressing their own needs because they are unhappy with the way in which the system addresses them. Peer self-help groups may demand information from professionals when many are still unwilling to share it, and in so doing challenge the status and power differences between professional and client.

Consciousness-raising plays an important role in the development of many self-help groups. Through talking together and sharing their experiences, members of these groups discover their shared ground and the common sources of oppression or indifference (Biklen 1983, pp. 193–4). Peer self-help groups may work to create their own alternative services or to change those already in operation (Biklen 1983, p. 195). In either case, they often demand greater control over services so that they may better meet their needs.

Unless they are appropriately funded, peer self-help groups may be encouraged by government in a way that exploits the community members who join them, particularly those who put considerable energy into organising and running them on a day-to-day basis. That is, governments may support peer self-help groups because they are a cheap option and because they assume the burden of responsibility for action in what are often difficult or previously ignored areas. Health workers need to reflect critically on suggestions to encourage the development of self-help groups, so as to ensure that these groups do not develop more for the benefit of the health system than the community itself.

In deciding whether a peer self-help group should be established, health workers must consider whether the people concerned actually want such a group — that is, whether felt need is present. As obvious as this may sound, on many occasions health workers establish self-help groups and then wonder why people do not participate. Clearly, community members will not participate in a group if they do not feel they need to do so. Attempts to impose self-help groups are likely to be unsuccessful, and may well set similar groups up to fail, once a community perception of a self-help group as failing has been established.

Another problem with some health workers' approaches to peer self-help groups is that they may sometimes support the idea of these groups being support groups, but are less supportive of, and even discourage, peer self-help groups that take on action group activities. However, supporting these groups for their support work only, while discouraging social action, amounts to a form of social control in which group members are expected to put all their energy into achieving tasks that could perhaps be achieved legitimately by the health system, and are not supported in their work for the necessary changes.

Health workers have an important role to play with self-help groups in supporting them and acting as consultants, when groups request this. They should act as resources, and not take over the decision-making process (Kearney 1991, p. 31). Developing a partnership between self-help groups and health workers may enable them to continue their work effectively. Like any good partnership, the relationship between health workers and self-help groups should be one of mutual respect.

The typical life of a group

Several theorists have proposed that groups typically go through a series of stages as they establish themselves, develop and ultimately wind down. Probably the most commonly used model is Tuckman's (1965) model of group development. It has been further developed by others and is known now as a five-stage model, suggesting that a group typically goes through a series of stages in its life — forming, storming, norming, performing and ending (or mourning). These stages describe the way in which the group goes about its activities (that is, the *process* of its behaviour). Groups will be attempting to get on with the business that brought them together at the same time as these processes are developing. The development of group process may, however, structure the way in which a group tries to do its business, and the effectiveness of the group may depend to a large extent on how it develops through the five stages. It is worthwhile, therefore, examining Tuckman's model, as it provides a useful framework for understanding behaviours that can commonly occur at different times in a group's life.

Despite the impression that Tuckman's (1965) model may give, it is important to acknowledge that the stages of a group's life do not necessarily occur in a neat straight line. Moreover, groups may not go through all these stages; for example, some groups may get stuck in the storming process, not resolve the power and control issues, and so not perform effectively. On another level, however, this series of stages may be experienced to some extent every time a group gets together (Brown 1992, p. 111). Tuckman's model provides a useful guide to what we might normally expect in the life of a group. However, it is not definitive, and other models also have merit and are worthy of examination (see, for example Sampson & Marthas 1990, or Bundey et al 1989). Also, as you examine groups with which you are involved, you will see the extent to which the life of individual groups varies in relation to those models, and you may like to add important points of your own. The following explanation of Tuckman's model is based on the summary given by Brown (1992, pp. 101–10).

Forming

When the group first comes together, and for some time afterwards, it may be little more than a collection of individuals, rather than a group with its own identity. People may be feeling apprehensive about joining and anxious about their role in the group and how they should perform. At this point, if the group has a designated leader, that person usually plays a significant role, the members of the group being reluctant to take responsibility for decision-making. Members rely on the leader to make decisions and control the direction of the activity at hand. At this time, they may be examining the group and their role in it to decide if it has something to offer them. Formal group leaders therefore have an important role to play in making clear what the aims of the group are, and in negotiating with the group regarding what it will set out to do and how it will do it. In those cases where there is no designated leader, the group may be tentative at this stage as a leader begins to emerge or as various people take up leadership positions.

Storming

In the storming stage of the group's life, people look for the role or roles they can play. Issues of power and control are often most prominent at this stage as group members jockey for position. At the same time, people may be afraid of losing their individuality and being absorbed into the group. Both these factors may cause the group to be quite fragile at this stage. The leader may need to ensure that dominant people are not permitted to take over and that all members have an opportunity to establish an equal role. This may take some skill and this stage may be the most difficult for the leader to deal with.

Norming

Once most of the issues of power and control have been sorted out, the group is in a position to develop a sense of cohesion and trust between members. Norms of appropriate behaviour are set so that people have a sense of where they stand and what is acceptable behaviour. As a result, group members may start to settle into the group. At this point its leader may need to harness the cohesion developed and use it to get the group working effectively on its tasks.

Performing

When members start taking responsibility for the group and its tasks, they are in the performing stage of its life. At this stage, there is a high level of cohesion and trust between members and the group is largely self-sufficient in relation to the leader. In many respects this stage is similar to the previous one: they differ only in the degree to which the group is performing its tasks and the level of self-sufficiency with which it is doing this.

Mourning

When the time comes for a group to come to an end, this will have an impact on it, even if it was convened to work for change and the ending of the group signifies success (as, for example, in the case of a community action group working to resist the development of a highway through their town). In this final stage of the group, it is important for it to evaluate its achievements and deal with any unfinished business. Some members may want to postpone the end of the group because they may have benefited a great deal from being a group member and may want to continue enjoying the company of other members and the sense of achievement that the group may have been experiencing. Having some form of ritual ending, such as having a meal together or carrying out a 'group closure' activity (see Pfeiffer & Jones, 1974–1985) may help the group to finalise its activities and members to acknowledge its ending.

Elements of successful group work

Johnson and Johnson (1997, p. 31) suggest that an effective group is one that accomplishes its goals, maintains good working relationships and develops in response to changing circumstances. Groups are more likely to be effective when:

- goals are clear and relevant to all group members;

- communication is accurate and clear, and two-way;

- participation and leadership are shared among members;

- decision-making procedures suit the issue being dealt with;

- power and influence are shared, based on expertise not power;

- controversy is encouraged, and creativity and problem-solving promoted;

- conflicts are resolved constructively.

(Johnson & Johnson 1997, pp. 32–4)

In observing a group, therefore, and deciding which aspects of its operations are effective and which may need improving, several issues are worth examining.

The task, maintenance and individual activities of the group

The activities that a group performs can be roughly divided into three types: those that get the group's task done; those that maintain the life of the group and therefore may help it to get its tasks done; and those that individuals perform to look after their own needs. It is important that groups address these sets of activities. If members try to push through to accomplish their tasks while ignoring the needs of individuals, the group may soon become ineffective. If, on the other hand, a group concentrates on maintaining itself, people may communicate effectively and enjoy meetings for a while, but may leave the group without having addressed the issue that brought them to it in the first place. They may leave feeling frustrated at the group's lack of achievement.

Of course, not all activities fit neatly into task functions or maintenance functions. Some activities may have components of both, and whether an activity is a task or maintenance function of a group may vary depending on the context and the particular group. For example, a support group's task activities may be the development of friendship and support networks, an activity that may be regarded in another type of group as having a maintenance function. To succeed, all groups need to address both their task functions and their maintenance functions, although there is no set proportion of activities that should be assigned to either category. What is important is for each group to strike a balance between the two types of activities. This balance will depend on the reason each group is meeting and, to some extent, on the individual needs of people in each group. You could ask yourself the following questions when observing task, maintenance and individual activities in a group:

- Who keeps the group from getting too far away from its task?
- Who asks the group for suggestions about how to deal with a problem?
- Does anyone summarise group discussion?
- Does anyone try to involve people who do not seem to be participating (Bundey et al 1989, pp. 101–2)?
- Does the group take time out to talk socially and find out how everyone is doing?
- Do the needs of any individuals in the group dominate?

Leadership

The pattern of leadership within a group is well worth examining, as it will tell us a great deal about how the group operates and how involved members are. Many people assume that the originator of the group is the only person who should exhibit leadership behaviours, but this is not so. Even in a group where a worker has some responsibility for it, if the group is to be effective, its leadership should be shared. You could ask yourself the following questions when observing the leadership patterns in a group:

- What leadership behaviours are exhibited in the group?
- Is leadership shared by members of the group, or does one person maintain control?
- Who exhibits leadership behaviours and who does not?

Power and influence

Power and influence are very much linked to leadership in a group. Indeed, if the people with the power and influence in a group are not its leaders, conflict may result. However, people with power and influence may not be those who talk the most or are the most active in the group. Bundey et al (1989, p. 100) point out that some people may have a great deal of influence, but say little; however, when they do speak, others take notice. You could ask yourself the following questions when observing power and influence in a group:

- Are there any people in the group whose opinions are listened to very carefully?
- Are there any people whose opinions are ignored?
- Are people with influence helping the group to achieve its goals?
- Are there conflicts between people with influence?

Decision-making

There are several aspects of decision-making that need to be considered when observing group process. They are:

- *when* decisions are made (timing);

- *how* decisions are reached (process);

- *who* is responsible (who monitors the decision-making process);

- *what* issues are to be decided.

(Bundey et al 1989, p. 40)

When decisions are made reflects a number of important elements of the group process. In a formal health education group, for example, this might include examining what decisions the group leader makes before the group actually starts, thus preventing the whole group from being involved in those decisions. In community action groups it might include consideration of whether important decisions are left until the end of long and arduous meetings, when people may not be as fresh and capable of good decision-making, or when people with other commitments have had to leave. Conversely, decisions taken early in meetings may leave people feeling there was inadequate discussion.

How decisions are made may determine what degree of ownership is felt by group members over these decisions and help determine their level of satisfaction with the group's performance.

You could ask yourself the following questions when observing decision-making in a group:

- How are decisions made in this group?
  - by one person?
  - by a small dominant group?
  - by simple majority?
  - by consensus?
- Who controls the decision-making procedures in a group?
- Are there issues that feature prominently in the group over which it has no decision-making power?

Group goals

A key issue in determining whether people feel involved in a group is the extent to which they share the group's goals. If the goals of an individual do not match the goals of the group, it is unlikely that he or she will be committed to it. Once again, this is just as relevant for community groups as for groups participating in health education activities. In either case, if someone or a small group of people dominate the goal-setting process, others can be left out of the group or drop out because of lack of commitment. In formal health education groups, this can happen when the group leader alone establishes the goals of the group without involving members in the process. The goals of the group might then suit no one in the group, and might reflect only the group leader's ideas of what people want. What a waste of energy this is when simply determining or clarifying group goals together could prevent this!

You could ask yourself the following questions when observing goal-setting in a group:

- Does the group have clear goals?
- Who was involved in establishing them?
- Who 'owns' goals that are set?
- Are there members of the group who do not seem to share the group goals?

Communication

Patterns of communication in a group are extremely important. Distribution of leadership, participation, power and control, and conflicts of interest, will all be reflected in observable patterns of communication. Communication is both verbal and non-verbal and occurs between individuals and between an individual and the group. It has a key role in facilitating the group's achievement of its tasks and group members' comfort and sense of belonging.

You could ask yourself the following questions when observing communication in a group:

- Who talks and to whom?
- Who keeps the interaction going in the group?
- Are people silent, and if so, how does the group respond (Bundey et al 1989, p. 46)?
- Do people address the whole group when they talk or just some people?
- What non-verbal communication is happening?
- How powerful are the non-verbal messages?
- Is anyone giving mixed messages?
- Is more being not said than said?

Rules and norms

Many groups will establish appropriate rules of behaviour or ground rules to guide their activities. For example, it might be decided that only one person will speak at any one time, that only the spokesperson will speak publicly for the group or that discussions at group meetings are confidential. In addition to the rules themselves, what is important is how they were developed. Did the group as a whole decide on them and agree with them, or were they imposed on the group by a leader?

In addition to these explicit rules by which the group operates, there may be a number of norms guiding the group, of which group members may or may not be aware (Bundey et al 1989, p. 103). Norms are implicit rules that guide the activities of the group, often more strongly than the explicit rules. They influence the group powerfully, and can either support its activities or hinder its progress, depending on the norms themselves and what the group is trying to achieve. Some examples of group norms are that it is acceptable to turn up to group meetings 15 minutes late because they will not begin on time; that it is acceptable to talk about each other when no one else is around; that it is acceptable to interrupt each other during discussions and dominate discussion; or that it is unacceptable to disagree with someone else in the group.

In deciding whether a norm is unhelpful, it is important to look carefully at what is happening and what role it plays in the group's behaviour overall. For example, what may at first glance seem like an unhelpful norm may actually act as a valuable means of releasing tension. Laughter and games interrupting meeting procedure may be one example of this. It is vital that cultural norms also be considered. For instance, what may seem like an unhelpful norm of people consistently being late for group meetings may stem from particular cultural views of time in which being ruled by the clock is not as strong as it is in other cultures. In these cases, it is more likely to be the group leader, not the group, that will need to do the adapting.

However, in instances when unhelpful norms are minimising the group's ability to function, it will be necessary for the group leader to deal with the issue. This will mean making the group aware of what is happening, since it may not be conscious of the norm operating. Sometimes this will be enough: individuals will recognise how they are contributing to the norm and will agree to change their behaviour. If this does not happen, the group as a whole will need to decide how best to deal with it. Perhaps they will decide to leave things as they are and accept the consequences, or they may establish new ground rules and agree to stick to them. Alternatively, the norm may have arisen because a particular aspect of the group did not suit some group members, and the group may therefore decide to make the appropriate changes. For example, if people are consistently arriving late, it may be that the starting time for meetings needs to be altered to fit in with other commitments that people have. You could ask yourself the following questions when observing rules and norms in a group:

- What are the rules guiding behaviour in the group?
- Which of these are 'written' (rules) and which are 'unwritten' (norms)?
- Which seem to be supporting the group's activities and which seem to be hindering its progress?
- Are there any rules and norms that are hindering the group's progress and that group members do not seem to be aware of?

Controversy and creativity

Controversy can be extremely important to the life of a group. From it come new ideas and challenges to people's thinking. Unfortunately, people sometimes think that controversy is bad and to be avoided at all costs, and so do not allow it to be explored. Not only does this deprive the group of the opportunity to develop new and innovative solutions to the problems they are addressing, it can also run the risk of damaging the group. Janis (1982) has highlighted the great danger posed by 'groupthink' if controversy is not allowed to exist in a group.

'Groupthink' is described as a process that can occur when disagreement and creativity are stifled, and it results in extremely poor decisions, often out of touch with reality. It has been highlighted as the cause of some of the disastrous decisions made in political history. It typically occurs when the group has a strong directive leader, when criticism within the group is stifled and when opportunities for criticism from outside the group are removed. As a result, uncritical acceptance of the leader's opinions leads to extremely poor, even dangerous, decisions. Janis (1982, cited by Johnson & Johnson 1997, pp. 256–8) has outlined eight symptoms of groupthink:

1. Self-censorship. Group members censor themselves by not voicing any concerns about the issue being discussed.

2. Illusion of unanimity. Because of the lack of discussion, group members assume that everyone else is in agreement about the issue.

3. Direct pressure on dissenters. If anyone does speak out, pressure is brought to bear on that person to conform.

4. 'Mind guards'. Some particular group members take on the role of discouraging objections.

5. Illusion of invulnerability. Members assume that the group is in a powerful position and cannot be criticized by outsiders. This results in very risky decisions.

6. Rationalization. Group members rationalize the decision taken, in order to justify to themselves the position adopted by the group.

7. Illusion of morality. The group does not consider the ethical issues involved, and assumes that it is morally above reproach.

8. Stereotyping. Group members stereotype critics or competitors ('they are all stupid') in order to rationalize any outside opposition.

Groupthink provides an extreme example of what can happen to a group and its decision-making when creativity and controversy are discouraged. Many people have experienced at least mild forms of groupthink and been concerned about its impact. You could ask yourself the following questions when observing controversy and creativity in a group:

- How do the others respond when a group member makes an unusual suggestion or disagrees with the group leader?
- Does the group use processes to encourage creative thinking among its members (for example brainstorming)?

Conflicts of interest

If controversy in a group is extreme, it may be that real conflicts of interest are present. Perhaps members of a community action group are there for very different reasons, so that the group cannot agree on an action plan. Perhaps a worker acting as group leader is in a group because of his or her agency's expectations, and not because of a personal commitment to helping people facing the particular issue being addressed. In any case, when conflicts of interest are not handled well, they can damage a group and hurt individuals involved in it. It is therefore vital for group leaders to be able to recognise conflicts of interest and, where possible, structure activities to minimise the damage caused by those conflicts. The possibility of conflicts of interest is one reason why clarifying the group's goals and involving everybody in their establishment are so important. These may not be enough to prevent conflicts of interest but they are an important start. You could ask yourself the following questions when observing conflict in a group:

- Are there issues that always bring out anger?
- Is the group working through conflicts that arise or are these a barrier to action?

- Are there any people who seem to be always disagreeing and who are unable to allow others' viewpoints?
- How does the rest of the group respond to this?

This brief overview of the various elements of group dynamics should provide you with a standpoint from which to observe these elements at work. Being able to observe these dynamics in operation will enable you in many cases to steer the group away from unproductive patterns towards those that better enable the group to achieve its goals.

Hints for working with groups

There are several practical points that may make working with groups a more positive process for both facilitators and group members. These have been developed on the basis of the experience of people working with groups over a number of years. The following hints for working with groups have been developed from Ewles and Simnett (1999, pp. 242–59).

Numbers

In considering the optimal size of a group, the first consideration will be the purpose for which the group is meeting. If it is a public meeting designed to canvass opinion on an issue, the actual size of the group may not influence effectiveness. If it is a structured meeting, where members of several interested parties need representation, the size of the group may be determined by the number of such parties.

If, on the other hand, the group is a health education group built on the principle of maximum participation by its members, it will be important to keep it to a manageable size. In such cases, the optimal size of a group is regarded as being between 8 and 12 people. If there are fewer than eight people in a group, people may feel exposed and be unwilling to participate. Moreover, an insufficient number of ideas may be generated in a problem-solving group. However, if there are more than 12 people in a group, it is difficult for everyone to get involved, and often the louder members will dominate.

If you need to have more than 12 people in a group, consider whether you can split it up into smaller groups for discussion and activities. Alternatively, it may be worthwhile running two separate groups alongside each other. Which solution to choose will depend on the reason the group is meeting (can the topic 'cope' with a large group?) and the amount of resources you have (can you afford to run the same group twice?). If, however, you are dealing with a sensitive topic, it may be appropriate to have a group of fewer than eight people in order to enable people to speak comfortably about the topic. In these cases, you may also consider whether it is more appropriate to discuss the topic on a one-to-one basis.

Timing

The length of time that a group meets for is very important in determining whether members feel it is valuable or not. Groups need to be together long enough to break the ice, settle down and achieve something, but not so long that people begin to get bored or feel they are wasting their time. Generally, between an hour and an hour-and-a-half is a reasonable amount of time. Breaks or changes in the group's activity will enable it to stay fresh for that length of time, or even longer if necessary. However, meetings lasting more than one-and-a-half hours would need to be well planned, and you would need a good reason to justify them. Planning the length of meetings with the participants will increase the likelihood that the duration planned is realistic and fits in with the other needs of group members.

The day and time that the group meets will have a considerable bearing on who will attend. There are some commonsense rules you can follow to ensure that the timing does not prevent people from attending. For example, after school in the afternoon may not be a good time to run a single parents' support group unless childcare is available. Meetings between 5.30 p.m. and 7 p.m. may be unpopular, as this tends to be meal time for many people.

All the planning in the world, however, will not enable you to prevent clashes with the other commitments that members of each particular group may have. It, therefore, makes good sense to check at the group's first meeting whether the day and time suit members and, if they do not, to negotiate a day and time that suit most of them. Not only does this increase the likelihood that people can attend the group, it also makes it quite clear that the group belongs to everyone, not just the group leader. Furthermore, you may want to experiment with different meeting times to maximise attendance and ensure that people who want to attend the groups are not consistently missing out because of poor timing.

Location

Location can also be negotiated. It is important that group members feel comfortable in the venue. Obviously, if people feel threatened, they are unlikely to continue going to the group. For example, many Aboriginal people have had negative experiences in hospitals, and may not feel comfortable in a hospital or community health centre. If there is no local Aboriginal Medical Service, the local Aboriginal Land Council offices may be a comfortable place to meet.

Remember that hospitals and, to a lesser extent, community health centres, have a history of being authoritarian and of being places where people lose control over themselves. It may be difficult for these associations to be broken and so, in the meantime, if there is any doubt, find a more neutral place. Church halls, Country Women's Association halls, youth clubs, senior citizens' centres, Aboriginal Land Council offices and people's homes are just some examples of possible meeting places. Which venue is most appropriate will depend very much on the members of the group.

Another important point about location is that it needs to be accessible to group members. Organising a group to meet in a venue that is not accessible by public transport, or wheelchair, is likely to prevent some people from being able to attend.

Seating

If a group is to work successfully, all members need to feel that they have an equal right to participate. Comfortable seating, arranged so that everyone can see and hear each other is likely to be most effective. However, until group members get to know one another, barriers such as tables are sometimes useful because they stop people feeling exposed or threatened.

The position of the facilitator is important. They may sit opposite shy people in order to encourage them to speak, or next to someone who is talkative in order to minimise eye contact with that person, enabling others in the group to participate.

Getting the group started

How the group is established and the atmosphere that is created when it first meets will help determine whether or not people will go to future meetings. It is, therefore, important to start the group in a way that 'breaks the ice' and enables people to feel comfortable in their surroundings and with each other. If you are organising a group meeting for community development or action work, this may be done fairly informally through introductions and discussion of the particular issues involved. However, for an educational or support group, it might be done more formally.

Icebreakers

Several things can be done at the beginning of a group's life, and at other times when necessary, to break the ice and help relax people into the group. These icebreakers may provide an opportunity for people to introduce themselves to one another in a fun way or discuss their reasons for being involved with the group and what they want to accomplish. There are several resources containing examples of icebreaker activities that can be useful in various groups (for example, West 1997). Some icebreaker activities can also serve as goal-setting activities, when they provide people with an opportunity to discuss why they have joined the group.

Introducing the group

Once the ice is broken and people are settled in you can introduce the group and its goals. If you have asked people during the icebreaker to tell you what they want to achieve from the group, you can now all use this information to plan together the group goals. You may find at this time that your own goals for the group go out the window to some extent, and the group together plans its goals.

By the time you have finished the introduction, members should have an understanding of the group and what it will achieve, and should have had an opportunity to change the group plan so that it more accurately meets their needs.

Experiential activity

Having met one another and determined which issues will be covered during the group's life, group members should leave the first meeting also having had a taste of what the group will be doing. You might therefore involve the group in an activity that begins its formal life or demonstrates just what you will achieve. For example, a stress management group might discuss the particular stressors of its members and do a relaxation exercise. In this way, members are able to leave the first meeting with some sense of whether the group is likely to be beneficial for them or not, and whether or not they plan to return.

Facilitating group discussion

Very often people plan to have a discussion in a group, but they do not plan how it will actually happen. They assume that if they say, 'Let's discuss . . . ' a discussion will just begin. Unfortunately, the times when that will happen are more the exception than the rule. Most times, it is necessary to structure activities that will enable a discussion to develop (Ewles & Simnett 1999, p. 253). You may not need them, but more often than not you will. It will be necessary to have an idea of group members' attitudes to the topic before launching into discussion, so that you have a sense of the best approach to take. Can you be provocative in order to encourage a vigorous debate, or do you need to begin gently and lead the group into the controversial areas? You will need to bear this in mind when planning discussion. Ewles and Simnett (1999, pp. 253–5) suggest that the activities discussed below may be useful in encouraging discussion. *↓ group discussion*

Using trigger materials

Show a film, read a personal account, or play a game that touches on the issues you hope to cover. If it is slightly controversial, it will motivate people to discuss the issues. Then ask specific questions to draw out the pertinent issues. Make sure that you plan a set of questions before the event and that these are open-ended, so that you do not simply receive only 'yes' or 'no' answers.

Debate

Break the group into two, provide both sides with information if necessary, give them time to prepare and then have them debate the issue. Of course, if you want to encourage participation you may be better to keep the debate informal. Having group members argue the position they disagree with is one way of enabling them to clarify their views and hear the views of their 'opponents'.

Brainstorming

Brainstorming is a way of pooling everyone's ideas and coming up with innovative ones, especially if you are trying to find solutions to a problem. It could be used, for example, to come up with ways to change the attitudes of local government councillors towards childcare facilities, convince businesses to become environmentally responsible, devise effective over-eating avoidance tactics or plan stress-release activities into a normal working day.

The typical strategy for brainstorming is as follows:

- put the problem or issue to the group;
- ask participants to think up as many ideas as possible, without judging their own or other people's ideas;
- accept all suggestions and write them down; and

- keep going until all ideas are exhausted and people cannot think of anything else.

What you do next depends on the reason for the brainstorming. If the group was trying to find the most appropriate solution to a problem, the next step would be to prioritise the suggestions made. This may require group members simply to vote, or there may be lengthy discussion, depending on the issue and the philosophy of the group. If the brainstorming was designed to answer a question, you may simply want to group the answers into similar categories.

Rounds

Rounds ensure that everyone has an equal opportunity to participate. They can therefore be used both to encourage shy group members to speak and to prevent dominant group members from monopolising conversation. Ewles and Simnett (1999, p. 254) suggest four rules that are necessary if rounds are to be successful:

1. no interruptions until each person has finished his [or her] statement;

2. no comments on anybody's contribution until the full round is complete (i.e. no discussion, praise, interpretation, criticism or I-think-that-too type of remark);

3. anyone can choose not to participate. Give permission, clearly and emphatically, that anyone who does not want to make a statement can just say 'pass'. This is very important for reinforcing the principle of voluntary participation; and

4. it does not matter if two or more people in the round say the same thing. People should stick to what they wanted to say even if someone has said it already; they do not have to think of something different.

Rounds can be valuable for beginning and ending sessions and getting feedback, or as a measurement of the entire group's opinion.

Buzz groups

Breaking the group into smaller groups to discuss a key issue may enable everyone to participate more fully in the group. As a rule, these small groups need only occur for relatively short periods of time, after which they can report back to the main group.

Conclusion

This chapter has briefly reviewed the role of education in health promotion and discussed some of the key principles to be considered from a Primary Health Care approach. Two-way communication and respect, learning based around needs identified by people themselves and active learning form a foundation for health literacy. On the whole, health workers already have much scope within their traditional roles to incorporate education readily into their work, to do so in a way that enables people to take greater control over their lives, and to use education as a springboard to other health-promotion strategies when these are of value.

Awareness of group process is an extremely useful component of working effectively with groups, whether they are work teams, social action groups, participants in an education group or members of a family. Working with groups in a supportive, enabling way, rather than a limiting or controlling way, is an important part of work to promote health using a Primary Health Care approach.

Medical approaches to health promotion

In Chapter 7 we move to the far end of the continuum of health-promotion approaches outlined in Chapter 1 and examine some of the medical approaches to health promotion. There are a range of strategies used in this approach, including social marketing, immunisation, individual risk factor assessment and screening. If these strategies are underpinned by a Primary Health Care philosophy, then medical approaches to health promotion fit best with the Ottawa Charter for Health Promotion action area of reorientation of health care.

In Chapter 1 we discussed the medical model of health promotion, which is known as selective Primary Health Care. As we said in that chapter, it is a more limited form of Primary Health Care because the principles of social justice, equity, community control and working for social changes that impact on health and wellbeing, do not necessarily form the foundation of this approach. The approaches in selective Primary Health Care concentrate on disease and usually ensure that control over health is maintained by health professionals who do not necessarily take the social context of people's lives into consideration.

This is not arguing against the importance of addressing specific diseases. Selective Primary Health Care has produced important gains. Clearly we must address those diseases that cause human suffering and death. However, as we said in Chapter 1, by only addressing those illnesses, we risk perpetually attempting to address the end result of the problem instead of addressing the root causes of the diseases themselves or the social conditions that perpetuate disease and other suffering.

At the global level, the WHO's approach to surveillance of infectious diseases internationally does appear to work from the foundations of Primary Health Care principles. The WHO focuses on resource-poor countries, and supports the strengthening of national capacity for 'alert and response' through a multi-disease or integrated approach.

At the national level, social marketing is an example of how national governments might become involved in health promotion. The focus of the campaign and development of the strategy may or may not be underpinned by Primary Health Care philosophy.

215

At the local level, medical approaches to health promotion are usually carried out in primary care services, such as community health centres and with primary care providers such as domiciliary nurses, general medical practitioners and allied health professionals. These services do not necessarily foster Primary Health Care principles of social justice, consumer control over decision-making or collaboration with other health and welfare workers to deal effectively with health issues.

Social marketing

Social marketing can be defined as 'the design and implementation of programs aimed at increasing the voluntary acceptance of social ideas or practices' (Egger et al 1999, p. 32). Whilst social marketing is usually associated with use of the mass media, it can be used in any communication medium. Social marketing aims to influence people's values, attitudes and behaviour by encouraging individuals to make healthy choices. It therefore uses the mass media as an information tool to advise or motivate individuals. While they are seen as individual approaches because they focus on individual behaviour change, social marketing strategies are usually aimed at a large well-defined audience. Social marketing involves the application of marketing approaches, developed to sell commercial products, to 'sell' health-enhancing ideas (Egger et al 1993, p. 32). Social marketing is built on recognition of the powerful influence of the mass media on the choices that people make. Social marketing really came into the public agenda in Australia in the 1970s with the use of 'Norm' and the 'Life. Be in it' campaign. This occurred following the recognition of the relationship between so-called 'lifestyle' behaviours and epidemiological health outcomes and the realisation that health-promotion practitioners were not necessarily the most effective way of communicating health messages to wider audiences (Egger et al 1993). As the term 'social marketing' suggests, a significant function, in addition to providing health information, is the 'selling' of a social idea; bringing about gradual social change. For example, the concept of 'safe sex' being everyone's responsibility has widely permeated society following the initial publicity about the spread of HIV and AIDS. Previously, the topic of sexual behaviour was considered to be a personal and private matter, not discussed in public forums. However see Insight 7.1 for a summary of a health promotion project with a social marketing focus. The 'WayOut' project won a 2004 State Government of Victoria Public Health excellence award for innovation in the capacity building category. Social marketing campaigns typically involve an organised set of communication activities, such as:

- *Advertising*: perhaps most notable as well-funded national campaigns about key social health issues, such as safe driving and smoking cessation. Campaigns conducted by the Transport Accident Commission (TAC) and the Anti-Cancer Council — QUIT and Sunsmart — have achieved prominence.
- *Publicity materials*: mass media campaigns that have a memorable logo or catchy slogan such as the red tick (✔) of approval for 'heart safe' foods or 'Slip Slop Slap' for sun protection, have promoted wide awareness.
- *Edutainment*: this is an under-recognised role of the media in promoting or changing social awareness about various issues. Specific themes,

---

Insight 7.1 WayOut: Central Victorian Youth and Sexual Diversity

The main aim of the WayOut project is to redress the isolation, stigma and discrimination that same-sex attracted young people may face as studies show that life for same-sex attracted young people can be very difficult. Since commencement, our project was committed to young people's participation in the design and delivery of services. Through networks in one shire we established our first local working committee of young people, all aged under 25 years. The group decided that it would be open to all young people, irrespective of their sexuality, who shared our aim of challenging homophobia. Same-sex attracted young people are not necessarily identifiable and, indeed, may be going to great lengths to remain invisible, particularly in rural areas such as ours.

The young people in our committee decided that the best way to reach others was to 'flood' the environment with merchandise that included positive messages about sexual diversity and/or slogans to challenge homophobia. The group were confident that young people in particular 'love free stuff' and we could get our messages out by distributing free stickers, T-shirts and posters etc. The group subsequently designed a very innovative range of products and they proved enormously successful. Below is an example of the group's work.

We have also produced pens and badges with the 'We're all human, Fight Homophobia' slogan and an information card for same-sex attracted young people, their family and friends. Our most recently completed resource is a 10-minute DVD/video called 'Homophobia Exposed' which is being used as a resource to raise awareness in schools, community groups and a range of human service agencies.

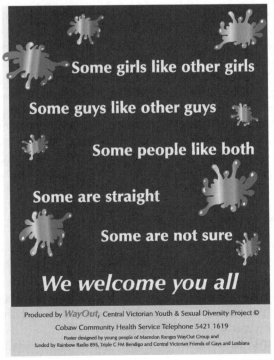

Some girls like other girls

Some guys like other guys

Some people like both

Some are straight

Some are not sure

We welcome you all

Produced by *WayOut*, Central Victorian Youth & Sexual Diversity Project ©
Cobaw Community Health Service Telephone 5421 1619
Poster designed by young people of Macedon Ranges WayOut Group and
funded by Rainbow Radio 89.5, Triple C FM Bendigo and Central Victorian Friends of Gays and Lesbians

such as respect for people suffering mental health problems, or the issue of domestic violence, are crafted into television series and films. Health-promotion professionals provide advice in script development. (For an excellent example of the successful use of edutainment in social marketing see the comprehensive description of the *Soul City* multimedia edutainment program that was developed in South Africa which incorporates health and development issues into television and radio drama serials; Goldstein et al 2004.) Detailed evaluation of this program and the associated resources has demonstrated the effectiveness of the approach when the focus moves away from individual behaviour to interpersonal and social change (Scheepers et al 2004).

In addition, campaigns may be augmented by editorial comment or sponsorship, billboards, brochures and other 'give-aways' or 'handouts' such as stickers, T-shirts, caps etc.

Those who support social marketing in health promotion believe that it can contribute positively if it is part of an integrated health-promotion program and if too much is not expected of it, given the context in which it is being used. Social marketing activities may be aimed at individuals, networks, organisations and societal levels. They are most effective when they are combined with inter-personal and community-based events to enhance health options. Media interventions alone, without complementary health education and community development approaches, are likely to have little impact on behaviour (Redman et al 1990).

It is important to bear in mind that the advertising industry itself conducts considerable market research and targets its advertising very specifically to the groups it wishes to convince. Health workers simply do not have the resources or the skills to match these activities. This is an important point because it alerts health workers to the problems inherent in trying to emulate (and undo) the larger campaigns run by the advertisers. On many occasions it will be more appropriate for a health worker to draw on the expertise of a graphic artist or advertising agency than to prepare materials 'in-house'. However, at other times, especially where the budget is small, workers may need to get their message across by developing their own media resources. Two issues arise here: the need to draw on the expertise of those in the field when planning major advertising campaigns, and the need to work very carefully when running small social marketing campaigns or using the social marketing approach to support other health-promotion work.

Benefits of social marketing

Social marketing approaches can have a number of benefits for communities that may enable them to make sustained change in social conditions that enhance health.

- National awareness campaigns can be 'tagged' onto local community-driven activities, thus gaining greater awareness of the issue, and enhancing the credibility of a local project.
- They can be used to reflect community values and create a sense of ownership towards significant issues in a community.

- As outlined in the previous chapter, knowledge is itself enabling and empowering. Thus, social marketing messages should provide an 'action plan' informing the person what to do if they decide to take action on the issue.
- They can bring forth a groundswell in networks seeking change in an issue affecting the community.
- They can enhance understanding of complex issues using short, accessible and memorable messages, especially to groups who may not access more traditional health education activities.

Can we sell health like we sell tangible commercial products?

A significant challenge for social marketing approaches is that most commercial products offer instant gratification (and long-term risk), whereas the benefits of health behaviour change are often delayed. One recent attempt to help balance the influence of unhealthy and healthy advertising in Australia has been the banning of some unhealthy advertising; most notably, tobacco advertising. However, for an impact to be made on unhealthy advertising overall, there would need to be considerable legislative control of advertising. This would be likely to be vigorously opposed, because it would be regarded as seriously eroding people's expectations about freedom of speech and freedom of choice. Targeted health behaviours are often at odds with social pressures. For example, harm minimisation approaches contrast with strong teenage peer pressure to drink to excess.

Legislative control of advertising raises ethical questions about the right of the state to take over the life of the individual. This is by no means a simple issue; after all, it is argued that mass media advertising itself manipulates people's free choice, often beyond recognition (Connell 1977, pp. 195–6). In addition, health risk behaviours are often complex and involve several determinants, as we have outlined in earlier chapters. Short messages are necessarily simplistic and cannot account for the complexities in individual situations.

Finally, millions of dollars are spent annually on advertising unhealthy, but profitable, products. Health workers, even when they are supported by national media campaigns, are in no position to match the extent to which unhealthy products are marketed — they simply do not have the same financial resources at their disposal (Eisenberg 1987, p. 110). However, social marketing strategies can be a form of advocacy directed at policy-makers, systems and social structures just as readily as they can be directed at the individual (State Government of Victoria 2003). Proponents of social marketing argue that it can be used effectively in a way that supports Primary Health Care work and is empowering for those it is designed to assist. For example, it can be used as a reminder of healthy behaviours and can therefore be supportive of other health-promotion strategies. It can inform the public about the importance of new health policy or legislation at the same time that those changes are being developed. The principles of Primary Health Care, however, are not an inherent component of social marketing, and so it is up to each individual health worker to ensure that he or she uses social marketing in a way that supports the principles of Primary Health Care.

A question of ethics in social marketing

The whole notion of social marketing does not sit comfortably with everyone. The tactics advertising companies use, are often held to be unethical because they are based on the idea of influencing people's choices, often without their awareness. Using the same tactics, and therefore trying to beat advertisers at their own game, does have some ethical problems.

Much media advertising is built on unhealthy stereotypes of people, and much social marketing seems to accept these unquestioningly, rather than challenge them. There is, therefore, much work to be done in challenging these stereotypes, which themselves can contribute to narrow views of health and normality and reduced feelings of self-worth in individuals. If social marketing builds on these stereotypes, rather than challenging them, the overall health benefit from any messages may be limited.

Key criticisms

The key criticisms of social marketing are:

- Stereotyping — in order to generate wider appeal the 'ideal' type is used (young, blonde, beautiful). The 'target' audience for the message may not associate themselves and their situation with the message.

- It may ignore the social, economic and environmental determinants of health. Messages are usually short and cannot accommodate wider social issues. This has potential to reinforce the disadvantage of disadvantaged groups, and raises the potential of 'victim-blaming' [discussed in more detail in the previous chapter].

- It has a single issue focus, rather than emphasising holistic wellbeing.

- Social marketing, despite its applicability at social and policy levels, is generally used as an individual, behaviour-change strategy.

(State Government of Victoria 2003)

Analysing the audience

Successful social marketing campaigns achieve their aim of creating awareness of an issue or bringing about change because they understand the characteristics of their audience; their knowledge, attitudes, values and beliefs. Gathering information to clearly understand the audience enables the strategy to be specifically targeted at a small, fairly homogenous priority audience. The aim is to address and build on existing knowledge and beliefs and to correct misconceptions that are impeding adoption of healthier actions. Using a planning model, such as the Health Belief Model (see Chapter 6), at this stage of planning will enable a broad understanding of the audience segment. Good preparation, making use of research data and pilot-testing ideas with the audience, such as using focus groups, is essential to ensure the expected effects are achieved. 'Segmenting' the audience in this way will mean the strategy is likely to 'reach' the priority group, saving money and effort entailed in a 'one-size-fits-all approach', and it will help prevent the possibility of failing to engage with the group(s) you want to reach most.

Who is your primary audience? These are the key things you need to know about your audience in order to create the right message for them. For social marketing at social or policy levels, the themes would need to be modified accordingly.

Demographic characteristics

- Age range, gender balance, work characteristics, income and education levels, where they live and work, and specific cultural characteristics.

Behavioural characteristics

- What behaviour is currently putting them at risk?
- What reinforces the existing behaviours?
- Do they have perceptions about the risk or seriousness associated with their current behaviour?
- Do they have perceptions about the costs and benefits of the desired change?

Psychographic characteristics

- What are their values and beliefs about the issue or behaviour?
- What are their main and preferred sources of health information — their media preferences?
- What or who influences their readiness to change an existing behaviour?

Identifying the key messages

Literature and demographic analysis will identify the priority issues that are the focus of social marketing messages. From this analysis, a small number of key succinct statements (no more than five), which are the most relevant points to be conveyed to the audience, need to be developed. Attention to the wording to ensure it is appropriate to the audience is important.

Setting social marketing objectives

SMART objectives were emphasised in Chapter 6; that is, the importance of clearly defining what the activity will achieve. Social marketing objectives will be primarily concerned with raising awareness or knowledge about an issue, to produce favourable attitudes to a desirable change, to influence social norms within the priority audience, to influence public opinion to be in line with changing social values, and to produce modest behaviour change. It is very easy to set objectives that are too 'grand' for the style of message and/or the spread of the message. Health communication objectives will need to link to a wider social agenda (such as national health priority area) or a community-based initiative. In this way, a strategy for a wider purpose will generate objectives for a social marketing campaign.

Consider possible communication options

Planners need to select the mode of communication most likely to reach the priority audience. This decision needs to be balanced by budget considerations. Where possible, consider the multiplier benefits of 'tagging' a local campaign onto a national social marketing strategy. For example, have a local 'Healthy Eating' campaign on 'National No-diet Day'. A very specifically targeted message may produce a good return if it can reach the desired audience.

Make use of any 'free' opportunities for raising awareness about the issue, such as 'Letters to the Editor' and editorials in newspapers, social service announcements on radio and television, and news segments in agency newsletters. Some of these options may only be available in partnership with paid advertising. Consider whether the paid advertising will in fact reach the priority audience. Mass circulation newspapers have a very low readership in some audience segments.

Consider the following options:

- Newsletters — identify how frequently a newsletter is published, what the publication requirements are and whether the readership fits with your strategy.
- Press releases — sometimes a press release is published 'as is', especially when photographs are provided at the time of submission, or a photo opportunity is identified. More details about writing a press release are provided in the next section.
- Internet sites — a website may be the mode of information-seeking most used by some audiences. Consider using this audience in the development phase.
- Posters — these will contain the key messages in a form that attracts attention to the specific audience that is sought. They should not be too complicated, but should contain contact information relevant to the theme.
- Static displays — displays that are designed to interest a passing audience are useful at venues where people congregate, such as shopping centres and farming field days. Interest is enhanced when there is an additional 'hook' to attract the audience, such as screenings or 'give-aways'. These sites can also be very useful for market research about social issues and community values.
- Brochures, pamphlets and fact sheets — distribution can be in hard-copy or via email. They may be used to engage participants and/or to provide more detailed health information that supports a social marketing campaign. They should always contain contact information. More detail about their preparation is provided in the next section.
- Promotional material — distributed free or for sale can be produced relevant to the characteristics of the market. Young audiences are very fond of free items, such as stickers, writing pads, pens, fridge magnets, bookmarks, T-shirts, drink bottles and so on. The items are often costly to produce, but the advantage is that the message is retained. Consider engaging the audience in selection, design and production of the materials.
- Advertising — print, television, radio or online options may be considered. Consider cost and audience preferences.

Skills in using the mass media

Working effectively with the mass media requires skill. As with any other specialty, it is wise to seek out the support and advice of experts when planning a major media campaign. The following hints are suggested to help you develop an effective working relationship with local media outlets.

Preliminary work

An important first step in using the mass media is establishing contact with the people who make the decisions in local newspapers, radio stations and television stations, as well as the writers and production people (Weiss & Kessel 1987, p. 40). Getting to know all these people may increase the chance of your articles or stories being accepted. Find out how to present the stories so that they are more likely to be accepted. They may also be able to provide some valuable advice on how to improve media presentation skills. Find out about the deadlines for copy. It can be very frustrating to miss the deadline and to have the story run too late for other elements of the project.

Check the local paper and radio station to see if particular journalists or interviewers seem to have an interest in health issues, and then establish a working relationship with them. Working with those people will be much more useful, since they are the ones most likely to be interested in these projects. They may also be more inclined to call for information about other issues should they need it. Establishing an ongoing relationship in this way can be useful for both health workers and media people.

A word of warning, however. Check the workplace protocol for media releases. Many health agencies require all contact with the mass media, and all media resources, to be approved and overseen by the chief executive officer. If that is the case, use the correct channels and prepare the material sufficiently in advance to enable it to be reviewed and passed on.

What makes an item newsworthy?

It is important to present stories for the news in a manner that is newsworthy. Elements that help make an item newsworthy (Levey 1983, cited by Weiss & Kessel 1987, p. 40) include:

- Information — the item will need to give information that is new to people or provide a new angle on what they know.
- Timeliness — the item will need to be presented at a time that fits in with other local or national events. Indeed, part of the skill in producing newsworthy items is in taking advantage of other events that have already proved newsworthy by 'dovetailing' into them. If your item is to be timely, it will also need to be presented far enough ahead of any action in which you are encouraging people to become involved, so that they have the opportunity to become involved if they wish to.
- Significance and relevance — the item will need to present material that is significant and relevant to the lives of the audience. If the relevance is not likely to be obvious to the whole of the audience, the item should outline the significance of the issues discussed.
- Scope — the item will need to be relevant to many community members or a significant group in the community.
- Interest — the item will need to be interesting to the audience. Weiss and Kessel (1987, p. 40) suggest that items can be made more newsworthy by involving a famous person, linking the story to a national or historical issue, or presenting the story with interesting photographs or cartoons. It

is important to note, however, that these things need to be done with some sensitivity or they may backfire (see Insight 7.2).

- Human interest — the item is more likely to be newsworthy if it is made directly relevant to the lives of ordinary people or the life of the community.
- Uniqueness — the item is more likely to be newsworthy if it presents an angle not found in other stories about the issue.

The more of the above elements presented, the more likely it is that the item will be accepted for publication. Remember, however, that these are a guide only, and an item that really stands out on one or two of these points may be more newsworthy than an item that just satisfies each point. Since decisions about newsworthiness are made more on the 'feel' of the editor than the application of any equation, the way in which the story is presented and how it appeals to the editor will be a key factor.

Insight 7.2 Do media campaigns motivate people or put them under added pressure?

The practice of using famous people as role models in media campaigns on arthritis is generally accepted, but does their use motivate those of us who have arthritis, or does it just put unnecessary pressure on us? I think the latter is the case and, as an arthritis activist, researcher and lobbyist with a long personal experience of rheumatoid arthritis, I believe the practice needs to be questioned.

There is a lack of awareness of the impact on people with arthritis, when the achievements of television personalities or sportsmen are continually emphasised during fundraising campaigns. Their achievements certainly help to raise funds, but with the reports of these 'Super Cripps' doing remarkable things despite their arthritis, comes the implication that we should be emulating them, and that is impossible for many of us. Getting out of bed in the morning is a major achievement for some people with arthritis, and these people in particular can do without the 'buck up and go out' treatment presented by current media campaigns.

Our society's obsession with competition and achievement is inappropriate when people are sick. It is also inappropriate to use male role models when arthritis predominantly affects women. In the Arthritic Women's Task Force's video 'Women with rheumatoid arthritis: don't take us at face value', one of the women talks about the arthritis posters, which depict the achievements of a famous AFL footballer, and the resulting pressures on her also to be an achiever. Those pressures are usually exerted by well-meaning relatives, friends and neighbours, who are impressed by the media campaigns. They do not understand the difference between rheumatoid arthritis and the milder forms of arthritis and fail to realise the seriousness of her illness. They just look at her face and do not see the rest.

This is probably an even greater problem for women whose arthritis has not yet reached the obvious stage. They do not look sick and, if their husbands do not understand what rheumatoid arthritis is like, or if their husbands have deserted them, the pressures to achieve, according to male perceptions of achievement, are especially distressing. These women are already aware that they are considered to be inadequate underachievers; having media pressure put on them, particularly when they are trying to cope with a major flare-up of their arthritis and care for their homes and children at the same time, only increases their problems.

There is another aspect of the practice of using famous people in media campaigns that should be questioned. That is the failure of the media and the fundraising organisations to recognise the fact that some of these people are doing irreparable harm to their bodies in their determination to achieve stardom and that they are not, in fact, good role models for people with arthritis to emulate. The pressures on television personalities and sportspeople to perform to a very high standard are just as destructive as the pressures on us to emulate them, and it is distressing to see how soon famous people are forgotten when they are no longer able to perform.

It is extremely difficult for people with arthritis to object to or challenge the way media campaigns are carried out because the famous people, the fundraisers, the media and the community at large all believe that they are helping us. The concept of charity is deeply rooted in our culture, and we are seen as ungrateful when we question the way it is dispensed. The fact that no one asked us whether we wanted that sort of media campaign or whether we want to be treated as objects of charity is overlooked in a sea of hurt feelings.

The needs of a great many people are met when they participate in a media fundraising campaign. It makes them feel good and, until they question the real impact of their actions on us, or until we, the people with arthritis, become politically active consumers, I think the failure of media campaign organisers to recognise the difference between motivation and pressure (the latter exemplified by the threatening slogan 'Move it or Lose it') will persist.

Joan Byrne
Consumer and arthritis activist

Another key factor will be when a story is submitted and what other stories have come in that day. An excellent story may be rejected if it arrives on the editor's desk at the same time as stories about a forthcoming political battle, a bus crash and a rags-to-riches lottery win. In such a case, you may need to wait a few days and resubmit your story. Furthermore, some days are easier for having stories accepted because they are less likely to be days when the media have many stories to deal with. Beauchamp (1986, p. 76) suggests that Fridays are invariably bad days to submit items, and so avoid it unless it is something that will stop the presses. One additional technique that has been used with success, particularly in regional areas, is to arrange sponsorship of health-promotion activities by mass media outlets. Box 7.1 provides health workers with some general rules to use as a guide before submitting a letter to the editor.

Writing to persuade: writing letters and media releases

The key to success when writing a media release, a letter to the editor of a newspaper or a letter to a member of parliament, is to write persuasively. Rather than merely letting a journalist know that an important event is soon to occur or that a particular issue warrants discussion, and hoping that he or she will write an article about it, submit a media release. This increases the chance that the story will run, because most of the work has already been done for the journalist. Moreover,

> **Box 7.1 Hints for writing letters to the editor**
>
> - Check the newspaper to which you are writing for any guidelines on presentation of letters.
> - Type or write clearly, using double spacing and leaving a wide margin.
> - Be as brief as possible, examining the length of letters previously published may be a useful guide.
> - Keep your sentences short and sharp.
> - Present constructive criticism, rather than simply being critical.
> - Avoid using too much emotional language.
> - If you wish to have your letter published anonymously, you can request this, but you will still need to supply your name and address, explaining why you want your name withheld.
> - If your letter does not appear, you can contact the letters editor to find out why. It is not unusual for letters to take a number of weeks to be published.

(Source: based on Beauchamp, K. 1986 *Fixing the Government: Everyone's Guide to Lobbying in Australia.* Penguin, Melbourne, pp. 64–7)

the media release itself may provide the information that convinces the journalist that the issue is a valuable one and a newsworthy item. There may have been many times when journalists have rejected potential news items simply because they did not have enough information at their fingertips. Similarly, present your views on an issue to members of a community. Writing a letter to the editor of a local or major newspaper may be a useful way to get a message across. If a good argument is presented, and presented in a way that is interesting, the letter is more likely to be published.

Writing persuasively takes some practice but there are a few simple steps to follow to increase the chance that your written material will present a persuasive argument. Keep in mind, also, the elements of a newsworthy item. Firstly, write clearly and simply, so that the message is understood. Robert Gunning (cited in Anderson & Itule 1988, p. 39) has suggested 'ten principles of clear writing', which provides a useful guide:

1. Keep sentences short, on the average.
2. Prefer the simple to the complex.
3. Prefer the familiar word.
4. Avoid unnecessary words.
5. Put action into your verbs.
6. Write the way you talk.
7. Use terms your reader can picture.
8. Tie in with your reader's experience.
9. Make full use of variety.
10. Write to express not impress.

As well as being clearly written, the media release or letter will need to be well structured. Wrigley and McLean (1990) suggest four steps in the development of persuasive writing. They are:

1. get the reader's attention;

2. arouse the reader's interest;

3. motivate the reader to take action; then

4. tell the reader what action to take.

Get the reader's attention

Wrigley and McLean (1990, pp. 238–9) suggest two ways in which to get the reader's attention: use an attractive layout, and make the content relevant to the reader. The layout of the document will give the reader an idea of whether he or she wants to read it, and this is therefore very important. It includes a title that grabs the reader's attention, together with the use of headings and white space to help break up the document. These will be discussed in more detail below. Making the content relevant to the reader starts with being clear about whom the article is intended for, and writing with that audience in mind. Writing to the reader (by saying 'you' and 'your'), focusing on people, using graphics where appropriate and keeping your message simple and clear will all help.

Arouse the reader's interest

The reader's interest will be aroused through the title and the first paragraph of the document, which, like any good introduction, should summarise what the document will tell the reader. Writing in a 'journalistic' style means that the most important or newsworthy point is stated first, which is contrary to the usual 'academic' style, where the background and rationale for the topic are provided first.

Motivate the reader to take action

Present a succinct summary of the issues in a way that helps the reader to work through the facts and come to an opinion. This can be done by arranging information in a logical order, explaining where necessary and documenting any new or contentious information that is presented.

Tell the reader what action to take

Although putting all the above into practice may have convinced the reader that your message is valid, the aim is often to do more than that. If the aim is to encourage people to act on an issue, tell them what action they can take. If this isn't done, they may feel more informed when they have finished reading, but no more sure of what to do. It is important, then, that they know what they can do to make a difference.

Using photographs

Whether you are submitting a press release to a journalist or simply asking him or her to cover a particular issue, providing a photograph, or advising of a photo opportunity, will help your story in two ways. Firstly, it will increase the chance that your story will be published, because it will be a more interesting piece for the newspaper to print with a photograph nearby. Secondly, because your story has visual appeal, more people are likely to read it when it appears in the paper. Photographs can attract a reader and persuade just as successfully as words, and sometimes even more so. If you are providing a photograph, it will need to be of high quality and preferably black and white, although a sharply contrasted colour photo may be acceptable.

Preparing for a radio or television interview

Radio and television interviews are useful means of getting across a message to a wide audience. However, the pace is usually fast, and complex issues are often not given the depth they may require. Because of the fast pace, preparation for such an interview is important.

Wherever possible, present the interviewer with a list of the questions that need to be asked to cover the topic. Clarify the basic points with the interviewer beforehand. There is nothing worse than a two-minute interview disappearing without the message being put across because the interviewer did not understand a basic point and subsequently asked irrelevant questions.

In addition to presenting the interviewer with questions, prepare the answers, even on familiar topics. It is very easy to become nervous and forget the message. Also, because of the pace, the most important things must go first. There is no shame in not doing totally off-the-cuff interviews; indeed, only very experienced interviewees can usually get away with them.

If it is not possible to prepare questions beforehand, discuss what the interviewer plans on asking you. Use this discussion as an opportunity to suggest other appropriate questions. Interviewers usually appreciate any suggestions that will improve the quality of the interview.

Find out if the interview is going to be pre-taped or live. If it is pre-taped, there will be an opportunity for it to be edited if necessary. This is wise and it may be possible to request that the interview be pre-taped. Many interviewers will be happy to oblige if it is possible, but a word of warning — *never* assume that something that is said is 'off the record'.

Always make eye contact with the interviewer. Maintaining eye contact with the interviewer, rather than continually reading notes, is enough to help keep your voice sounding conversational rather than monotone. Talking directly to the interviewer as much as possible will help keep your voice interesting.

Controversial issues and media interviews

Since health issues can so often involve differences of opinion, it is a good idea to go into every interview expecting the unexpected! The important thing to remember when being interviewed on a controversial topic is to stay focused on the issue and not get caught up in the controversy that is being created. This takes some self-discipline but is well worth it if you do not want to cloud the issues.

Preparing health information materials

Using the media to support or strengthen a personal health message is increasingly part of health-promotion work. It is vital, therefore, to be able to critically review these materials to determine whether they are appropriate. If nothing suitable is available, the following general principles may guide the way in which local materials are produced for maximum effect.

Written materials

Written materials, such as brochures, posters and booklets, can provide useful reinforcement for other health information materials and enable people to take information home with them. With any written materials, a few key elements can make the difference between a readable, appealing document and one that does not invite the potential reader to go beyond a casual glance. These are:

- the use of white space;
- a variety of print sizes;
- readable language; and
- drawings and photographs to help the words used come alive.

White space

White space is simply the amount of empty space left in the document. It is very important because, without adequate white space, a document can seem crowded and difficult to read. Space between words and paragraphs helps potential readers to see that the document is unlikely to swamp them, and will help them to work their way through it.

Variety of print sizes

Varying the print size and style, through the use of headings and different type fonts, makes the words on the page interesting and again helps to break up text. Headings that stand out also act as a summary of the document for people flipping through it, and so enable them to see if they would like to continue reading.

Readable language

Of course, no amount of variety in print size will counteract words that are difficult to understand or unreadable by the people your materials are supposedly designed for. So many written materials produced for health education contain language that makes the information in them inaccessible to many people. Several formulas for assessing the readability of education materials have been suggested (see, for example, Hawe et al 1990, pp. 70–2).

Involving some of the people you are designing the materials for in the development process will ensure that the materials are readable. It will also ensure that the materials are appropriate and acknowledge the expertise of these people in issues related to their own lives. Schwab et al (1992) and Neuhauser et al (1998) provide an example of how this process was implemented in the preparation of a *Wellness Guide*. Through involving a group of potential consumers of the *Wellness Guide* in reviewing a draft of the guide, and responding when these community members identified a range of problems from a consumer's perspective, the developers were able to produce a final product whose impact far exceeded their original idea, and which had real meaning for the community.

Drawings and photographs

Drawings and photographs are key ingredients in written health education materials. Indeed, there are times when they may appropriately represent all the 'writing' in the document. The old saying 'A picture is worth a thousand words' is relevant here. Drawings and photographs may tell the reader a great deal more than words alone could do, and this is the case not only for people who have difficulty in reading, but for all readers. Drawings and photographs help to make sense of any words, and may clarify things that are expressed with difficulty in words. They also give the document appeal and break up any writing in much the same way as white space.

A word of caution about drawings, however. Ensure that they make sense to the people you are presenting the material for. Drawings, like words, have readability levels. Health workers have a range of knowledge about matters of health and illness, and it is easy to forget how much of this is not shared by members of the community.

General guidelines for 'take-home' health information material

You will all be familiar with the 'display board' of pamphlets and brochures in many health agencies. You will also have noticed that some are much more 'user-friendly' than others; they are more attractive or enticing to select, and/or they convince you to read the detail. At times you may be called upon to design a health education brochure or material to advertise a forthcoming health education or community activity. Drawing on the 'ten principles of clear writing' presented previously, the following guidelines may be useful when preparing take-home material.

1. Work in partnership with members of your prospective audience to select and design the style of material and develop the wording.

2. Be as concise as you can to present the simplest possible message, using simple language. Get rid of any wasted words.

3. Short sentences help you develop an argument; they help the flow and are easier to fit into the layout of pamphlets.

4. Avoid jargon because it limits the audience and it dates the material.

5. Avoid too many definitions and too much background.

6. Use headings as 'signposts' and use a verb in the headings.

7. 'Road-test' the material with other prospective clients of the resource.

8. Get feedback from cultural minority groups and others who do not understand the topic.

9. Allow plenty of time, prepare a draft, leave it, then return to edit it.

10. Check for completeness — ensure it provides contact details, links to relevant agencies, and details of time and location where relevant.

11. Consider the requirements for agency or sponsor logo. Size and placement are important to agencies. Unauthorised use or alteration may be subject to legal penalty. Agency logo placement and size may also need to reflect the 'size' of their sponsorship of the social marketing strategy.

Audiovisual materials

Videos and audio tapes can provide useful health education in a form that is often more interesting than written materials and accessible to people who do not have good literacy skills. They may also be preferred by those people who learn more readily through listening and watching than through reading.

Amateur videos may be quite successful if made by members of the group whose needs are being addressed, and can be very useful teaching tools. Materials produced by community members themselves are more likely to address a group's needs and be acceptable to it. However, producing a video is expensive. It is possible, though, to keep the costs down by engaging a producer to take on the role of consultant.

Adapting material from state or national campaigns to your local area

There are times when health workers are asked to implement a campaign developed at a regional or national level. Materials may be provided as part of that program. These materials will need to be assessed for suitability to the local conditions. If they are not, they may be able to be adapted. Hints for preparing media releases are provided in Box 7.2.

Box 7.2 Hints for preparing media releases

- Present the release in typewritten form on A4 paper, double spaced, typed on one side only and with a wide margin.
- Use letterhead paper, so that the organisation presenting the release is clearly identifiable.
- Ensure that the release is clearly dated, or that the date for publication of the material is given.
- Clearly mark the document with the heading 'Media Release'.
- Use plain language, and short, sharp sentences.
- Keep the release short — no more than two pages.
- Suggest an attractive title.
- Include quotations from relevant people.
- Include a contact name and phone number (and be prepared to be contacted).

(Source: based on Flood, M. and Lawrence, A. 1987 *The Community Action Book*. NSW Council of Social Services, Sydney, pp. 84–5; and Beauchamp, K. 1986 *Fixing the Government: Everyone's Guide to Lobbying in Australia*. Penguin, Melbourne, pp. 71–2)

Immunisation, screening, individual risk factor assessment and surveillance

We now move to the furthest end of the continuum of health-promotion approaches and examine some of the remaining medical approaches to health promotion. This includes immunisation, screening and individual risk factor assessment. As we have said, these strategies may not be underpinned by a Primary Health Care philosophy. The four best known medical approaches to health promotion are immunisation, screening, individual risk factor assessment and surveillance. They have emerged as population-based strategies.

✝ Immunisation

There are national immunisation programs in many countries that aim to reduce the spread of vaccine-preventable diseases across targeted populations. In Australia, for example, the program targets infants, children, adolescents and seniors for inoculations against diseases such as hepatitis B, diphtheria and tetanus in infants, measles, mumps and rubella in children, and influenza in seniors.

To control a vaccine-preventable disease, a sufficient pool of people must be immunised against the disease to prevent spread of that disease in the population. There have been some spectacular results in this regard, such as the global eradication of smallpox.

It must be remembered that political will to support programs to address the disease, and substantial resources, are required to achieve this type of result, and even then, in Australia, for example, where there is a national immunisation program, Plant (1995 in Baum 2002) reports that immunisation programs have not been able to reach a sufficient pool of people to prevent the spread of some diseases. This is despite legislation in some states requiring evidence of vaccination status before entering school, and also, the efforts of members of the Australian Technical Advisory Group on Immunisation who advise the national government and assisted the National Health and Medical Research Council to produce *The Australian Immunisation Handbook* (2003). This book provides health professionals with guidance about vaccines and diseases and vaccine practice. This begs the question, 'What else needs to be done?'

The responsibility for providing immunisation programs in Australia rests with Environmental Health Officers and Maternal and Child Health Nurses in local government, and with private general medical practitioners. General (medical) practitioners have identified structural barriers within their practice to engaging in health-promotion activities. These barriers include lack of initial and continuing education in health promotion, low financial incentives and lack of time in consultations (James et al 2003; Baum 2002). Considerable effort has been made by many local governments to increase the immunisation rates in their municipality. These strategies include asking parents what needs to be done to facilitate attendance at immunisation sessions. Family friendly times and venues have emerged to meet the needs of some communities as a result of including the community in the planning of these programs. This has resulted in increased immunisation rates within these municipalities.

✝ Screening

Screening is a medical approach to health promotion where a health professional or agency advertises a service and promises a result (Cochrane 1972 in Robinson & Elkan 1996). The decision to provide a screening service is determined following a cost benefit analysis.

The aim of a screening procedure in health promotion is to identify specific conditions in targeted groups before symptoms appear. 'Screening involves the systematic use of a test or investigatory tool to detect individuals at risk of developing specific disease that is amenable to prevention or treatment' (State

Government of Victoria 2003, p. 45). Priorities for screening differ from country to country. Common health-promotion screening procedures in Australia include childhood screening for hearing and eyesight problems, screening for breast and cervical cancer in women, and screening for hypertension in adults. Screening criteria have been developed to guide governments and health services in their decision-making about providing screening services.

Screening criteria includes information about the disease, the test, follow-up and treatment, and the cost (Robinson & Elkan 1996). The disease, for example, must be one that has a definite effect on length or quality of life and the progression from the latent or early symptomatic stage of the disease must be well understood. The test must be safe, simple, reasonably accurate and acceptable to the providers and population. False positive results and false negative results can cause immeasurable damage to the individual. Follow-up and treatment procedures must be in place and acceptable. Follow-up for positive results must be available quickly and treatment for early detection effective. The cost of screening a population or sub-group of the population, follow-up and treatment must be something the community can afford (Robinson & Elkan 1996).

Screening may also occur for risk factors such as family history, nutrition and physical activity. It has been considered important to maximise the opportunity for disease prevention at the point of screening. Health professionals may conduct a risk factor assessment and provide information to individuals about risk factors for a range of diseases. Screening and risk factor assessments are often used as an engagement strategy or within an integrated disease prevention strategy. For example, Papanicolaou smear screening may be a strategy to provide women with information about risk factors for diseases other than cervical cancer.

Individual risk factor assessment

The aim of a risk factor assessment is similar to screening procedures; that is, to identify specific factors in targeted groups before symptoms appear. 'Individual risk factor assessment involves a process of detecting the overall risk of a single disease or multiple diseases. These can include biological, psychological and behavioural risks' (State Government of Victoria 2003, p. 45). Many assessment checklists have been developed for health professionals to assist them in identifying specific diseases such as the potential for cardiovascular disease. Self-administered tools exist but it is thought that 'for tools requiring diagnostic interpretation, individuals should be referred to qualified professional staff' (State Government of Victoria 2003, p. 45).

Effectiveness of these interventions

Evidence from studies that alerted us to the possibility that medical and behaviour-change interventions in health promotion had limitations was from Rose and Marmot (1981), who found that the main risk factors for coronary heart disease, for example, cholesterol, smoking, blood pressure and others combined, explained considerably less than half of the difference in mortality between different ranks of the civil service in Britain (Baum 2001, p. 319). This led many to question the efficacy of screening and risk factor assessment programs.

Controversy over screening and risk factor assessment procedures continues. For example, while the benefits of mammography screening for women over 50 years of age have been demonstrable, there is no evidence that breast self-examination is effective in reducing mortality from breast cancer (Weller 1997 in Baum 2002, p. 317). Further, there is little evidence that screening followed by an educational intervention has an impact on risk factors (Baum 2000, p. 317).

> ... relevant information, such as information about the increased risk of diagnosis with screening, is often counterintuitive. Benefits are relatively rare and often delayed, and the screening process can involve a whole series of interventions. The harms of screening are poorly understood by the public, and screening tests are often viewed uncritically.
>
> (Barratt et al 2004, pp. 507–10)

Screening decisions are complex, and according to Barratt et al (2004, pp. 507–10):

- leads to over-detection and over-treatment;
- may include invasive follow up investigations and treatments;
- harm is immediate and benefits are delayed;
- few people experience benefits from screening compared with the number who would be expected to benefit from most treatments;
- individual values and preferences are critical to screening decision-making;
- evidence base for screening decision aids is often limited;
- public attitude is that early detection and or prevention must be good;
- little regulation is in place to protect consumers from aggressive marketing, and there may be strong financial incentives to get people to participate in screening.

Decision aids for policy-makers, health professionals and consumers have been suggested by Barratt et al (2004, pp. 507–10) and include:

- present the chances of having pseudo-disease as well as clinically important disease detected by screening;
- give information about the whole of the early detection and treatment process;
- present balanced information about the cumulative chance of benefits and harms over equivalent time frames;
- present very small numbers by using large and consistent denominators, for example, outcomes per 1000 or per 10 000 people screened;
- screening decision aids need to accommodate flexibility in labelling the outcomes of screening as benefits or harms;
- explicitly declare where high quality evidence is lacking; use ranges or some other method to convey uncertainty in numerical estimates;
- explain that there is a choice and the reasons why people might decide to decline screening;
- information about financial gains to the organisation offering the screening test may need to be included in decision aids.

✳ Surveillance

Surveillance can be part of the Primary Health Care approach to health promotion. The WHO recognises that governments have a responsibility for the health of their peoples, which can be fulfilled only by the provision of adequate health and social measures (WHO 1948). The WHO addresses issues such as the unequal development in different countries in the promotion of health and control of disease, especially communicable disease.

The increasing threats to public health posed by epidemic-prone and emerging infections, led the World Health Assembly in 2001 to adopt the resolution 'global health security — epidemic alert and response' which made specific recommendations about surveillance and response to the WHO and its member states (WHO 2004e).

Animal pathogens are 'jumping species' more easily due to deforestation and urban sprawl that bring humans and animals in closer contact and as a result new epidemics are emerging. Globalisation, climate change, the growth of mega-cities and the explosive increase in international travel are increasing the potential for the rapid spread of infections (WHO 2004e).

Many of these epidemics, such as cholera and meningitis, recurrently challenge health systems in countries with limited resources. Others, such as influenza and dengue, have an increasing potential to create new pandemics. The emergence and rapid spread of drug-resistant tuberculosis and malaria increase treatment costs (WHO 2004e).

Every country should be able to detect, verify rapidly and respond appropriately to epidemic-prone and emerging disease threats when they arise, to minimise their impact on the health of the population (WHO 2004e).

Global health security needs the involvement of many collaborators; no single entity can bring it about on its own. Formal and informal networks collect and analyse information, and develop resources and tools to assist countries to implement activities.

Working with its partners, the WHO Department of Communicable Disease Surveillance and Response (the CSR) aims to reach global health security following three strategic directions: contain known risks, respond to the unexpected and improve preparedness (WHO, 2004e).

- Contain known risks — the CSR focuses on the leading epidemic-prone and emerging diseases, such as cholera, dysentery, influenza, meningococcal meningitis, plague, viral haemorrhagic fevers (Ebola, Lassa), 'mad cow' disease, anthrax and others.
- Respond to the unexpected — rapid, effective response to outbreaks relies on timely alert and response mechanisms. CSR's epidemic intelligence system gathers and verifies outbreak information daily from around the world and coordinates international responses to outbreaks of global importance.
- Improve preparedness — focusing particularly on resource-poor countries, CSR provides tools, expert assistance and carefully tailored training to enhance skills in laboratory diagnosis, field epidemiology and public health mapping.

Conclusion

The medical model of health promotion is a more limited form of Primary Health Care because the principles of social justice, equity, community control and working for social change that impact on health and wellbeing, are not necessarily taken into consideration. Disease is the focus of these approaches and control over health is usually maintained by health professionals. There are a range of strategies used, including social marketing, immunisation, individual risk factor assessment, surveillance and screening. However, evidence from many studies have alerted us to the possibility that medical and behaviour-change interventions in health promotion have limitations.

Nevertheless, the mass media have a powerful influence on people's lives and the manner in which they view the world. Using the mass media within the Primary Health Care philosophy to promote health is therefore of considerable potential value. Whether it be attempting to re-frame health issues in the public eye to raise awareness of public policy issues through media advocacy, or working to encourage a positive health idea or behaviour through social marketing, the mass media offers considerable scope in the promotion of health. As with other health-promotion strategies, there is much to be gained by working in partnership with community members when working with the mass media, and being mindful of the fact that media coverage of health issues, even successful media coverage, is not an end in itself, but a means to achieve health-promoting change.

Screening programs for specific diseases and risk factors in targeted populations are not an end in themselves either. Screening programs have had mixed success. Screening is most successful when the program is part of an integrated approach to health promotion. Furthermore, the disease must be one that has a definite effect on length or quality of life and the progression from the latent or early symptomatic stage of the disease is understood.

Despite the limitations, medical approaches to health have produced important gains. International and national immunisation programs have reduced the spread of vaccine-preventable diseases across targeted populations. Internationally and nationally these programs do appear to work from the foundations of Primary Health Care. Similarly, the approach to surveillance of infectious diseases appears to work from these foundations. The WHO focuses on resource-poor countries, and supports the strengthening of national capacity for 'alert and response' through an integrated approach.

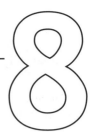

Using the Ottawa Charter for Health Promotion

In this chapter we highlight the key points from the preceding chapters and provide you with some questions that you may ask yourself in your practice as a health worker. The questions arise from the Ottawa Charter for Health Promotion and how the action areas from the charter can guide practice within the socio-ecological, behavioural and medical approaches to health promotion.

It will have become progressively clearer that this book has provided you with an introduction to the knowledge about particular approaches you can take in promoting health and the skills you can use. We have also introduced you to some fundamental concepts concerning the determinants of wellness and illness. This knowledge tells us where we need to be concentrating our efforts as health workers in promoting health.

Key themes in promoting health

The social determinants of health are the key influences on people's experience of life. There is strong evidence that the mal-distribution of society's material and social resources is a determinant of ill health, along with racism, poverty and social exclusion (Wise and Hearn 2004). Degradation of the physical environment is a result of these and exacerbates the problem of ill health further. These determinants need to be taken into account; they need to underpin our actions. We encourage health workers to keep the 'iceberg' model in mind as a guide to practice.

> There is no longer any doubt that the health of populations can be improved significantly by the active efforts of multiple people, communities, and organisations including government and non-government and private sectors. There is also no longer any doubt that the processes used to bring about change — the active engagement of people and communities in making their own choices

237

about priorities and about solutions — are critical to bring about sustained and sustainable changes. The evidence is strong.

(Wise & Hearn 2004, p. 91)

In promoting health, the values, especially that of equity, underpin practice. A socially just society is a healthier society, physically, economically, spiritually, emotionally and environmentally. These values are exemplified in concepts such as empowerment and cultural safety. International frameworks such as the Declaration of Alma-Ata and the Universal Declaration of Human Rights provide guidelines for their implementation. However, these values may not be the values of those in power and, further, the evidence may be ignored by those in power, so enabling people to become healthy and stay healthy will be a political activity.

Whatever the issue is, we may need one or all of the action areas of the Ottawa Charter to guide our practice, or one or all of the approaches that were advocated in Chapter 1 to address the issue. To be effective, it is highly likely that more than one area will be called for. Empowerment happens, and social justice is achieved, when people are enabled to make changes in the context of their lives that enhance their health, in its broadest sense. Health workers can be advocates to influence policy at all levels through formal lines of authority. Health-promotion work involves advocating on behalf of vulnerable community groups for the desired changes to be enshrined in policy. Policy within government or agencies can be used as 'leverage' to bring about change in the social environment, management systems and structures, and to provide rationale for actions in support of the community.

Success in health promotion is dependent upon:

- examining the values that guide the development of healthy public policy;
- examining power in communities and challenging the misdistribution of power;
- raising the consciousness of communities to the determinants of health; and
- working inclusively, respectfully, collaboratively and flexibly.

At all stages and in all activities health workers who value the wisdom, experience and contributions of community members, will be successful in promoting health all of the time. A community's effective participation may be in the hands of health workers.

We are not saying that working for change to promote health is easy. There are challenges in working within communities and with health workers. Health workers can be part of the problem. Hitler wasn't a health worker but he was a 'rabid anti-smoker, a vegetarian, a vigorous exerciser, a greenie and the original member of the animal rights movement' (Galbally 2004, p. 191). Some health workers are megalomaniacs who want to control the agenda. In any given situation we urge health workers to examine the distribution of power first. A change in this distribution will always be the biggest challenge.

Working with vulnerable groups within communities may not be easy either. 'Community groups can be exclusive, elitist, hierarchical and clogged up with the same old faces . . . They can be racist, sexist, ageist, able-bodyist, homophobic, and exclude new blood and new visions' (Galbally 2004, p. 288). Critical consciousness-raising is the key to change here.

238

Ways of working in health promotion

Public health practice involves working with a range of different individuals and communities in a diverse range of settings. The ways of working in health promotion imply a set of values, approaches and strategies as follows:

- working *with* individuals, communities and populations;
- *in* settings such as workplaces, schools, sporting venues and the arts;
- *within* socio-ecological, behavioural and medical models;
- *around* issues including risk conditions such as discrimination, poverty, and natural resource depletion, psychosocial risk factors such as social exclusion, behavioural risk factors such as poor nutrition, and physiological risk factors such as stress;
- *by* policy development, community action for social change, health education, health information, screening and surveillance; and
- *using* frameworks such as the Ottawa Charter for Health Promotion to guide you.

Where do you go from here?

To keep developing your skills and expertise in the area of health promotion you can:

- Use the information here to develop your skills. Put the ideas into practice and see which ones work for you and the community within which you work.
- Keep reading about the areas covered in this book. Each area is based on sound theory and practice. As you develop your background in the areas, you'll be more effective in developing your own theory and practice.
- Talk with your colleagues. Discuss your ideas, your successes and your failures, with anyone who is interested to learn with you.
- Ask questions. Successful people draw on the expertise of others.
- Share your learning professionally, by joining professional associations, attending conferences and presenting papers on your work. So many people who do great work fail to recognise how many people would like to hear about their work and learn from it.
- Work together, supporting and encouraging each other and promoting the health of the team. A great many of the strategies described in this book need to be implemented within health organisations first. Developing the self-efficacy of everyone in the team is vital. Too often health workers write each other off, ignoring the strong socialisation processes that have impacted on each other. Work together, support and encourage each other and promote the health of the team. The ripples of this work will be felt far beyond the confines of the organisation and you will be able to establish a team environment that will achieve so much more than that which individuals alone may achieve.
- Continue working to keep the development of a Primary Health Care system on the agenda, and to ensure that the system develops towards a greater emphasis on the promotion of health. An important component of this will be working for the continuing reorientation of undergraduate and

postgraduate education of health workers and others whose actions impact on health towards a Primary Health Care approach.

The rhetorical questions in the following sections, within the action areas of the Ottawa Charter, are posed to encourage health workers to reflect upon the impact of their actions. They provide practice goals for health workers to aspire to. Specific guidance to achieving them is contained within the various chapters of the book.

Using the Ottawa Charter for socio-ecological approaches

Build healthy public policy
- What are the organisational constraints that would impact on your capacity to adopt a socio-ecological approach to the issue?
- What changes need to be made to ensure fairness?

Create supportive environments
- Is the community in control of identifying the problem, deciding on priorities for action and strategies, and deciding what success will mean?
- Would the use of a health-promotion planning framework, such as PRECEDE, create broader action for change?
- Is the worker working *with* the community — not on or for them?
- Are community members being provided with opportunities to know what is happening in their community and the project?

Strengthen community action
- Has the community been assisted to identify a clear goal?
- Is there a concrete benefit that is clearly evident and desired by community members?
- Is the worker's role enabling rather than managing?
- Can people's life experience be used as a form of advocacy?
- Are there opportunities for fun along the way?
- Have the community's achievements been celebrated?

Develop personal skills
- Have the assets within the community been recognised?
- Is it possible to reorient personal support and crisis management as the initial step in wider social action?
- Is funding used to facilitate the development of transferable and useful skills?

Reorient health services
- Is the health agency able to take a long-term view about social change?
- Are other non-health agencies working together towards the community goal?
- Are agencies in the community flexible enough to deal with a stronger and more skilled community?

The Ottawa Charter as a community assessment tool

Build healthy public policy

- Are there policies that disadvantage people in the community who are already vulnerable or disadvantaged?
- Would a change in policy make it easier for some to be healthy?
- Is policy working to the advantage of those who are already in positions of authority or power?
- Are you able to act as advocate for change that can be enshrined in agency or government policy?
- Are appropriate human ethics procedures being followed — are the rights of community members being protected?
- Does the proposal and its procedures make false promises to community members — are they expecting more than can be delivered?

Create supportive environments

- Is a health-promotion planning framework being used as a guide for data-gathering which reflects a social view of health?
- Are you hearing the voices of all sections of the community?
- Are the processes of assessment excluding some, because of language, locality or other forms of barriers?
- How are you treating people who are 'different'?
- Are you enabling all to learn from the process of assessment?
- Can you ensure that community members will not become scapegoats if decisions do not work out as planned?

Strengthen community action

- Who defined the need?
- Are all community members being consulted?
- Is their participation more than tokenism?
- Can the community strengthen their claims by using research and epidemiological data?
- Are all community members able to understand the assessments findings, and do they all know where to find them?
- Is the community itself leading the decision-making?

Develop personal skills

- Are there opportunities to gain new skills?
- Can you act as a mentor?
- Can the health worker facilitate skills in accessing other relevant information?

Reorient health services

- Are funds being allocated ethically, given the priorities identified in the community assessment?
- Is a new planning cycle based on the outcomes of previous activities?
- Can health promotion be put on the agenda more often?

- Is there an agency agreement or a policy statement that enables support for the most vulnerable community members?
- Is there a focus on providing an environment of support, rather than individual behaviour change?

The Ottawa Charter as an evaluation tool

Build healthy public policy

- Can national, state and local policy priorities provide a rationale for the activities of a program or project?
- Are there agency protocols for funding evaluation procedures and personnel?

Create supportive environments

- Who is participating in the evaluation?
- Is the evaluation process reflecting the profile of participants?
- Were participants in the evaluation consulted about the nature and process of the evaluation — did they make the decisions?
- What methods have been used to enable all interested people to participate in the evaluation — how did they learn about it? Can their confidentiality be maintained?

Strengthen community action

- Are validated data-gathering and community action strategies being used?
- Does the rationale for the project clearly set out the importance of community engagement and capacity building?
- Is the process of engaging the community members documented in program objectives?
- Can the 'software' of community participation be documented and valued?
- Can the community showcase its skills to others?

Develop personal skills

- Are community members supported to consider evaluation at the time actions are being planned?
- Are objectives written from the perspective of the community or program participants?
- Are the objectives SMART?
- Who is conducting the evaluation — can it be undertaken by community members?
- Are they adequately supported so they are not set up to fail?

Reorient health services

- Whose 'needs' is the evaluation serving — the funding agency's, the agency staff or community members?
- Who, in a position of influence, can the evaluation report be sent to?
- Is a process set up where the findings of the evaluation can be acted on to bring about change?

Using the Ottawa Charter for behavioural approaches

Build healthy public policy

- Are health information strategies supported by national and state health-promotion priority areas?
- Are strategies directed at people who have the power to change the context of people's lives — where they live, work and play?

Create supportive environments

- Will use of a health education planning framework enhance focus on a social model of health, rather than the medical model?
- Do the strategies take account of the context of people's lives — are they enabling?
- Are you very sure the strategies do not amount to 'victim blaming'?

Strengthen community action

- Have the community members requested the advice or information?
- Did community members decide what content should be in the advice and what format it should take?
- Is health advice accompanied by an 'action plan' that is achievable for even the most disadvantaged and vulnerable recipients of the message?
- Are there opportunities for peer education or 'train-the-trainer'?

Develop personal skills

- Do health information and behaviour-change approaches have a mentoring role?
- Do health information strategies take account of the context of people's lives?
- Do the approaches draw on and value the wisdom of the community?
- Does participation allow each person to enhance their self-esteem?
- Is people's participation in decision-making more than mere tokenism?
- Are participants able to develop personal and transferable skills by taking part in the activity?
- Could participants be the next round of educators?

Reorient health services

- Can you make the behaviour-change approach more health promoting; that is, can it address social, environmental and emotional determinants of illness?
- Are the health information strategies directed at capacity building for policy-makers and agency management?

Using the Ottawa Charter for medical approaches

Build healthy public policy

- Are screening and immunisation services supported in agency policy?

Create supportive environments

- Is health screening an option in work settings?
- Are screening, assessment and early intervention services accessible to those who traditionally under-utilise the services?
- Does the agency have positive engagement strategies to reach out to community members?
- Are recruitment resources accessible in terms of readership, language, circulation and media sources?
- Are staff members non-judgmental and positively supportive towards those who are 'different'?
- Are the services affordable for all?

Strengthen community action

- Are there opportunities for community members to give advice about preferences for service modifications?

Develop personal skills

- Do people understand their role in making the service effective?
- Is there sufficient time for explanation and education?
- Does information provide for the cultural safety of services users?

Reorient health services

- Is the service health promoting?
- Is there a clear rationale for the benefit of the strategy based on epidemiological and economic outcomes?
- Is the service accessible and affordable to vulnerable groups?

Effective reorientation of the health care system to a focus on the promotion of health and the needs of the community will only come from a concerted effort by health workers and community members. Do not underestimate the importance of your role in this process. You can make a difference, and we wish you all the best in your health-promotion work.

Appendix one

The Declaration of Alma-Ata

On 12 September 1978, at Alma-Ata in Soviet Kazakhstan, representatives of 134 nations agreed to the terms of a solemn declaration pledging urgent action by all governments, all health and development workers, and the world community to protect and promote the health of all the people of the world. The climax of a major International Conference on Primary Health Care, jointly sponsored by WHO and UNICEF, this declaration stated:

1. The conference strongly reaffirms that health, which is a state of complete physical, mental and social wellbeing, and not merely the absence of disease or infirmity, is a fundamental human right and that the attainment of the highest possible level of health is a most important worldwide social goal whose realization requires the action of many other social and economic sectors in addition to the health sector.

2. The existing gross inequality in the health status of the people, particularly between developed and developing countries as well as within countries, is politically, socially and economically unacceptable and is, therefore, of common concern to all countries.

3. Economic and social development, based on a New International Economic Order, is of basic importance to the fullest attainment of health for all and to the reduction of the gap between the health status of the developing and developed countries. The promotion and protection of the health of the people is essential to sustained economic and social development and contributes to a better quality of life and to world peace.

4. The people have the right and duty to participate individually and collectively in the planning and implementation of their health care.

5. Governments have a responsibility for the health of their people which can be fulfilled only by the provision of adequate health and social measures. A main social target of governments, international organizations and the whole world community in the coming decades should be the attainment by all peoples of the world by the year 2000 of a level of health that will permit them to lead a socially and economically productive life. Primary Health Care is the key to attaining this target as part of development in the spirit of social justice.

6. Primary Health Care is essential health care based on practical, scientifically sound and socially acceptable methods and technology

made universally accessible to individuals and families in the community through their full participation and at a cost that the community and country can afford to maintain at every stage of their development in the spirit of self-reliance and self-determination. It forms an integral part both of the country's health system, of which it is the central function and main focus, and of the overall social and economic development of the community. It is the first level of contact of individuals, the family and community with the national health system, bringing health care as close as possible to where people live and work, and constitutes the first element of a continuing health care process.

7. Primary Health Care:

    i. reflects and evolves from the economic conditions and socio-cultural and political characteristics of the country and its communities, and is based on the application of the relevant results of social, biomedical and health services research and public health experience;

    ii. addresses the main health problems in the community, providing promotive, preventive, curative and rehabilitative services accordingly;

    iii. includes at least: education concerning prevailing health problems and the methods of preventing and controlling them; promotion of food supply and proper nutrition; an adequate supply of safe water and basic sanitation; maternal and child health care, including family planning; immunization against the major infectious diseases; prevention and control of locally endemic diseases; appropriate treatment of common diseases and injuries; and provision of essential drugs;

    iv. involves, in addition to the health sector, all related sectors and aspects of national and community development, in particular agriculture, animal husbandry, food, industry, education, housing, public works, communication and other sectors; and demands the coordinated efforts of all those sectors;

    v. requires and promotes maximum community and individual self-reliance and participation in the planning, organization, operation and control of Primary Health Care, making fullest use of local, national and other available resources, and to this end develops through appropriate education the ability of communities to participate;

    vi. should be sustained by integrated, functional and mutually supportive referral systems, leading to the progressive improvement of comprehensive health care for all, and giving priority to those most in need;

    vii. relies, at local and referral levels, on health workers, including physicians, nurses, midwives, auxiliaries and community workers as applicable, as well as traditional practitioners as needed, suitably trained socially and technically to work as a health team and to respond to the expressed health needs of the community.

8. All governments should formulate national policies, strategies and plans of action to launch and sustain Primary Health Care as part of a

comprehensive national health system and in coordination with other sectors. To this end, it will be necessary to exercise political will, to mobilize the country's resources and to use available external resources rationally.

9. All countries should cooperate in a spirit of partnership and service to ensure Primary Health Care for all people since the attainment of health by people in any one country directly concerns and benefits every other country. In this context the joint WHO/UNICEF report on Primary Health Care constitutes a solid basis for the further development and operation of Primary Health Care throughout the world.

10. An acceptable level of health for all the people of the world by the year 2000 can be attained through a fuller and better use of the world's resources, a considerable part of which is now spent on armaments and military conflicts. A genuine policy of independence, peace, détente and disarmament could and should release additional resources that could well be devoted to peaceful aims and in particular to the acceleration of social and economic development of which Primary Health Care, as an essential part, should be allotted its proper share.

The International Conference on Primary Health Care calls for urgent and effective national and international action to develop and implement Primary Health Care throughout the world and particularly in developing countries in a spirit of technical cooperation and in keeping with a New International Economic Order. It urges governments, WHO and UNICEF, and other international organizations, as well as multilateral and bilateral agencies, non-governmental organizations, funding agencies, all health workers and the whole world community to support national and international commitment to Primary Health Care and to channel increased technical and financial support to it, particularly in developing countries. The conference calls on all the aforementioned to collaborate in introducing, developing and maintaining Primary Health Care in accordance with the spirit and content of this declaration.

(Source: World Health Organization 1978 The Declaration of Alma-Ata. *World Health*. August/September 1988, pp. 16–17)

Appendix two

The Ottawa Charter for Health Promotion

The first International Conference on Health Promotion, meeting in Ottawa this 21st day of November 1986, hereby presents this CHARTER for action to achieve Health for All by the year 2000 and beyond.

This conference was primarily a response to growing expectations for a new public health movement around the world. Discussions focused on the needs in industrialized countries, but took into account similar concerns in all other regions. It built on the progress made through the Declaration on Primary Health Care at Alma-Ata, the World Health Organization's Targets for Health for All document, and the recent debate at the World Health Assembly on inter-sectoral action for health.

Health promotion

Health promotion is the process of enabling people to increase control over, and to improve, their health. To reach a state of complete physical, mental and social wellbeing, an individual or group must be able to identify and to realize aspirations, to satisfy needs, and to change or cope with the environment. Health is, therefore, seen as a resource for everyday life, not the objective of living. Health is a positive concept emphasizing social and personal resources, as well as physical capacities. Therefore, health promotion is not just the responsibility of the health sector, but goes beyond healthy lifestyles to wellbeing.

Prerequisites for health

The fundamental conditions and resources for health are peace, shelter, education, food, income, a stable ecosystem, sustainable resources, social justice and equity. Improvement in health requires a secure foundation in these basic prerequisites.

Advocate

Good health is a major resource for social, economic and personal development and an important dimension of quality of life. Political, economic, social, cultural, environmental, behavioral and biological factors can all favor health or be harmful to it. Health promotion action aims at making these conditions favorable through advocacy for health.

Enable

Health promotion focuses on achieving equity in health. Health promotion action aims at reducing differences in current health status and ensuring equal opportunities and resources to enable all people to achieve their fullest health potential. This includes a secure foundation in a supportive environment, access to information, life skills and opportunities for making healthy choices. People cannot achieve their fullest health potential unless they are able to take control of those things which determine their health. This must apply equally to women and men.

Mediate

The prerequisites and prospects for health cannot be ensured by the health sector alone. More importantly, health promotion demands coordinated action by all concerned: by governments, by health and other social and economic sectors, by non-governmental and voluntary organizations, by local authorities, by industry and by the media. People in all walks of life are involved as individuals, families and communities. Professional and social groups and health personnel have a major responsibility to mediate between differing interests in society for the pursuit of health.

Health promotion strategies and programmes should be adapted to the local needs and possibilities of individual countries and regions to take into account differing social, cultural and economic systems.

Health-promotion action means:

Build healthy public policy

Health promotion goes beyond health care. It puts health on the agenda of policy makers in all sectors and at all levels, directing them to be aware of the health consequences of their decisions and to accept their responsibilities for health.

Health promotion policy combines diverse but complementary approaches including legislation, fiscal measures, taxation and organizational change. It is coordinated action that leads to health, income and social policies that foster greater equity. Joint action contributes to ensuring safer and healthier goods and services, healthier public services, and cleaner, more enjoyable environments.

Health promotion policy requires the identification of obstacles to the adoption of healthy public policies in non-health sectors, and ways of removing them. The aim must be to make the healthier choice the easier choice for policy makers as well.

Create supportive environments

Our societies are complex and interrelated. Health cannot be separated from other goals. The inextricable links between people and their environment constitutes the basis for a socio-ecological approach to health. The overall guiding principle for the world, nations, regions and communities alike, is the need to encourage reciprocal maintenance — to take care of each other, our communities and our natural environment. The conservation of natural resources throughout the world should be emphasized as a global responsibility.

Changing patterns of life, work and leisure have a significant impact on health. Work and leisure should be a source of health for people. The way society organizes work should help create a healthy society. Health promotion generates living and working conditions that are safe, stimulating, satisfying and enjoyable.

Systematic assessment of the health impact of a rapidly changing environment — particularly in areas of technology, work, energy production and urbanization — is essential and must be followed by action to ensure positive benefit to the health of the public. The protection of the natural and built environments and the conservation of natural resources must be addressed in any health promotion strategy.

Strengthen community action

Health promotion works through concrete and effective community action in setting priorities, making decisions, planning strategies and implementing them to achieve better health. At the heart of this process is the empowerment of communities, their ownership and control of their own endeavors and destinies.

Community development draws on existing human and material resources in the community to enhance self-help and social support, and to develop flexible systems for strengthening public participation and direction of health matters. This requires full and continuous access to information, learning opportunities for health, as well as funding support.

Develop personal skills

Health promotion supports personal and social development through providing information, education for health and enhancing life skills. By so doing, it increases the options available to people to exercise more control over their own health and over their environments, and to make choices conducive to health.

Enabling people to learn throughout life, to prepare themselves for all of its stages and to cope with chronic illness and injuries is essential. This has to be facilitated in school, home, work and community settings. Action is required through educational, professional, commercial and voluntary bodies, and within the institutions themselves.

Reorient health services

The responsibility for health promotion in health services is shared among individuals, community groups, health professionals, health service institutions and governments. They must work together towards a health care system which contributes to the pursuit of health.

The role of the health sector must move increasingly in a health promotion direction, beyond its responsibility for providing clinical and curative services. Health services need to embrace an expanded mandate which is sensitive and respects cultural needs. This mandate should support the needs of individuals and communities for a healthier life, and open channels between the health sector and broader social, political, economic and physical environmental components.

Reorienting health services also requires stronger attention to health research as well as changes in professional education and training. This must lead to a change of attitude and organization of health services, which refocuses on the total needs of the individual as a whole person.

Moving into the future

Health is created and lived by people within the settings of their everyday life; where they learn, work, play and love. Health is created by caring for oneself and others, by being able to take decisions and have control over one's life circumstances, and by ensuring that the society one lives in creates conditions that allow the attainment of health by all its members.

Caring, holism and ecology are essential issues in developing strategies for health promotion. Therefore, those involved should take as a guiding principle that, in each phase of planning, implementation and evaluation of health promotion activities, women and men should become equal partners.

Commitment to health promotion

The participants in this conference pledge:

- to move into the arena of healthy public policy, and to advocate a clear political commitment to health and equity in all sectors;
- to counteract the pressures towards harmful products, resource depletion, unhealthy living conditions and environments, and bad nutrition; and to focus attention on public health issues such as pollution, occupational hazards, housing and settlements;
- to respond to the health gap within and between societies, and to tackle the inequities in health produced by the rules and practices of these societies;
- to acknowledge people as the main health resource; to support and enable them to keep themselves, their families and friends healthy through financial and other means, and to accept the community as the essential voice in matters of its health, living conditions and wellbeing;
- to reorient health services and their resources towards the promotion of health; and to share power with other sectors, other disciplines and most importantly with people themselves;
- to recognize health and its maintenance as a major social investment and challenge; and to address the overall ecological issue of our ways of living.

The conference urges all concerned to join them in their commitment to a strong public health alliance.

Call for international action

The Conference calls on the World Health Organization and other international organizations to advocate the promotion of health in all appropriate forums and to support countries in setting up strategies and programs for health promotion.

The Conference is firmly convinced that if people in all walks of life, non-governmental and voluntary organizations, governments, the World Health Organization and all other bodies concerned join forces in introducing strategies for health promotion, in line with the moral and social values that form the basis of this CHARTER, Health for All by the Year 2000 will become a reality.

This CHARTER for action was developed and adopted by an international conference, jointly organized by the World Health Organization, Health and Welfare Canada and the Canadian Public Health Association. Two hundred and twelve participants from 38 countries met from November 17 to 21, 1986, in Ottawa, Canada to exchange experiences and share knowledge of health promotion.

The Conference stimulated an open dialog among lay, health and other professional workers, among representatives of governmental, voluntary and community organizations, and among politicians, administrators, academics and practitioners. Participants coordinated their efforts and came to a clearer definition of the major challenges ahead. They strengthened their individual and collective commitment to the common goal of Health for All by the Year 2000.

This CHARTER for action reflects the spirit of earlier public charters through which the needs of people were recognized and acted upon. The CHARTER presents fundamental strategies and approaches for health promotion which the participants considered vital for major progress. The Conference report develops the issues raised, gives concrete examples and practical suggestions regarding how real advances can be achieved, and outlines the action required of countries and relevant groups.

The move towards a new public health policy is now evident worldwide. This was reaffirmed not only by the experiences but by the pledges of Conference participants who were invited as individuals on the basis of their expertise. The following countries were represented: Antigua, Australia, Austria, Belgium, Bulgaria, Canada, Czechoslovakia, Denmark, Eire, England, Finland, France, German Democratic Republic, Federal Republic of Germany, Ghana, Hungary, Iceland, Israel, Italy, Japan, Malta, Netherlands, New Zealand, Northern Ireland, Norway, Poland, Portugal, Romania, St. Kitts-Nevis, Scotland, Spain, Sudan, Sweden, Switzerland, Union of Soviet Socialist Republics, United States of America, Wales and Yugoslavia.

(Source: World Health Organization 1986 *The Ottawa Charter for Health Promotion.*
World Health Organization, Geneva)

Appendix three

Universal Declaration of Human Rights

On 10 December 1948 the General Assembly of the United Nations adopted and proclaimed the Universal Declaration of Human Rights, the full text of which appears in the following pages. Following this historic act the Assembly called upon all Member countries to publicize the text of the declaration and 'to cause it to be disseminated, displayed, read and expounded principally in schools and other educational institutions, without distinction based on the political status of countries or territories'.

Preamble

Whereas recognition of the inherent dignity and of the equal and inalienable rights of all members of the human family is the foundation of freedom, justice and peace in the world,

Whereas disregard and contempt for human rights have resulted in barbarous acts which have outraged the conscience of mankind, and the advent of a world in which human beings shall enjoy freedom of speech and belief and freedom from fear and want has been proclaimed as the highest aspiration of the common people,

Whereas it is essential, if man is not to be compelled to have recourse, as a last resort, to rebellion against tyranny and oppression, that human rights should be protected by the rule of law,

Whereas it is essential to promote the development of friendly relations between nations,

Whereas the peoples of the United Nations have in the Charter reaffirmed their faith in fundamental human rights, in the dignity and worth of the human person and in the equal rights of men and women and have determined to promote social progress and better standards of life in larger freedom,

Whereas Member States have pledged themselves to achieve, in co-operation with the United Nations, the promotion of universal respect for and observance of human rights and fundamental freedoms,

Whereas a common understanding of these rights and freedoms is of the greatest importance for the full realization of this pledge,

Now, Therefore THE GENERAL ASSEMBLY proclaims THIS UNIVERSAL DECLARATION OF HUMAN RIGHTS as a common standard of achievement for all peoples and all nations, to the end that every individual and every organ of society, keeping this Declaration constantly in mind, shall strive by teaching and education to promote respect for these rights and freedoms and by progressive measures, national and international, to secure their universal and effective recognition and observance, both among the peoples of Member States themselves and among the peoples of territories under their jurisdiction.

Article 1.
All human beings are born free and equal in dignity and rights. They are endowed with reason and conscience and should act towards one another in a spirit of brotherhood.

Article 2.
Everyone is entitled to all the rights and freedoms set forth in this Declaration, without distinction of any kind, such as race, color, sex, language, religion, political or other opinion, national or social origin, property, birth or other status. Furthermore, no distinction shall be made on the basis of the political, jurisdictional or international status of the country or territory to which a person belongs, whether it be independent, trust, non-self-governing or under any other limitation of sovereignty.

Article 3.
Everyone has the right to life, liberty and security of person.

Article 4.
No one shall be held in slavery or servitude; slavery and the slave trade shall be prohibited in all their forms.

Article 5.
No one shall be subjected to torture or to cruel, inhuman or degrading treatment or punishment.

Article 6.
Everyone has the right to recognition everywhere as a person before the law.

Article 7.
All are equal before the law and are entitled without any discrimination to equal protection of the law. All are entitled to equal protection against any discrimination in violation of this Declaration and against any incitement to such discrimination.

Article 8.
Everyone has the right to an effective remedy by the competent national tribunals for acts violating the fundamental rights granted him by the constitution or by law.

Article 9.

No one shall be subjected to arbitrary arrest, detention or exile.

Article 10.

Everyone is entitled in full equality to a fair and public hearing by an independent and impartial tribunal, in the determination of his rights and obligations and of any criminal charge against him.

Article 11.

(1) Everyone charged with a penal offence has the right to be presumed innocent until proved guilty according to law in a public trial at which he has had all the guarantees necessary for his defence.

(2) No one shall be held guilty of any penal offence on account of any act or omission which did not constitute a penal offence, under national or international law, at the time when it was committed. Nor shall a heavier penalty be imposed than the one that was applicable at the time the penal offence was committed.

Article 12.

No one shall be subjected to arbitrary interference with his privacy, family, home or correspondence, nor to attacks upon his honour and reputation. Everyone has the right to the protection of the law against such interference or attacks.

Article 13.

(1) Everyone has the right to freedom of movement and residence within the borders of each State.

(2) Everyone has the right to leave any country, including his own, and to return to his country.

Article 14.

(1) Everyone has the right to seek and to enjoy in other countries asylum from persecution.

(2) This right may not be invoked in the case of prosecutions genuinely arising from non-political crimes or from acts contrary to the purposes and principles of the United Nations.

Article 15.

(1) Everyone has the right to a nationality.

(2) No one shall be arbitrarily deprived of his nationality nor denied the right to change his nationality.

Article 16.

(1) Men and women of full age, without any limitation due to race, nationality or religion, have the right to marry and to found a family. They are entitled to equal rights as to marriage, during marriage and at its dissolution.

(2) Marriage shall be entered into only with the free and full consent of the intending spouses.

(3) The family is the natural and fundamental group unit of society and is entitled to protection by society and the State.

Article 17.

(1) Everyone has the right to own property alone as well as in association with others.

(2) No one shall be arbitrarily deprived of his property.

Article 18.

Everyone has the right to freedom of thought, conscience and religion; this right includes freedom to change his religion or belief, and freedom, either alone or in community with others and in public or private, to manifest his religion or belief in teaching, practice, worship and observance.

Article 19.

Everyone has the right to freedom of opinion and expression; this right includes freedom to hold opinions without interference and to seek, receive and impart information and ideas through any media and regardless of frontiers.

Article 20.

(1) Everyone has the right to freedom of peaceful assembly and association.

(2) No one may be compelled to belong to an association.

Article 21.

(1) Everyone has the right to take part in the government of his country, directly or through freely chosen representatives.

(2) Everyone has the right of equal access to public service in his country.

(3) The will of the people shall be the basis of the authority of government; this will shall be expressed in periodic and genuine elections which shall be by universal and equal suffrage and shall be held by secret vote or by equivalent free voting procedures.

Article 22.

Everyone, as a member of society, has the right to social security and is entitled to realization, through national effort and international co-operation and in accordance with the organization and resources of each State, of the economic, social and cultural rights indispensable for his dignity and the free development of his personality.

Article 23.

(1) Everyone has the right to work, to free choice of employment, to just and favorable conditions of work and to protection against unemployment.

(2) Everyone, without any discrimination, has the right to equal pay for equal work.

(3) Everyone who works has the right to just and favorable remuneration ensuring for himself and his family an existence worthy of human dignity, and supplemented, if necessary, by other means of social protection.

(4) Everyone has the right to form and to join trade unions for the protection of his interests.

Article 24.

Everyone has the right to rest and leisure, including reasonable limitation of working hours and periodic holidays with pay.

Article 25.

(1) Everyone has the right to a standard of living adequate for the health and wellbeing of himself and of his family, including food, clothing, housing and medical care and necessary social services, and the right to security in the event of unemployment, sickness, disability, widowhood, old age or other lack of livelihood in circumstances beyond his control.

(2) Motherhood and childhood are entitled to special care and assistance. All children, whether born in or out of wedlock, shall enjoy the same social protection.

Article 26.

(1) Everyone has the right to education. Education shall be free, at least in the elementary and fundamental stages. Elementary education shall be compulsory. Technical and professional education shall be made generally available and higher education shall be equally accessible to all on the basis of merit.

(2) Education shall be directed to the full development of the human personality and to the strengthening of respect for human rights and fundamental freedoms. It shall promote understanding, tolerance and friendship among all nations, racial or religious groups, and shall further the activities of the United Nations for the maintenance of peace.

(3) Parents have a prior right to choose the kind of education that shall be given to their children.

Article 27.

(1) Everyone has the right freely to participate in the cultural life of the community, to enjoy the arts and to share in scientific advancement and its benefits.

(2) Everyone has the right to the protection of the moral and material interests resulting from any scientific, literary or artistic production of which he is the author.

Article 28.

Everyone is entitled to a social and international order in which the rights and freedoms set forth in this Declaration can be fully realized.

Article 29.

(1) Everyone has duties to the community in which alone the free and full development of his personality is possible.

(2) In the exercise of his rights and freedoms, everyone shall be subject only to such limitations as are determined by law solely for the purpose of securing due recognition and respect for the rights and freedoms of others and of meeting the just requirements of morality, public order and the general welfare in a democratic society.

(3) These rights and freedoms may in no case be exercised contrary to the purposes and principles of the United Nations.

Article 30.

Nothing in this Declaration may be interpreted as implying for any State, group or person any right to engage in any activity or to perform any act aimed at the destruction of any of the rights and freedoms set forth herein.

(Source: United Nations Department of Public Information, Office of the High Commissioner for Human Rights. Online. Available: http://www.unhchr/udhr/lang/eng.htm [accessed 17 September 2004])

Appendix four

The Earth Charter

Preamble

We stand at a critical moment in Earth's history, a time when humanity must choose its future. As the world becomes increasingly interdependent and fragile, the future at once holds great peril and great promise. To move forward we must recognize that in the midst of a magnificent diversity of cultures and life forms we are one human family and one Earth community with a common destiny. We must join together to bring forth a sustainable global society founded on respect for nature, universal human rights, economic justice, and a culture of peace. Towards this end, it is imperative that we, the peoples of Earth, declare our responsibility to one another, to the greater community of life, and to future generations.

Earth, our home

Humanity is part of a vast evolving universe. Earth, our home, is alive with a unique community of life. The forces of nature make existence a demanding and uncertain adventure, but Earth has provided the conditions essential to life's evolution. The resilience of the community of life and the wellbeing of humanity depend upon preserving a healthy biosphere with all its ecological systems, a rich variety of plants and animals, fertile soils, pure waters, and clean air. The global environment with its finite resources is a common concern of all peoples. The protection of Earth's vitality, diversity, and beauty is a sacred trust.

The global situation

The dominant patterns of production and consumption are causing environmental devastation, the depletion of resources, and a massive extinction of species. Communities are being undermined. The benefits of development are not shared equitably and the gap between rich and poor is widening. Injustice, poverty, ignorance, and violent conflict are widespread and the cause of great suffering. An unprecedented rise in human population has overburdened ecological and social systems. The foundations of global security are threatened. These trends are perilous — but not inevitable.

The challenges ahead

The choice is ours: form a global partnership to care for Earth and one another or risk the destruction of ourselves and the diversity of life. Fundamental changes are needed in our values, institutions, and ways of living. We must realize that when basic needs have been met, human development is primarily about being more, not having more. We have the knowledge and technology to provide for all and to reduce our impacts on the environment. The emergence of a global civil society is creating new opportunities to build a democratic and humane world. Our environmental, economic, political, social, and spiritual challenges are interconnected, and together we can forge inclusive solutions.

Universal responsibility

To realize these aspirations, we must decide to live with a sense of universal responsibility, identifying ourselves with the whole Earth community as well as our local communities. We are at once citizens of different nations and of one world in which the local and global are linked. Everyone shares responsibility for the present and future wellbeing of the human family and the larger living world. The spirit of human solidarity and kinship with all life is strengthened when we live with reverence for the mystery of being, gratitude for the gift of life, and humility regarding the human place in nature.

We urgently need a shared vision of basic values to provide an ethical foundation for the emerging world community. Therefore, together in hope we affirm the following interdependent principles for a sustainable way of life as a common standard by which the conduct of all individuals, organizations, businesses, governments, and transnational institutions is to be guided and assessed.

Principles

I. Respect and care for the community of life

1. Respect Earth and life in all its diversity.

   a. Recognize that all beings are interdependent and every form of life has value regardless of its worth to human beings.

   b. Affirm faith in the inherent dignity of all human beings and in the intellectual, artistic, ethical, and spiritual potential of humanity.

2. Care for the community of life with understanding, compassion, and love.

   a. Accept that with the right to own, manage, and use natural resources comes the duty to prevent environmental harm and to protect the rights of people.

   b. Affirm that with increased freedom, knowledge, and power comes increased responsibility to promote the common good.

3. Build democratic societies that are just, participatory, sustainable, and peaceful.

   a. Ensure that communities at all levels guarantee human rights and fundamental freedoms and provide everyone an opportunity to realize his or her full potential.

    b. Promote social and economic justice, enabling all to achieve a secure and meaningful livelihood that is ecologically responsible.

4. Secure Earth's bounty and beauty for present and future generations.

    a. Recognize that the freedom of action of each generation is qualified by the needs of future generations.

    b. Transmit to future generations values, traditions, and institutions that support the long-term flourishing of Earth's human and ecological communities.

II. Ecological integrity

5. Protect and restore the integrity of Earth's ecological systems, with special concern for biological diversity and the natural processes that sustain life.

    a. Adopt at all levels sustainable development plans and regulations that make environmental conservation and rehabilitation integral to all development initiatives.

    b. Establish and safeguard viable nature and biosphere reserves, including wild lands and marine areas, to protect Earth's life support systems, maintain biodiversity, and preserve our natural heritage.

    c. Promote the recovery of endangered species and ecosystems.

    d. Control and eradicate non-native or genetically modified organisms harmful to native species and the environment, and prevent introduction of such harmful organisms.

    e. Manage the use of renewable resources such as water, soil, forest products, and marine life in ways that do not exceed rates of regeneration and that protect the health of ecosystems.

    f. Manage the extraction and use of non-renewable resources such as minerals and fossil fuels in ways that minimize depletion and cause no serious environmental damage.

6. Prevent harm as the best method of environmental protection and, when knowledge is limited, apply a precautionary approach.

    a. Take action to avoid the possibility of serious or irreversible environmental harm even when scientific knowledge is incomplete or inconclusive.

    b. Place the burden of proof on those who argue that a proposed activity will not cause significant harm, and make the responsible parties liable for environmental harm.

    c. Ensure that decision making addresses the cumulative, long-term, indirect, long distance, and global consequences of human activities.

    d. Prevent pollution of any part of the environment and allow no build-up of radioactive, toxic, or other hazardous substances.

    e. Avoid military activities damaging to the environment.

7. Adopt patterns of production, consumption, and reproduction that safeguard Earth's regenerative capacities, human rights, and community wellbeing.

   a. Reduce, reuse, and recycle the materials used in production and consumption systems, and ensure that residual waste can be assimilated by ecological systems.

   b. Act with restraint and efficiency when using energy, and rely increasingly on renewable energy sources such as solar and wind.

   c. Promote the development, adoption, and equitable transfer of environmentally sound technologies.

   d. Internalise the full environmental and social costs of goods and services in the selling price, and enable consumers to identify products that meet the highest social and environmental standards.

   e. Ensure universal access to health care that fosters reproductive health and responsible reproduction.

   f. Adopt lifestyles that emphasize the quality of life and material sufficiency in a finite world.

8. Advance the study of ecological sustainability and promote the open exchange and wide application of the knowledge acquired.

   a. Support international scientific and technical cooperation on sustainability, with special attention to the needs of developing nations.

   b. Recognize and preserve the traditional knowledge and spiritual wisdom in all cultures that contribute to environmental protection and human wellbeing.

   c. Ensure that information of vital importance to human health and environmental protection, including genetic information, remains available in the public domain.

III. Social and economic justice

9. Eradicate poverty as an ethical, social, and environmental imperative.

   a. Guarantee the right to potable water, clean air, food security, uncontaminated soil, shelter, and safe sanitation, allocating the national and international resources required.

   b. Empower every human being with the education and resources to secure a sustainable livelihood, and provide social security and safety nets for those who are unable to support themselves.

   c. Recognize the ignored, protect the vulnerable, serve those who suffer, and enable them to develop their capacities and to pursue their aspirations.

10. Ensure that economic activities and institutions at all levels promote human development in an equitable and sustainable manner.

    a. Promote the equitable distribution of wealth within nations and among nations.

    b. Enhance the intellectual, financial, technical, and social resources of developing nations, and relieve them of onerous international debt.

    c. Ensure that all trade supports sustainable resource use, environmental protection, and progressive labor standards.

    d. Require multinational corporations and international financial organizations to act transparently in the public good, and hold them accountable for the consequences of their activities.

11. Affirm gender equality and equity as prerequisites to sustainable development and ensure universal access to education, health care, and economic opportunity.

    a. Secure the human rights of women and girls and end all violence against them.

    b. Promote the active participation of women in all aspects of economic, political, civil, social, and cultural life as full and equal partners, decision makers, leaders, and beneficiaries.

    c. Strengthen families and ensure the safety and loving nurture of all family members.

12. Uphold the right of all, without discrimination, to a natural and social environment supportive of human dignity, bodily health, and spiritual wellbeing, with special attention to the rights of indigenous peoples and minorities.

    a. Eliminate discrimination in all its forms, such as that based on race, color, sex, sexual orientation, religion, language, and national, ethnic or social origin.

    b. Affirm the right of indigenous peoples to their spirituality, knowledge, lands, and resources, and to their related practice of sustainable livelihoods.

    c. Honor and support the young people of our communities, enabling them to fulfil their essential role in creating sustainable societies.

    d. Protect and restore outstanding places of cultural and spiritual significance.

IV. Democracy, non-violence, and peace

13. Strengthen democratic institutions at all levels, and provide transparency and accountability in governance, inclusive participation in decision making, and access to justice.

    a. Uphold the right of everyone to receive clear and timely information on environmental matters and all development plans and activities which are likely to affect them or in which they have an interest.

    b. Support local, regional and global civil society, and promote the meaningful participation of all interested individuals and organizations in decision making.

    c. Protect the rights to freedom of opinion, expression, peaceful assembly, association, and dissent.

    d. Institute effective and efficient access to administrative and independent judicial procedures, including remedies and redress for environmental harm and the threat of such harm.

    e. Eliminate corruption in all public and private institutions.

    f. Strengthen local communities, enabling them to care for their environments, and assign environmental responsibilities to the levels of government where they can be carried out most effectively.

14. Integrate into formal education and life-long learning the knowledge, values, and skills needed for a sustainable way of life.

    a. Provide all, especially children and youth, with educational opportunities that empower them to contribute actively to sustainable development.

    b. Promote the contribution of the arts and humanities as well as the sciences in sustainability education.

    c. Enhance the role of the mass media in raising awareness of ecological and social challenges.

    d. Recognize the importance of moral and spiritual education for sustainable living.

15. Treat all living beings with respect and consideration.

    a. Prevent cruelty to animals kept in human societies and protect them from suffering.

    b. Protect wild animals from methods of hunting, trapping, and fishing that cause extreme, prolonged, or avoidable suffering.

    c. Avoid or eliminate to the full extent possible the taking or destruction of non-targeted species.

16. Promote a culture of tolerance, non-violence, and peace.

    a. Encourage and support mutual understanding, solidarity, and cooperation among all peoples and within and among nations.

    b. Implement comprehensive strategies to prevent violent conflict and use collaborative problem solving to manage and resolve environmental conflicts and other disputes.

    c. Demilitarize national security systems to the level of a non-provocative defence posture, and convert military resources to peaceful purposes, including ecological restoration.

    d. Eliminate nuclear, biological, and toxic weapons and other weapons of mass destruction.

e. Ensure that the use of orbital and outer space supports environmental protection and peace.

f. Recognize that peace is the wholeness created by right relationships with oneself, other persons, other cultures, other life, Earth, and the larger whole of which all are a part.

The way forward

As never before in history, common destiny beckons us to seek a new beginning. Such renewal is the promise of these Earth Charter principles. To fulfil this promise, we must commit ourselves to adopt and promote the values and objectives of the Charter.

This requires a change of mind and heart. It requires a new sense of global interdependence and universal responsibility. We must imaginatively develop and apply the vision of a sustainable way of life locally, nationally, regionally, and globally. Our cultural diversity is a precious heritage and different cultures will find their own distinctive ways to realize the vision.

We must deepen and expand the global dialog that generated the Earth Charter, for we have much to learn from the ongoing collaborative search for truth and wisdom.

Life often involves tensions between important values. This can mean difficult choices. However, we must find ways to harmonize diversity with unity, the exercise of freedom with the common good, short-term objectives with long-term goals. Every individual, family, organization, and community has a vital role to play. The arts, sciences, religions, educational institutions, media, businesses, non-governmental organizations, and governments are all called to offer creative leadership. The partnership of government, civil society, and business is essential for effective governance.

In order to build a sustainable global community, the nations of the world must renew their commitment to the United Nations, fulfil their obligations under existing international agreements, and support the implementation of Earth Charter principles with an international legally binding instrument on environment and development.

Let ours be a time remembered for the awakening of a new reverence for life, the firm resolve to achieve sustainability, the quickening of the struggle for justice and peace, and the joyful celebration of life.

(Source: *The Earth Charter*. Online. Available: www.earthcharter.org [accessed 24 September 2004])

Appendix five

Some useful internet sites

There is a wide range of valuable information of relevance for health promotion on the worldwide web. Below are some website addresses that may be useful to people working in Primary Health Care and health promotion. This list is by no means meant to be definitive. Rather, it is intended as a starting point, to encourage you to explore the web and to get a taste of the information that can be of use to you in working to promote health. Many of the sites also have links to other useful sites, so this really is designed as a beginning only.

Commonwealth sites

Australian Indigenous Health InfoNet

http://www.healthinfonet.ecu.edu.au/

The Australian Indigenous Health InfoNet brings together a wide range of information on indigenous health issues. It contains a bibliographical database, with information on Aboriginal and Torres Strait Islander health publications and unpublished material from 1915, a discussion group for those wishing to discuss issues and share information related to indigenous health, and an online journal, the *Aboriginal and Torres Strait Islander Health Bulletin*. Links are provided to related internet sites, as well as to relevant documents and journals.

Australian Institute of Health and Welfare

http://www.aihw.gov.au

The Australian Institute of Health and Welfare (AIHW) site provides a wide range of information on the AIHW, its publications, major health-and-welfare-related conferences and workshops. Most AIHW publications are available free of charge from the website, such as the *Australian Burden of Disease and Injury Study*. In addition, it contains a 'data cubes' section, which provides agreed sets of data items for health and welfare statistics, and links to a number of related organisations.

Commonwealth Department of Health and Aged Care

http://www.health.gov.au

The Commonwealth health site provides a range of information about the department, including current campaigns and provides a search engine with which to explore the material here. Linked into this website are a wide variety of

266

departmental, portfolio agencies (Australian and international) as well as State and Territory Health Departments.

Consumers' Health Forum of Australia

http://www.chf.org.au

The Consumers' Health Forum site provides all the necessary information about the Consumers' Health Forum, its freely accessible publications, and details of membership. In addition, it includes links to a range of health-related and health consumer-related sites.

Health *Insite*

http://www.healthinsite.gov.au

This Commonwealth internet initiative brings together a wide range of links to information sources for a variety of health issues, life stages and population groups. The site contains expert views, quizzes, links to health-related news and a monthly newsletter.

Public Health Association of Australia

http://www.phaa.org.au

The site of this professional association includes information about Public Health Association conferences and campaigns, and information about the Association's refereed journal (*Australian and New Zealand Journal of Public Health*) and newsletter. It also contains specific information for members only. There are also links to international and Australian health-related professional, government and community organisations.

State and territory health departments

These websites of the various state and territory government health departments around Australia contain a wide range of information of direct relevance to each state and territory, including local priorities, policies and other publications. Many of them also have links to other useful sites.

ACT Health

http://www.health.act.gov.au

Of note on this site is the link to the ACT Health Library services. There are also links to ACT Research and University health-related groups.

Department of Health and Community Services, Northern Territory

http://www.health.nt.gov.au/

This site includes the Caring for our Children newsletter, link to Menzies School of Health and a comprehensive list of links to health improvement strategies in the Northern Territory. Available through this site is the *Public Health Bush Book*, a resource to support health workers who work with Aboriginal communities in rural/remote areas.

Department of Human Services, Victoria

http://www.dhs.vic.gov.au

Linked to this website are a variety of Victorian state government strategies. For example, the Better Health Channel (http://www.betterhealth.vic.gov.au) is an online information service for health topics, services and healthy eating. This site also links to the Victorian Government Health Information website (www.health.vic.gov.au) which provides comprehensive information on a variety of health topics.

Department of Health, South Australia

http://www.health.sa.gov.au

This site contains a link to the South Australian Women's and Children's Hospital public health seminars, and a range of information publications.

Department of Health and Human Services, Tasmania

http://www.dchs.tas.gov.au

This site provides a range of information for a variety of services and health-related topics. Of interest are links to a range of online resources.

NSW Health

http://www.health.nsw.gov.au

Of note on this site is the page for the Collaborative Centre for Aboriginal Health Promotion. As well as providing consumer information this site offers a range of assistance for health professionals. For example, the link to the Multicultural Health Communication Service website (www.mhcs.nsw.gov.au) assists professionals to communicate with non-English speaking communities.

Queensland Health

http://www.health.qld.gov.au/

This site provides links to health information sites and links to program education/ workshop sessions in Queensland.

Western Australia Department of Health

http://www.health.wa.gov.au

Of note on this site is the Disaster Preparedness and Management page as well as the link to Healthway (www.healthway.wa.gov.au), a funding body for programs that promote health.

Other sites

Amnesty International Australia

http://www.amnesty.org.au

The Amnesty International site provides access to much material of relevance to those wishing to learn more about Amnesty's work or become more actively involved. It contains the latest information on current and urgent human rights issues and campaigns.

Australian Health Promotion Association

http://www.healthpromotion.org.au

The site of this professional association includes information about health-promotion conferences and campaigns, and information about the Association's journal (*Health Promotion Journal of Australia*, with abstracts available) and newsletter. It also contains specific information for members only.

Community Aid Abroad

http://www.caa.org.au

The site of Community Aid Abroad includes news of current issues and details of conferences and ongoing campaigns. It also includes material on ethical business, and provides a range of suggestions on how individuals may become involved in Community Aid Abroad activities. This site also has access to a wide variety of related publications.

Earth Charter Initiative

http://www.earthcharter.org/

The Earth Charter document and related initiatives can be viewed on this site, out-lining shared international sustainable global development values and principles. The site provides information specific to education, local communities, youth and business.

Health Canada

http://www.hc-sc.gc.ca/

The Canadian Government's health department site provides a range of information about the department. Information is available for specific groups about lifestyle, diseases and conditions, and health protection. Of interest are links to the Canadian Health Network (health information site) and the Canada Health Portal (health and services information).

International Union of Health Promotion and Education

http://www.iuhpe.org/

This site provides information about the global organisation, its publications, projects and access to the organisation's online journal (*Reviews of Health Promotion & Education On-line*). The site also outlines current and future events, such as the World Conference on Health Promotion and Education. This site has a wide variety of links to international health-promotion and education organisations.

National Health and Medical Research Council (NH&MRC)

http://www.nhmrc.gov.au

The NH&MRC site provides a range of information about the Research Council, its research priorities, publications and health advice. Of note is the information available on ethical issues in health and research.

Prometheus information

http://www.prometheus.com.au

This site provides access to the HealthWIZ (Australia's National Social Health Data Library, http://www.healthwiz.com.au/), the computer-based database containing a wide range of health information, and HEAPS (Health Education and Promotion System), a health-promotion project and research activity database.

Social Health Atlas of Australia

http://www.publichealth.gov.au/atlas.htm

This site provides access to the Social Health Atlas of Australia, outlining demographic data and disparities that exist in health and health service access for each state and territory.

The Health Report (Radio National)

http://www.abc.net.au/rn/talks/8.30/helthrpt/index/hralphaidx.htm

Provides an alphabetical index to interview transcripts (from previous editions of the Health Report) conducted with key health researchers in a range of areas, including references to journal publications.

United Nations Human Rights

http://www.un.org/rights/

The UN Human Rights site provides information about the organisation and human rights action. There are links to the Universal Declaration of Human Rights, information about treaties, the International Criminal Tribunal for the former Yugoslavia, as well as links to a variety of human rights organisations, committees and databases.

United Nations Sustainable Development

http://www.un.org/esa/sustdev/

The UN Sustainable Development site provides information about the department, its priority activities and groups, the Commission on Sustainable Development and sustainable development issues. The site has a comprehensive listing of the department's documents, publications, media releases and organisational links.

Victorian Health Promotion Foundation (VicHealth)

http://www.vichealth.vic.gov.au

The site of VicHealth provides information and publications on population health, particularly priority areas for health improvement in Victoria. A range of publications are available on this site. Of note is the link to the Cochrane Health Promotion and Public Health Field (www.vichealth.vic.gov.au/cochrane), an evolving site for debate and reviews of effective health promotion and public health interventions. This site also provides a comprehensive list of health-promotion links, including research centres.

World Health Organization

http://www.who.int/en/

This site provides all the latest information about aspects of the World Health Organization's work, including its policies, the work of the various Collaborating Centres (some of which focus on health promotion, injury prevention and Primary Health Care, for example) and health topics of current interest. It also provides links to research tools, such as the WHO's Library database (WHOLIS).

Research centres

Australian Centre for Health Promotion

http://www.health.usyd.edu.au/achp

This site details professional development courses, and highlights current research activity and publications from the centre. There are links to many Australian and international health-promotion organisations. Of note are the links to sites for globalisation and health.

Center for Health Promotion, University of Toronto, Canada

http://www.utoronto.ca/chp/

This site provides information about the centre and health promotion generally. The site outlines a range of Canadian and international projects, including best practice initiatives. A range of publications can be sourced through this site, including a health-promotion series and an annotated bibliography of selected health-promotion titles.

South Australian Community Health Research Unit (SACHRU)

http://www.sachru.sa.gov.au

The SACHRU site provides information about the unit's functions, publications and online newsletter. The site profiles innovative research projects, such as the Project Evaluation Wizard (PEW), a software tool for program evaluation. The site also outlines training and professional development workshops and seminars.

Field-specific sites of interest

Australian Clearinghouse for Youth Studies

http://www.acys.utas.au/index.html

This is an information service for those in the youth field. The site contains an online newsletter, and content summaries of its peer reviewed journal *Youth Studies Australia*. There are extensive links to databases, information topics, youth studies courses, discussion groups, youth organisations and much more.

Australian Women's Health Network

http://www.awhn.org.au

This site outlines current issues and reforms related to women's health, details of conferences and current women's health research activity. There are many useful links, particularly to an email list for representatives from organisations not represented nationally.

Centre for Culture, Ethnicity and Health

http://www.ceh.org.au

This site outlines the activities of the centre and provides links to multilingual health information websites. This site also includes a searchable library catalogue, and further multicultural information resources under the headings of health promotion, health links, rural health and acute health.

References

Aitkin, D. 1985 ' "Countrymindedness": the spread of an idea', *Australian Cultural History*. 4, pp. 34–41

Alinsky, S. 1972 *Rules for Radicals*. Vintage Books, New York

Anderson, D. A. and Itule, B. D. 1988 *Writing the News*. Random House, New York

Arnstein, S. 1971 'Eight Rungs on the Ladder of Citizen Participation', in Cahn, E. S. and Passett, B. A. (eds), *Citizen Participation: Effecting Community Changes*. Praeger Publishers, New York

Ashton, J. 1990 'Healthy Cities: an Overview of the International Movement', in Australian Community Health Association (eds), *Making the Connections: People, Communities and the Environment*. Papers From the First National Conference of Healthy Cities Australia. Australian Community Health Association, Sydney, NSW

Atkin, C and Wallack, C. 1990 *Mass Communication and Public Health: Complexities and Conflicts*. Sage Publications, Newbury Park, Cal

AtKisson, A. 1999 *Believing Cassandra. An Optimist Looks at a Pessimist's World*. Scribe Publications Pty Ltd, Melbourne, Vic

Auer, J. 1988 *Exploring Legislative Arrangements For Promoting Primary Health Care in Australia*. Social Health Branch, South Australian Health Commission, Adelaide, SA

Auer, J., Repin, Y. and Roe, M. 1993 *Just Change: the Cost-Conscious Manager's Toolkit*. National Reference Centre for Continuing Education in Primary Health Care, University of Wollongong, Wollongong, NSW

Australian Institute of Health and Welfare (AIHW) 1998 *Australia's Health 1998: the Sixth Biennial Report of the Australian Institute of Health and Welfare*. AIHW, Canberra. Online. Available: http://www.aihw.gov.au/publications/health/ah96/ah96-x03.html [accessed 29 January 2004]

— 2002 *Australia's Health 2002*. AIHW, Canberra

— 2004 *Australia's Health 2004*. AIHW, Canberra

— 2004 *About Us*. Online. Available: http://www.aihw.gov.au/aboutus/index.html [accessed 29 January 2004]

Barratt, A., Trevena, L., Davey, H. M. and McCaffery, K. 2004 'Use of decision aids to support informed choices about screening', *British Medical Journal*. 329, pp. 507–10 (28 August)

Bartley, M. and Blane, D. 1997 'Socioeconomic determinants of health: Health and the life course: Why safety nets matter', *British Medical Journal*. 314, pp. 1194

Bates, E. and Linder-Pelz, S. 1990 *Health Care Issues*. Allen and Unwin, Sydney, NSW

Baum, F. 1990a 'The new public health: force for change or reaction?', *Health Promotion International*. 5(2), pp. 145–50

— 1990b 'Troublemakers for health?', In*Touch*. Newsletter of the Public Health Association. 7 (1), pp. 5–6

— 1992 'Researching community health: evaluation and needs assessment that makes an impact', in Baum, F., Fry, D. and Lennie, I. (eds) *Community Health: Policy and Practice in Australia*. Pluto Press/Australian Community Health Association, Sydney, NSW

— 1998 *The New Public Health: an Australian Perspective*. Oxford University Press, Melbourne, Vic

— 1999 'The role of social capital in health promotion: Australian perspectives', *Proceedings of the 11th National Health Promotion Conference*. Perth, WA

— 2000 'Social capital, economic capital and power: further issues for a public health agenda', *Journal of Epidemiology and Community Health*. 54(6), pp. 409–10

— 2002 *The New Public Health*, 2nd edn. Oxford University Press, South Melbourne, Vic

—   2004 *What Makes for Sustainable Health Cities Initiatives?: a Review of the Evidence from Noralunga After 16 Years*. Paper presented at the 18th World Conference on Health Promotion and Education, 26–30 April 2004, Melbourne, Vic

Baum, F. and Sanders, D. 1995 'Can health promotion and Primary Health Care achieve health for all without a return to their more radical agenda?', *Health Promotion International*. 10 (2), pp. 149–60

Beaglehole R. and Bonita R. 2004 *Public Health at the Crossroads. Achievements and Prospects*, 2nd edn. Cambridge University Press, New York

Beauchamp, K. 1986 *Fixing the Government: Everyone's Guide to Lobbying in Australia*. Penguin, Ringwood, Vic

Becker, M. H. (ed.) 1974 *The Health Belief Model and Personal Health Behaviour*. Charles B Slack, Thorofare NJ

—   1986 'The tyranny of health Promotion', *Public Health Review*. 14, pp. 15–25

Bedworth, A. and Bedworth, D. 1992 *The Profession and Practice of Health Education*. WC Brown, Dubuque, USA

Beillharz, L. 2002 *Building Community: The Shared Action Experience*. Solutions Press, Bendigo, Vic

Bello, W. 2002 *Deglobalization. Ideas for a New World Economy*. Zed Books, London

Bello, W. S., Cunningham, A. and Rau, B. 1994 *Dark Victory. The United States, Structural Adjustment and Global Poverty*. Pluto Press, London

Beresford, Q. 2000 *Governments Markets and Globalisation. Australian Public Policy in Context*. Allen and Unwin, Sydney, NSW

Biklen, D. P. 1983 *Community Organizing: Theory and Practice*. Prentice Hall, Englewood Cliffs, NJ

Blaxter, M. 1990 *Health and Lifestyles*. Tavistock/Routledge, London and New York

Bloom, A. 2000a 'Hospital co-locations: private sector participation in the hospital sector', in Bloom, A. L (ed.) *Health Reform in Australia and New Zealand*. Oxford University Press, Melbourne, Vic

—   2000b in Hilless, M. and Healy J. 2001 *Health Care Systems in Transition*. The European Observatory on Health Care Systems, Australia

Bloom, B. S. 1964 *Taxonomy Of Educational Objectives: the Classification of Educational Goals*. Longman Group, London

Botsman P. 1998 'Two Tier or New Frontier? The Challenge of Future Health Care Reform', *South West Health Care Papers*, No. 1. Division of Public Health/Centre for Health Outcomes and Innovations Research, University of Western Sydney, NSW

Bourdieu, P. 1974 'Structures, habitus, power: Basis for a theory of symbolic power', in Dirks, N. B., Eley, G. and Ortner, S. B. (eds), *Culture/Power/History. A reader in contemporary social theory*. Princeton University Press, Princeton, NJ, pp. 155–99

—   1986 'The forms of capital', in *Handbook of Theory and Research for the Sociology of Education*. J. Richardson (ed.). Greenwood Press, New York, pp. 241–58

Boutilier, M., Mason, R. and Rootman, I. 1997 'Community Action and Reflective Practice in Health Promotion Research', *Health Promotion International*. 12 (1), pp. 69–78

Bowling, A. 1997 *Research Methods in Health: Investigating Health and Health Services*. Open University Press, Buckingham

Boyden, S. V. 1987 *Western Civilisation in Biological Perspective: Patterns in Biohistory*. Clarendon Publishers, Oxford

Bradshaw, J. 1972 'The Concept of Social Need', *New Society*. 30 March, pp. 640–3

Braveman, P. B. and Gruskin, S. 2003 'Poverty, equity, human rights and health', *Bulletin of The World Health Organization*, WHO, Geneva

Braveman, P., Starfield, B. and Jack, G. H. 2001 'World Health Report 2000: how it removes equity from the agenda for public health monitoring and policy', *British Medical Journal*. 323, pp. 678–81

Brennan, A. 1992 'The Altona Clean Air Project', *Health Issues*. September, 32, pp. 18–20

Brown, A. 1992 *Groupwork*. Ashgate, Aldershot, Hampshire

Brown, L. 2002 *Eco-Economy: Building an Economy for the Earth*. W.W. Norton and Co, New York

Brown, V., Grootjans, J., Ritchie, J., Townsend, M., and Verrinder, G. K. (eds) 2005 *Sustainability and Health. Supporting Global Ecological Integrity in Public Health*. Allen and Unwin, Sydney, NSW

Browning, C. J. 1992 'Mass Screening in Public Health', in Gardner, H. (ed.) *Health Policy: Development, Implementation, and Evaluation in Australia*. Churchill Livingstone, Melbourne, Vic

Brundtland, G. 1988 *Our Common Future. Report of the World Commission on Environment and Development*. Oxford University Press, Oxford

Bryson, L. and Mowbray, M. 1981 'Community: the spray-on solution', *Australian Journal of Social Issues*. November, pp. 255–67

Bundey, C., Cullen, J., Denshire, L., Grant, J., Norfor, J. and Nove, T. 1989 *Group Leadership: a Manual About Group Leadership and a Resource for Group Leaders*. Western Sydney Area Health Promotion Unit, Westmead, Sydney, NSW

Butler, P. 1993 'Introduction', in Butler, P. and Cass, S. (eds), *Case Studies of Community Development in Health*. Centre for Development and Innovation in Health, Northcote, Vic

Butler, P. and Cass, S. 1993 *Case Studies of Community Development in Health*. Centre for Development and Innovation in Health, Melbourne, Vic

Callinicos, A. 2000 *Equality*. Polity Press, Cambridge

Carr, W. and Kemmis, S. 1986 *Becoming Critical: Knowing through Action Research*. Deakin University Press, Melbourne, Vic

Castles, F. G. (ed.) 1989 *The Comparative History of Public Policy*. Polity Press, Cambridge

Chamberlain, M. C. and Beckingham, A. C. 1987 'Primary Health Care in Canada: in Praise of the Nurse?', *International Nursing Review*. 34(6), pp. 158–60

Chapman, S. 1993 'Unravelling gossamer with boxing gloves: problems in explaining the decline in smoking', *British Medical Journal*. 307, pp. 429–32

Christie, D., Gordon, I. and Heller, R. 1987 *Epidemiology: an Introductory Text for Medical and Other Health Science Students*. New South Wales University Press, Sydney, NSW

Clark, D. B. 1973 'The concept of community: a re-examination', *The Sociological Review*. 21 (3), pp. 397–415

Coburn, D. 2000 'Income inequality, social cohesion and the health status of populations: the role of neo-liberalism', *Social Science and Medicine*. 51, pp. 135–46

Coleman, J. S. 1988 'Social capital in the creation of human capital', *American Journal of Sociology*. 94, pp. S95–S120

Colin, T. and Garrow, A. 1996 *Thinking, Listening, Looking, Understanding and Acting As You Go Along*. Council of Remote Area Nurses of Australia, Alice Springs, NT

Commonwealth of Australia 2003 *The Australian Immunization Handbook*, 8th edn. National Health & Medical Research Council, Canberra

Communique. Online. Available: http://www.healthsummit.org.au [accessed 18 November 2004]

Connell, R. 1977 *Ruling Class, Ruling Culture*. Cambridge University Press, Cambridge

Consumers' Health Forum 1999 *Guidelines for Consumer Representatives: Suggestions for Consumer or Community Representatives Working on Committees*. Consumers' Health Forum of Australia, Curtin, ACT

Couzos, S. and Murray, R. 2003 *Aboriginal Primary Health Care: An Evidence-Based Approach*. Oxford University Press, Melbourne, Vic

Cox, E. 1995 *A Truly Civil Society*. Australian Broadcasting Corporation, Melbourne, Vic

— 1998 'Measuring social capital as part of progress and well-being', in *Measuring progress: Is life getting better?* Eckersley, R. (ed.), CSIRO Publishing, Melbourne, Vic

Craig, G., Mayo, M. and Taylor, M. 2000 'Globalisation from below: implications for the *Community Development Journal*', *Community Development Journal*. 35(4) pp. 323–35

Crawford, R. 1977 'You are dangerous to your health: the ideology and politics of victim blaming', *International Journal of Health Services*. 7 (4), pp. 663–80

Curtis, S. and Taket, A. 1996 *Health and Societies: Changing Perspectives*. Edward Arnold, London

Daly, H. E. and Cobb, J. B. 1989 *For the Common Good: Redirecting the Economy Toward Community, the Environment and a Sustainable Future*. Beacon Press, Boston, Mas

de Vries, M. J. 1993 'A theoretical model for healing processes: rediscovering the dynamic nature of health and disease', in LaFaille, R. and Fulder, S. (eds), *Towards a New Science of Health*. Routlege, London and New York

Department of Human Services (DHS) Victoria. Primary Health Knowledge Base is the 'Clearing House' of Primary Health Care Information Relating to Public Health in the State of Victoria. Online. Available: http://hnb.dhs.vic.gov.au/rrhacs/phkb/phkb.nsf [accessed 29 January 2004]

Dudley, R. A. and Luft, H. S. 2001 'Managed care in transition', *New England Journal of Medicine*. (14), p. 344

Dunnet, S. C. 2004 'Current issues at the South Fremantle landfill site Western Australia', *Journal of Rural and Remote Environmental Health*. 3(1), pp. 40–51

Dwyer, J. 1989 'The politics of participation', *Community Health Studies*. 13(1), pp. 59–65

Earp, J. A. and Ennett, S. T. 1991 'Conceptual models for health education research and practice', *Health Education Research*. 6(2), pp. 163–71

Earth Charter. Online. Available: http://www.earthcharter.org/ [accessed 24 September 2004]

Earth Summit 2002 *Towards Earth Summit, 2002. Building Partnerships for Sustainable Development*. Briefing Paper on Health and Environment. Social Briefing No 3. Online. Available: http://www.earthsummit2002.org/es/issues/health/health.htm [accessed 11 February 2004]

Eckermann, A. K., Dowd, T., Martin, M., Nixon, L., Gray, R. and Chong, E. 1995 *Binan Goonj: Bridging Cultures in Aboriginal Health*. Department of Aboriginal and Multicultural Studies, University of New England, Armidale, NSW

Egger, G. Spark, R. and Lawson, J. 1999 *Health Promotion Strategies and Methods*. Mc Graw-Hill, Sydney, NSW

Egger, G., Donovan, R. and Spark, R. 1993 *Health and the Media: Principles and Practice for Health Promotion*. McGraw-Hill, Sydney, NSW

Eisenberg, L. 1987 'Value Conflicts in Social Policies for Promoting Health', in Doxiadis, S. (ed.), *Ethical Dilemmas in Health Promotion*. John Wiley and Sons, Chichester

Eng, E., Salmon, M. E. and Mullan, F. 1992 'Community empowerment: the critical base for primary health care', *Family and Community Health*. 15 (1), pp. 1–12

European Observatory on Health Systems and Policies 2004 Online. Available: http://www.who.dk/eprise/main/who/progs/obs/toppage [accessed 3 February 2004]

Ewles, L. and Simnett, I. 1995 *Promoting Health. A Practical Guide*, 3rd edn. Scutari Press, London

— 1999 *Promoting Health: a Practical Guide*. Baillière Tindall in association with the Royal College of Nursing, Edinburgh

Falk, I. and Kilpatrick, S. 2000 'What is social capital? A study of interaction in a rural community', *Sociologia Ruralis*. 40(1), pp. 87–110

Fawkes, S. 1997 'Aren't Health Services Already Promoting Health?', *Australian and New Zealand Journal of Public Health*. 21 (4), pp. 391–7

Feuerstein, M. T. 1986 *Partners in Evaluation: Evaluating Development and Community Programmes with Participants*. Macmillan, London

Flood, M. and Lawrence, A. 1987 *The Community Action Book*. NSW Council of Social services, Sydney, NSW

Foley, G (2000) *Understanding Adult education and Training*, 2nd edn. Allen and Unwin, Sydney, NSW

Freire, P. 1973 *Education for Critical Consciousness*. Sheed and Ward, London

Freudenberg, N. 1984 'Training health educators for social change', *International Quarterly of Community Health Education*. 5 (1), pp. 37–52

Fukuyama, F. 1995 *Trust. The Social Virtues and the Creation of Prosperity*. Hamish Hamilton, London

Gagné, R. M. 1985 *The Conditions of Learning and Theory Of Instruction*, 4th edn. Holt Reinhart & Winston, New York

Galbally, R. 2004. *Just Passions. The Personal is Political*. Pluto Press, North Melbourne, Vic

Gardner, H. 1995 'Interest groups and the political process', in Gardner, H. (ed.) *The Politics of Health. The Australian Experience*. Churchill Livingstone, Melbourne, Vic, pp. 184–215

Gilmore, G. D., Campbell, M. D. and Becker, B. 1989 *Needs Assessment Strategies for Health Education and Health Promotion*. Benchmark Press, Indianapolis, Ind

Glyn, A. and Miliband, D. (eds) 1994 *Paying for Inequality: the Economic Cost of Social Injustice*. IPPR/Rivers Oram Press, London

Goldstein, S, Japhet, G. Usdin, S. and Scheepers, E. 2004 'Soul City: a sustainable edutainment vehicle facilitating social change', *Health Promotion Journal of Australia*. 15(2), pp. 114–20

Green, L. W. 1980 'Healthy people: the Surgeon General's report and the prospects', in McNerney, W. J. (ed.), *Working for a Healthier America*. Ballinger, Cambridge, MA, pp. 95–110

Green, L. W. and Kreuter, M. W. 1999 *Health Promotion Planning: an Educational and Environmental Approach*. Mayfield Publishing Co, Mountain View, Cal

Guba, E. and Lincoln, Y. 1989 *Fourth Generation Evaluation*. Sage Publications, Newbury Park, Cal

Hancock, L. 1999 'Health, public sector restructuring and the market state', in Hancock, L. (ed.), *Health Policy in the Market State*. Allen and Unwin, Sydney, NSW, pp. 48–68

Hancock, T. 1998 'Caveat partner: reflections on partnership with the private sector', *Health Promotion International*. 13, (3), pp. 193–5

Harris, E. M., Wise, P., Hawe, P., Finlay, Y and Nutbeam, D. 1995 *Working Together: Inter-Sectoral Action for Health*. National Centre for Health Promotion, Commonwealth Department of Human Services and Health, AGPS, Canberra

Hawe, P. 1994 'Capturing the meaning of "community" ' in community intervention evaluation: some contributions from community psychology', *Health Promotion International*. 9 (3), pp. 199–210

— 1996 'Needs assessment must become more change-focused', *Australian and New Zealand Journal of Public Health*. 20(5), pp. 473–8

Hawe, P., Degeling, D. and Hall, J. 1990 *Evaluating Health Promotion: a Health Workers' Guide*. MacLennan and Petty, Sydney, NSW

Hawtin, M., Hughes, G. and Percy-Smith, J. 1994 *Community Profiling: Auditing Social Needs*. Open University Press, Buckingham

Healy, T. and Coté, S. 2001 *The Well-Being of Nations: the Role of Human and Social Capital*. Centre for Educational Research and Innovation, OECD, Paris

Heller, P. 1996 'Social capital as a product of class mobilization and state intervention: Industrial workers in Kerala, India', *World Development*. 24(6), pp. 1055–71

Henderson, D. 1995 'The revival of economic liberalism: Australia in an international perspective', *The Australian economic review*. pp. 59–85

Henderson, P. and Thomas, D. N. 1987 *Skills in Neighbourhood Work*. Allen and Unwin, London

Heron, J. 1999 *The Complete Facilitators Handbook*. Kogan Page Ltd, London

Hilless M. and Healy. J. 2001 *Health Care Systems in Transition: Australia*. The European Observatory on Health Care Systems. Online. Available: http://www.who.dk/eprise/main/who/progs/obs/toppage [accessed 3 February 2004]

Hoff, M. D. 1998 *Sustainable Community Development: Studies in Economic, Environmental, and Cultural Revitalization*. Lewis Publishers, Boca Raton, Fla

Honari, M. 1993 'Advancing health ecology: where to from here?', in Newman, N. (ed.), *Health and Ecology — a Nursing Perspective*. Proceedings of the First National Nursing the Environment Conference, Australian Nursing Federation, Melbourne, Vic

Hopkins, S. 1996 'Foreword', in McSwain, R. *Culture and Health Care: Culture, Settlement Experience and Lifestyle of Non-English Speaking Background People in Western Australia*. Multicultural Access Unit, Health Department of Western Australia, Perth, WA

Human Services, Victoria 1999 *Victorian Burden of Disease Study — Mortality, Morbidity*. Public Health and Development Division, Human Services, Victoria,. Online. Available: http://www.dhs.vic.gov.au/phd/9903009/index.htm [accessed 29 January 2004]

Ife, J. 2002 *Community Development. Community-Based Alternatives in an Age of Globalization*, 2nd edn. Longman, Sydney, NSW

Illich, I. 1975 *Limits to Medicine: Medical Nemesis: the Expropriation of Health*. Penguin, Harmondsworth

Jackson, T., Mitchell, S. and Wright, M. 1989 'The community development continuum', *Community Health Studies*, 13(1), pp. 66–73

James E. Talbot L. and Fishley, C. 2003 'Does external support from divisions increase preventive activities in rural Australian general practice?', *Australian Family Physician* 32(12), pp. 1044–6

Janis, I. L. 1982 *Groupthink: Psychological Studies of Policy Decisions and Fiascoes*. Houghton Mifflin Company, Boston

Johnson, D. W. and Johnson, F. P. 1997 *Joining Together: Group Theory and Group Skills*. Allyn and Bacon, Boston, MA

Johnstone, M. J. 1994 *Bioethics: a Nursing Perspective*. W. B. Saunders/Baillière Tindall, Sydney, NSW

Kalnins, I., McQueen, D. V., Backett, K. C., Curtice, L. and Currie, C. E. 1992 'Children, Empowerment and Health Promotion: Some New Directions in Research and Practice', *Health Promotion International*, 7(1), pp. 53–9

Kaplan, G. A., Pamuk, E. R., Lynch, J. W., Cohen, R. D. and Balfour, J. L. 1996 'Inequality in income and mortality in the United States: analysis of mortality and potential pathways', *British Medical Journal*. 20 April, 312, pp. 999–1003

Kawachi, I. and Kennedy, B. P. 1997 'Health and social cohesion: why care about income inequality?', *British Medical Journal*. 314, pp. 1037–40

Kawachi, I., Kennedy, B. P. and Wilkinson, R. 1999 'Crime: social disorganization and relative deprivation', *Social Science and Medicine*. 48(6), pp. 719–31

Kearney, J. 1991 'The Role of Self Help Groups: Challenging the System and Complementing Professionals', *Health* Issues. 28, pp. 29–31

Kickbusch, I. 1994 'An Overview to the Settings-Based Approach to Health Promotion', in *The Settings-Based Approach to Health Promotion: an International Working Conference in Collaboration with the World Health Organization Regional Office for Europe*. Conference report. Hertfordshire Health Promotion, Welwyn Garden City, Hertfordshire

Knowles, M. 1980 *The Modern Practice of Adult Education: From Pedagogy to Andragogy*. Cambridge Adult Educator, Cambridge

Labonté, R. 1986 'Social inequality and healthy public policy', *Health Promotion*. 1(3), pp. 341–51

— 1989a 'Community and professional empowerment', *Canadian Nurse*. March, pp. 23–8

— 1989b, 'Community empowerment: the need for political analysis', *Canadian Journal of Public Health*. 80, March/April, pp. 87–8

— 1997 *Power, Participation and Partnerships for Health Promotion*. VicHealth, Melbourne, Vic

— 1999 'Social capital and community development: practitioner emptor', *Australian and New Zealand Journal of Public Health*. 23(4), pp. 430–3

— 2004 'An unabashedly opinionated (but evidence-based) overview of globalisation's challenge to health', *VicHealth Letter*. (22), pp. 14–17

Labonté R. and Feather J. 1996 *Handbook on Using Stories in Health Promotion Practice*. Health Canada, Ottawa

Lalonde Report 1974 A new perspective on the health of Canadians. Marc Lalonde, Minister for Health and Welfare. Online. Available: http://www.hc-sc.gc.ca/hppb/phdd/pube/perintrod.htm [accessed 29 January 2004]

Leddy, S. and Pepper, J. M. 1989 *Conceptual Bases of Professional Nursing*. J. B. Lippincott, Philadelphia, Penn

Leeder, S. R. 2003 'Achieving equity in the Australian healthcare system', *Medical Journal of Australia*. 179(9), pp. 475–8

Lehmann, J. 2003 *The Harveys and Other Stories: Invitations to Curiosity*. St. Luke's Innovative Resources, Bendigo, Vic

Leventhal, H., Safer, M. A. and Panagis, D. M. 1984 'The impact of communications of the self regulation of health-beliefs, decisions and behaviour', *Health Education Quarterly*. 10(1), pp. 3–29

Lewin, K 1946 'Action research and minority problems', *Journal of Social Issues*. 2, pp. 34–46

LoBiondo-Wood, G. and Haber, J. 2002 Nursing Research: Methods, Critical Appraisal, and Utilization, 5th edn. Mosby, St Louis

Lowi, T. 1964 'American business, public policy, case studies and political theory', *World Politics*. 16, pp. 677–715

McArdle, J. 1999 *Community Development in the Market Economy*. Vista Publications, Melbourne, Vic

McCoppin, B. 1995 'The public service: from mandarins to managerialists', in Gardner, H. (ed.) *The Politics of Health. The Australian Experience*. Churchill Livingstone, Melbourne, Vic, pp. 88–107

McKenzie, J. F. and Jurs, J. L. 1993 *Planning, Implementing, and Evaluating Health Promotion Programs: a Primer*. Macmillan, New York

McKenzie, J. F., Neigher, B. L. and Smeltzer, J. L. 2005 *Planning, Implementing and Evaluating Health Promotion Programs: a Primer*, 4th edn. Pearson, San Franscisco, CA

McKenzie, J. F. and Smeltzer, J. L. 2001 *Planning Implementing and Evaluating Health Promotion Programs. a Primer*, 3rd edn. Allyn and Bacon, Boston, MA

Mc Kenzie, J. F., Neiger, B. L. and Smeltzer, J. L. 2005 *Planning, Implementing and Evaluating Health Promotion Programs. A primer*, 4th edn. Pearson, San Francisco, Cal

McKeown, T. 1979 *The Role of Medicine: Dream, Mirage or Nemesis?* Basil Blackwell, Oxford

MacKian S., Elliott H., Busby, H. and Popay, J. 2003 ' "Everywhere and nowhere": locating and understanding the "new: public health', *Health and Place*. 9(3), pp. 219–29

McMichael, A. J. 2001 *Human Frontiers, Environments and Disease: Past Patterns, Uncertain Futures*. Cambridge University Press, Cambridge

Markos, S. 1991 *Self Help Groups and the Role they Play in the Health Care System*. Health Issues Centre, Melbourne, Vic

Marmot, M. and Wilkinson, R. G. (eds) 1999 *Social Determinants of Health*. Oxford University Press, Oxford

Mathers, C. and Douglas, B. 1998 'Measuring Progress in Population Health and Wellbeing', in Eckersley, R. (ed.), *Measuring Progress: is Life Getting Better?* CSIRO Publishing, Melbourne, Vic

Mattessich, P. and Monsey, J. 1997 'Defining community and community engagement', cited in Child and Family Steering Committee on Community Governance, *2002 Policy Issue*, 12 June

Mies, M. 1983 'Towards a methodology for feminist research', in Bowles, G. and Dvelli Klein, R. (eds), *Theories of Women's Studies*, Routledge and Kegan Paul, London

Milio, N. 1988 *Making Policy: a Mosaic of Community Health Policy Development.* Department of Community Services and Health, AGPS, Canberra

Milio, N. 1990 'Healthy cities: the new public health and supportive research', *Health Promotion International.* 5 (3), pp. 291–7

Minas, I. H. 1990 'Mental health in a culturally diverse society', in Reid, J. and Trompf, P. (eds), *The Health of Immigrant Australia: a Social Perspective.* Harcourt Brace Jovanovich, Sydney, NSW

Minkler, M. 1991 'Improving health through community organization', in Glanz, K., Lewis, F. M. and Rimer, B. K. (eds), *Health Behavior and Health Education: Theory, Research and Practice.* Jossey Bass, San Francisco, Cal

— 1994. 'Ten commitments for community health education', *Health Education Research.* 9 (4), pp. 527–34

Minkler, M. and Cox, K. 1980 'Creating critical consciousness in health: application of Freire's Philosophy and methods to the health care setting', *International Journal of Health Services*, 10 (2), pp. 311–22

Moodie, R., Pisani, E. and de Castellarnau, M. 2000 'Infrastructure to promote health: The art of the possible', in *Fifth Global Conference on Health Promotion.* World Health Organization, Pan American Health Organization, Ministry of Health of Mexico 2000 Health Promotion, Bridging the Equity Gap, 5–9 June

Morehouse, W. (ed.) 1997 *Building Sustainable Communities: Tools and Concepts for Self-Reliant Economic Change.* The Bootstrap Press, New York, and Jon Carpenter Publishing, Charlbury

Mossialos, J. and Le Grand, E. 1999 in Hilless M. and Healy J. 2001 *Health Care Systems in Transition: Australia.* The European Observatory on Health Care Systems. Online. Available: http://www.who.dk/eprise/main/who/progs/obs/toppage [accessed 3 February 2004]

Naidoo, J. and Wills, J. 2000 *Health promotion. Foundations for practice.* Baillière Tindall, Edinburgh

National Aboriginal Health Strategy Working Party 1989 *A National Aboriginal Health Strategy.* Department of Aboriginal Affairs, AGPS, Canberra

National Expert Advisory Committee on Tobacco (NEACT) for the Ministerial Council on Drug Strategy (MCDS) 2000 *The National Tobacco Strategy.* Published by AusInfo for Commonwealth Department of Health and Aged Care, Canberra

National Health and Medical Research Council 2003 *The Australian Immunisation Handbook*, 8th edn. NHMRC, Canberra

Neuhauser, L., Schwab, M., Syme, S. L., Bieber, M. and Obarski, S. K. 1998 'Community participation in health promotion: evaluation of the *California Wellness Guide*', *Health Promotion International.* 13(3), pp. 211–22

Nutbeam, D. and Harris, E. 2004 *Theory in a Nutshell. A Practical Guide to Health Promotion Theories*, 2nd edn. Mc Graw-Hill, Sydney, NSW

Oakley, A. 1990 'Who's Afraid of the Randomized Clinical Trial? Some Dilemmas of the Scientific Method and "Good" Research Practice', in Roberts, H. (ed.), *Women's Health Counts.* Routledge, London and New York

Olson, M. 1982 *The Rise and Decline of Nations: Economic Growth, Stagflations and Social Rigidities.* Yale University Press, New Haven, Conn

Organisation for Economic Co-operation and Development 2000 in Hilless M. and Healy J. 2001 *Health Care Systems in Transition: Australia*. The European Observatory on Health Care Systems. Online. Available: http://www.who.dk/eprise/main/who/progs/ obs/toppage [accessed 3 February 2004]

— 2001 *The well-being of nations. The role of human and social capital*. Centre for Educational Research and Innovation, Organisation for Economic Co-operation and Development (OECD), Paris, France

Packer, J., Spence, R., Beare, E. 2002 'Building community partnerships: an Australian case study of sustainable community-based rural programmes', *Community Development Journal*. 37(4), October, pp. 316–26

Palfrey C. 2000 *Key Concepts in Health Care Policy and Planning: an Introductory Text*. Macmillan, Basingstoke

Palmer, G. R. and Short, S. D. 2000 *Health Care and Public Policy, an Australian Analysis*. Macmillan Education Australia, South Melbourne, Vic

Pfeiffer, J. W. and Jones, J. E. 1974–1985 *A Handbook of Structured Experiences for Human Relations Training*, volumes 1–10. University Associates, San Diego, Cal

Poland, B., Green, L. and Rootman, I. 2002 *Settings for Health promotion. Linking Theory and Practice*. Sage Publications, Newbury Park Cal

Polaschek, N. R. 1998 'Cultural safety. A new concept in nursing people of different ethnicities', *Journal of Advanced Nursing*. (27)3, pp. 452–7

Popay, J. 2000 'Social capital: the role of narrative and historical research', *Journal of Epidemiology and Community Health*. 54(6), pp. 401

Portes, A. 2000 'The two meanings of social capital', *Sociological Forum*. 15(1), pp. 1–12

Portes, A. and Landolt, P. 1996 'The downside of social capital', *The American Prospect*. 26, pp. 18–23

Posavac, E. J. and Carey R. G. 2003 *Program Evaluation Methods and Case Studies*, 6th edn. Prentice Hall, Englewood Cliffs, NJ

Primary Care Partnerships (PCP) *Strategy of the Department of Human Services (DHS)*. PCP, Victoria. Online. Available: http://hnb.dhs.vic.gov.au/rrhacs/phkb/phkb.nsf/ AllDocs/C15B8527F9F27E63CA256C5500211F74? [accessed 18 August 2004]

Productivity Commission 2003 *Social Capital: Reviewing the Concept and its Policy Implications*. Report No.89. AusInfo, Commonwealth of Australia, Canberra. Online. Available: www.pc.gov.au [accessed 18 August 2004]

Public Health Association of Australia 2003 Environmental Health Justice Policy. Online. Available: http://www.phaa.org.au [accessed 3 February 2004]

Pusey, M. 1998 'Incomes, standards of living and quality of life: preliminary findings from the "Middle Australia Project" ', in Eckersley, R. (ed.), *Measuring Progress: Is Life Getting Better?*, CSIRO Publishing, Melbourne, Vic

Putnam, R. 1993 *Making Democracy Work. Civic Traditions in Modern Italy*. Princeton University Press, Princeton, NJ

Putnam, R. D. 1995 'Bowling alone: America's declining social capital', *Journal of Democracy*. 6(1), pp. 65–78

Quinn, F. M. 1988. *The Principles and Practice of Nurse Education*, 2nd edn. Chapman and Hall, London

Raeburn, J. and Rootman, I. 1998 *People-Centred Health Promotion*. John Wiley and Sons, Chichester

Redman, S., Spencer, E. A. and Sanson-Fisher, R. W. 1990 'The role of mass media in changing health-related behaviour — a review of two models', *Health Promotion International*. 5, pp. 85–101

Rifkin, S. 1986 'Lessons from Community Participation in Health Programmes', *Health Policy and Planning*. 1(3), pp. 240–9

Rifkin, S. and Walt, G. 1986 'Why health improves: defining the issues concerning

"Comprehensive Primary Health Care" and "Selective Primary Health Care" ', *Social Science and Medicine.* 23(6), pp. 559–66

Rissel, C. 1991 'The tyranny of needs assessment in health promotion', *Evaluation Journal of Australia.* 3(1), pp. 26–31

Robinson, J. and Elkan, R. 1996 *Health Needs Assessment. Theory and Practice.* Churchill Livingston, Edinburgh

Rogers, E. M. 1995 *Diffusion of Innovations.* The Free Press, New York

Rose, G., and Marmot, M. 1981 'Social class and coronary heart disease', *British Heart Journal* 45, pp. 13–19

Rose, N. 1996 'The death of the social? Re-figuring the territory of government', *Economy and Society.* 25(3), pp. 327–56

Rothman, J. with Tropman, J. E. 1987 'Models of community organization and macro practice perspectives: their mixing and phasing', in Cox, F. M., Erlich, J. L., Rothman, J. and Tropman J. E., *Strategies of Community Organization.* F. E. Peacock, Itasca, Ill

Rubin, H. J. and Rubin I. S. 1992 *Community Organizing and Development*, 2nd edn. Allyn and Bacon, Boston, MA

Ryan, W. 1976 *Blaming the Victim.* Vintage Books, New York

Salisbury, R. and Heinz, J. 1970 'A theory of policy analysis and some preliminary applications', in Sharkansky, K. (ed.), *Policy Analysis and Political Science* Markham, Chicago

Sampson, E. E. and Marthas, M. 1990 *Group Process for the Health Professions.* Delmar, New York

Saunders, P. 2003 A *self reliant Australia: Welfare Policy for the 21st Century.* Centre for Independent Studies, Sydney, NSW

Sax, S. 1990 *Health Care Choices and the Public Purse.* Allen and Unwin, Sydney, NSW

Scheepers E., Christofides, N. J., Goldstein, S., Usdin, S., Patel, D. S. and Japhet, G. 2004 'Evaluating health communication — a holistic overview of the impact of Soul City IV', *Health Promotion Journal of Australia.* 15(2), pp. 121–33

Schwab, M., Neuhauser, L., Margen, S., Syme, S. L., Ogar, D., Roppel, C. and Elite, A. 1992 The Wellness Guide: Towards a New Model for Community Participation in Health Promotion. *Health Promotion International.* 7(1), pp. 27–36

Selener, D. 1997 *Participatory Action Research and Social Change.* The Cornell Participatory Action Research Network, Cornell University, Ithaca, New York

Sen, A. 1992 *Inequality Re-examined.* Russell Sage Foundation, New York

Sindal, C. and Dixon, J. 1990 'Creating supportive economic environments for health', in Australian Community Health Association (ed.), *Healthy Environment in the 90s: The Community Health Approach.* Papers from the 3rd National Conference of the Australian Community Health Association, Australian Community Health Association, Sydney, NSW

South Australian Community Health Research Unit 1991 *Planning Healthy Communities: a Guide to Doing Community Needs Assessment.* South Australian Community Health Research Unit, Bedford Park, SA

South Australian Health Commission 1988 *A Social Health Strategy for South Australia.* South Australian Health Commission, Adelaide, SA

State Government of Victoria 2002a *Municipal Public Health Planning Framework.* Online. Available: http://www.health.vic.gov.au/ [accessed 29 January 2004]

— 2002b *Victorian Tobacco Action Plan.* Department of Human Services, State Government of Victoria, Melbourne, Vic

— 2003a *Integrated Health Promotion Resource Kit.* Department of Human Services, State Government of Victoria, Melbourne, Vic

— 2003b *Integrated Health Promotion.* Primary and Community Health Branch, Public Health Branch, Rural and Regional Health and Aged Care Service Division. Department of Human Services, State Government of Victoria, Melbourne, Vic

— 2003c *Health Promotion Short Course Facilitators Guide. Module 1.* Department of Human Services, State Government of Victoria, Melbourne, Vic

Stephenson, C. 1996 *SF36 Interim Norms for Australian Data.* Australian Institute for Health and Welfare, Canberra

Stretton, H. and Orton, O. 1994 *Public Goods, Public Enterprise, Public Choice.* Macmillan, London

Suzuki, D. 2002 *Healthy Ecosystems Healthy People. Linkages between Biodiversity, Ecosystem Health and Human Health.* Keynote address, International Society for Ecosystem Health, Washington DC, 6–11 June 2002

Syme, S. L. 1997 'Individuals vs community interventions in public health practice: Some thoughts about a new approach', in *Health Promotion Matters: Newsletter of VicHealth.* Melbourne, Vic, (2), pp. 2–9

Syme, S. L. 1998 'Social and economic disparities in health: Thoughts about Intervention', *The Millbank Quarterly.* 76(3), pp. 493–505

Tassie, J. 1992 *Protecting the Environment and Health: Working Together for Clean Air on the Le Fevre Peninsula.* Le Fevre Peninsula Health Management Plan Steering Committee, Port Adelaide, SA

Teshuva, K., Kendig, H. and Stacey, B. 1997 Spirituality, health and health promotion in older Australians', *Health Promotion Journal of Australia.* 7(3), pp. 180–4

Thomson, N. (ed.) 2003 *The Health of Indigenous Australians.* Oxford University Press, Melbourne, Vic

Tones, K. and Green J. 2004 *Health Promotion. Planning and Strategies.* Sage, London

Tones, K. and Tilford, S. 1994 *Health Education: Effectiveness, Efficiency and Equity.* Chapman and Hall, London

Tones, K., Tilford, S. and Robinson, Y. 1990 *Health Education: Effectiveness and Efficiency.* Chapman and Hall, London

Tonts, M. 2000 'The restructuring of Australia's rural communities', in Pritchard, B. and McManus, P. (eds), *Land of Discontent. The Dynamics of Change in Rural and Regional Australia.* University of New South Wales Press, Sydney, NSW, Ch 4

Towards Earth Summit 2004 *Building Partnerships for Sustainable Development.* Briefing Paper on Health and Environment. Social Briefing No 3. Online. Available: http://www.earthsummit2002.org/es/issues/health/health.htm [accessed 11 February 2004]

Travis, J. W. and Ryan, R. S. 2004 *Wellness Workbook*, 3rd edn. Ten Speed Press, Berkeley, Cal

Tuckman, B. 1965 'Developmental sequence in small groups', *Psychological Bulletin.* 63, pp. 384–99

UNICEF 1992 cited in Werner, D., Sanders, D., Weston, J., Babb, S. and Rodriguez, B. 1997 *Questioning the Solution: The Politics of Primary Health Care and Child Survival.* Healthwrights, Palo Alto, Cal

United Nations 1992 *Rio Declaration on Environment and Development.* Report of the United Nations Conference on Environment and Development. Online. Available: http://www.un.org/esa/sustdev/documents/agenda21/index.htm [accessed 27 September 2004]

— 2003 *United Nations Development Program 2003.* Online. Available: http://www.undp.org/mdg/ [accessed 20th January 2004]

— 2004a *Universal Declaration of Human Rights.* Department of Public Information, Office of the High Commissioner for Human Rights. Online. Available: http://www.unhchr.ch/udhr/lang/eng.htm [accessed 17 September 2004])

— 2004b *Agenda 21.* Division for Sustainable Development, Department of Economic and Social Affairs. Online. Available: http://www.un.org/esa/sustdev/documents/agenda21/index.htm [accessed 27 September 2004]

Veenhoven, R. 1996 cited in Wearing, A. J. and Headey, B. 1998 'Who enjoys life and why: measuring subjective well-being', in Eckersley, R. (ed.), *Measuring Progress: Is Life Getting Better?* CSIRO Publishing, Melbourne, Vic

Verrinder, G. K. 2005 'Innovating', in *Sustainability and Health: Supporting Global Integrity in Public Health*. Allen and Unwin, Sydney, NSW

Verrinder, G. K., Nicholson, R. and Pickett, R. 2005 'Acting', in *Sustainability and Health: Supporting Global Integrity in Public Health*. Allen and Unwin, Sydney, NSW

VicHealth 2004 Victorian Health Promotion Foundation. Online. Available: www.vichealth.vic.gov.au/walkingschoolbus [accessed 20th January 2004]

Wadsworth, Y. 1997 *Everyday Evolution on the Run*. Allen and Unwin, Sydney, NSW

Walker, M. 1986 Community Development Lecture. Mitchell College of Advanced Education, Bathurst, 12 August

Walker, M. and Dixon, J. 1984 *Participation in Change: Australian Case Studies*. Mitchell College Of Advanced Education, Bathurst, NSW

Wallerstein, N. 1992 'Powerlessness, empowerment and health: implications for health promotion programs', *American Journal of Public Health*. January/February, 6(3), pp. 197–205

Wallerstein, N. and Bernstein, E. 1988 'Empowerment education: Freire's ideas adapted to health education. *Health Education Quarterly*. 15 (4), pp. 379–94

Wass, A. 1990 'The New Legitimacy of Women's Health: In Whose Interests?', in Smith, A. (ed.), *Women's Health in Australia*. Angie Smith, Armidale, NSW

— 2000 *Promoting Health: The Primary Health Care Approach*, 2nd edn. Saunders, Sydney, NSW

Wearing, A. J. and Headey, B. 1998 'Who enjoys life and why: measuring subjective well-being', in Eckersley, R. (ed.), *Measuring Progress: Is Life Getting Better?* CSIRO Publishing, Melbourne, Vic

Weiss, E. H. and Kessel, G. 1987 'Practical skills for health educators on using mass media', *Health Education*. June/July, pp. 39–41

Werner D., Sanders D., Weston J., Babb S. and Rodriguez, B. 1997 *Questioning the Solution: The Politics of Primary Health Care and Child Survival*. Healthwrights, Palo Alto, Cal

Werner, D. 1981 'The village health worker: lackey or liberator?', *World Health Forum*. 2 (1), pp. 46–68

West, E. 1997 *Icebreakers: Group Mixers, Warm-Ups, Energizers and Playful Activities*. McGraw-Hill, New York

Wilkinson, R. 1994 'Health, redistribution and growth', in Glyn, A. and Miliband, D. (eds), *Paying for Inequality: the Economic Cost of Social Injustice*. IPPR/Rivers Oram Press, London

— 1996 *Unhealthy Societies: the Afflictions of Inequality*. Routledge, London

Wilkinson, R. G., Kawachi, I. and Kennedy, B. P. 1998 'Mortality, the social environment, crime and violence', *Sociology of Health & Illness*. 20(5), pp. 578–97

Williams, S. 1986 'Community based finance', *Community Quarterly*. 8, pp. 4–10

Wilson, E. O. 2002 'The bottleneck', *Scientific American*. pp. 72–9 (February)

Wise, M. and Hearn, S. 2004 'The future of health promotion in Australia', *Health Promotion Journal of Australia*. 15(2) pp. 91–2

Woolcock, M. 1998 'Social capital and economic development: toward a theoretical synthesis and policy framework', *Theory and Society*. 27, pp. 151–208

World Bank 1993 *World Development Report 1993: Investing in Health*. Oxford University Press, Oxford

World Health Organization 1948 *World Health Organization Constitution*. Online. Available: http://www.who.int/en/ [accessed 21 January 2004]

— 1978 *Declaration of Alma-Ata*. Online. Available: http://www.who.int/hpr/NPH/docs/declaration_almaata.pdf [accessed 20 January 2004]

— 1986 *The Ottawa Charter for Health Promotion*. Online. Available: http://www.who.org [accessed 20 January 2004]

— 1988 *Education for Health: a Manual on Health Education in Primary Health Care*. WHO, Geneva

— 1995 Regional Guidelines — Development of Health-Promoting Schools. Online. Available: http://www.sofweb.vic.edu.au/hps/ [accessed 20 January 2004]

— 1997 'The Jakarta Declaration on Leading Health Promotion into the 21st Century', *Health Promotion International*. 12(4), pp. 261–4

— 1998 *The World Health Report 1998: Life in the 21st Century. A Vision for All*. WHO, Geneva

— 2000 'Health promotion, bridging the equity gap', at the *Fifth Global Conference on Health Promotion*. Pan American Health Organization, Ministry of Health of Mexico, 5–9 June

— 2003 *The World Health Report 2003. Shaping the Future*. WHO, Geneva

— 2004a *Jakarta Declaration*. Online. Available: www.who.int/hpr/NPH/docs/jakarta_declaration_en.pdf [accessed 27 September 2004]

— 2004b Conferences. Online. Available: http://www.who.int/hpr/ncp/hp.conferences.shtml [accessed 21 January 2004]

— 2004c *Belfast Declaration*. Online. Available: http://www.euro.who.int/healthy-cities [accessed 21 January 2004]

— 2004d Media releases. Online. Available: www.who.int/mediacentre/releases releases / 2004/pr21/en/ [accessed 21 January 2004]

— 2004e *Global Health Security — Epidemic Alert and Response*. Resolution adopted by the World Health Assembly, 2001. Online. Available: http://www.who.int/csr/alertresponse/en/ [accessed 15 October 2004]

World Health Organization and the Commonwealth Department Of Community Services and Health — Australia 1988 'Healthy Public Policy — Strategies for Action', in *Australian Nursing Federation 1990, Primary Health Care in Australia: Strategies for Nursing Action*. Australian Nursing Federation, Melbourne, Vic

Wrigley, J. and McLean, P. 1990 *Australian Business Communication*. Longman Cheshire, Melbourne, Vic

Index